DR. SHAPIRO'S

PICTURE PERFECT WEIGHT LOSS

The Visual Program for Permanent Weight Loss

Dr. Howard M. Shapiro

RODALE

Notice

This book is intended as a reference volume only, not as a medical manual. The information given here is designed to help you make informed decisions about your health. It is not intended as a substitute for any treatment that may have been prescribed by your doctor. If you suspect that you have a medical problem, we urge you to seek competent medical help.

Cover and interior design by Christina Gaugler
Cover and interior photographs by Kurt Wilson/Rodale Images, except pp. 4, 5, 12, 13, 56, 91, 112, 113, 124, 125, and 174, by Lou Manna
Food styling by Diane Vezza

Library of Congress Cataloging-in-Publication Data

Shapiro, Howard M., 1943–
   [Picture perfect weight loss]
   Dr. Shapiro's picture perfect weight loss : the visual program for permanent weight loss /
Howard M. Shapiro.
       p.   cm.
   Includes index.
   ISBN 1–57954–241–7   hardcover
   1. Weight loss.   I. Title: Doctor Shapiro's picture perfect weight loss.   II. Title.
RM222.2 .S469   2000
613.2'5—dc21   99–087668

Distributed to the book trade by St. Martin's Press

   4 6 8 10 9 7 5 3   hardcover

Visit us on the Web at www.preventionbookshelf.com, or call us toll-free at (800) 848-4735.

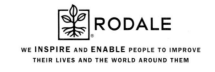

RODALE

WE **INSPIRE** AND **ENABLE** PEOPLE TO IMPROVE
THEIR LIVES AND THE WORLD AROUND THEM

ACKNOWLEDGMENTS

In writing this book, I have learned that authorship is a lot like medicine: Both are collaborative processes. I'm glad for this opportunity to acknowledge and thank the many people who helped make *Dr. Shapiro's Picture Perfect Weight Loss* a reality.

First and unquestionably foremost, I owe a debt of gratitude to nutritionist Phyllis Roxland. A friend and colleague of 20 years' standing, Phyllis was not only instrumental in formulating the principles of the weight-loss program, she also helped with every aspect of this book, often putting her personal life on hold to do so. I am thankful not only for the weekends sacrificed and the travel to and from Pennsylvania for numerous photo shoots but also for the dedication that kept me focused on the task at hand. This book simply would not have been possible without Phyllis Roxland.

In helping to shape and polish the book, writer Susanna Margolis and Ed Claflin, my editor at Rodale, offered intelligence and much-appreciated humor along with considerable professional expertise. They helped me express my thoughts—sometimes, it seemed, before they were even formulated in my mind—and they were a pleasure to work with. Kay von Bergen's creativity spurred my own and gave birth to the book's title, while her generous spirit sustained and supported the overall effort. My thanks also to Abbie Claflin, whose involvement in the book's creation was brief but memorable.

Mel Berger, my agent at the William Morris Agency, grasped the concept of the book early on and staunchly advocated the use of color photography, an element I believe is essential to the book's message.

Diane Vezza, ably assisted by Joan Parkin and Rose Holden, brilliantly styled the subjects of the photography, which were beautifully brought to life by photographer Kurt Wilson and his assistant, Troy Schnyder—all under the superb direction of James Gallucci, Rodale's photo editor.

In designing the book and cover and planning numerous photo shoots, senior book designer Christina Gaugler exhibited not just great talent but superb organizational savvy as well. I would also like to thank many others on the design and production staff, including

Leslie Keefe, Tom Aczel, Dan MacBride, Dale Mack, and Patrick Smith. A special thanks to Anne-Laure Lyon, friend and fashion stylist, whose keen eye and sense of style made such a difference to the cover photo.

As a first-time author, I felt warmly welcomed, encouraged, and supported by Rodale's incomparable publishing professionals. Easing my way into the world of books were Debora Yost, Darlene Schneck, Michael Ward, Brian Carnahan, Susan Massey, Karen Arbegast, Denyse Corelli, David Umla, Lisa Andruscavage, Vicki DaSilva, Kate Stuckert, Jackie Dornblaser, and Cathy Strouse. Senior copy editor Amy Kovalski was a paradigm of patience during many reviews of copy and layout. In the area of direct-response promotion, my thanks go to expert photographer Hilmar and to Eric Betuel, Karen Follweiler, and Brian Clifford.

I am particularly grateful to Cindy Ratzlaff for the great confidence she showed in planning and implementing publicity for the book. She was ably assisted by a superb trade-book marketing and promotion team that includes Renee James, Shannon Gallagher, and Mary Lengle.

Jerry Pendergast of Jerry's Caterers provided important factual data about airline food and menu creation, giving me an inside look I could not have gotten elsewhere.

The staff in my New York office deserves—and gets—my deepest thanks. On a daily basis, they dealt with my sometimes frantic effort to be both physician and author. They consistently exhibited equanimity of spirit while supporting the effort in very practical terms. I extend my most heartfelt gratitude to office staffers Gerri Pietrangolare, Alexandra Lotito, Shanette Vega, and Catherine Fallon; to nutritionist Marcia Cohen; to psychologists Dr. Stephanie Secolsky, Dr. Norman Wyloge, and Linda Charnes, MFT; and to physical therapist Yuri Usher. A special thank-you to Susan Amato, CSW, for her contributions to the chapters on the psychology of weight loss, and for her ongoing support of this project and her enthusiastic participation.

Support and enthusiasm were also offered in great measure by my brother, Michael Shapiro, and my sister, Marilyn McLaughlin. I am grateful to them both. I am also grateful to my dogs, Willow and Barkley, for uncharacteristically failing to eat the manuscript of the book.

Finally, I want to thank my patients—all those I have worked with over the past 21 years, and especially those who agreed to be interviewed and photographed for this book. You have been the proving ground for the principles of *Dr. Shapiro's Picture Perfect Weight Loss* program, and your enthusiasm, dedication, and commitment to those principles—as well as the successes you've achieved—have quite simply been my inspiration.

New York, November 1999

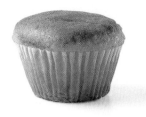

Look and Lose!
Do you think eating a corn muffin is saving calories? See page 126.

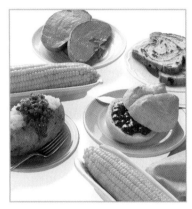

Look and Lose!
Instead of a square of corn bread, reach for all of this! See page 135.

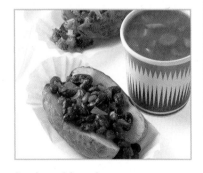

Look and Lose!
Need lunch on the run? See page 155 for your best choice.

Contents

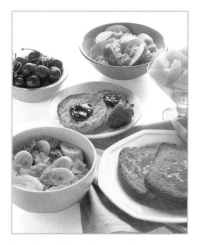

Look and Lose!
What's for breakfast?
See page 131.

Look and Lose!
Could you eat all this? Probably not, but if you eat one fat-free, sugar-free muffin, you're getting the same number of calories. See page 5.

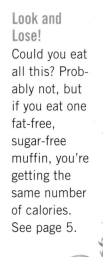

YES, IT'S OKAY TO EAT!

*F*ed up with diets?

You're not alone.

For nearly 20 years, I have specialized in weight control at my practice in mid-Manhattan. In addition to being the financial, shopping, and theater capital of the United States, New York City is also the diet capital.

Many of my patients are celebrities in the worlds of media, entertainment, and fashion. You can easily imagine how important it is to look great if you're in the limelight much of the time. For them, looking attractive and stylish is a job requirement. Of course they want to lose weight, feel healthy, and look terrific for personal reasons. But even more compelling than that are their professional reasons. This is something that *has* to happen for the sake of their careers.

Others are leaders in business and politics. To look powerful and in control, they have to appear healthy and fit. For them as well, losing weight is a very serious business.

I used to think New Yorkers were unique in their weight concerns. But of course they're not. Millions of people across America want to lose weight. And they're searching for the best way to do it.

When Diets Don't Do It

I've met thousands of people who were fed up with diets. These are people who vowed "Never again!"—and meant it. Many of the people who come through my door have tried four or five diets, and some have tried dozens. Many are hardened and cynical survivors of yo-yo dieting, that infamous and health-sapping pattern of drastically losing weight while dieting only to put it on again as soon as the diet is over.

And yet these hardened skeptics are still willing to visit a "weight-loss doctor."

Why?

The fact is, these people come to me because they don't want the same kind of diets they've tried before. Indeed, they're ready to run from those kinds of diets. They want a weight-loss plan that doesn't leave them feeling deprived, hungry, and unhappy. They're asking for some way to help them lose weight and keep it off while they continue with their busy, active lifestyles.

Even though weight loss is vital to their careers and their futures, it doesn't mean that it's easier for these people than it is for you and me. The only difference is that they can't

1

afford to fail. To lose weight and keep it off, many of them are willing to pay thousands of dollars. They get personal counseling, and my staff works with each person individually. But the secrets to their weight-loss successes, the reasons why they have succeeded and recommend me to others, are all in this book.

While you won't get personal coaching and counseling from this book, I can assure you that you will be able to get many of the same weight-loss benefits from it. You'll feel better, you'll look better, and you won't have to go through the heartbreaking cycle of losing weight only to gain it back again.

Best of all, you don't have to stop eating.

Once you've developed Food Awareness Training—using the techniques in this book—you'll never have to count calories or grams of fat. You don't have to think about all the food that "thin people can eat." You don't have to avoid restaurants or dodge dinner invitations.

After Food Awareness Training, one look is all it takes to help you make your choices. Weight loss becomes automatic because you react automatically.

I know this takes some explaining, but first, I'd like to give you some understanding of what lies behind this remarkable program.

Look—No Bad Foods!

Soon after I opened my weight-loss clinic, I made a discovery that has affected everything I've done since. I discovered a simple truth: No single weight-loss program can work for everyone.

Of course, we'd all like an easy solution to the problem of losing weight. Many people have spent a lot of time and money trying to figure out how. Some have even put their health at risk in search of the quick magic fix. Early in my practice, I began to encounter people who had been on many varieties of strange diets. Some ate extremely large or small quantities of food. Others tried bizarre combinations. Still others pursued programs that included pills and injections.

But I didn't have a "Dr. Shapiro Diet," and I still don't. When people leave my office, they don't carry handouts listing the foods that they should and shouldn't eat at various times of the day. I never ask patients to alter their usual routines, and that's probably a good thing, since most of them can't. As you've probably discovered yourself, you can't quit your job or change your family or cancel holidays just because you need to lose weight. Weight loss—or maintenance—needs to be something that happens while you're still getting on with your life.

I don't tell my patients what they can't eat or shouldn't eat. Instead, I talk about the choices that they can make. I ask them to subscribe to a few principles that, I believe, are the essential components of successful weight loss.

- **Any reason for eating is okay.** For years, people on diets were told: "Eat only when you're hungry." Research has shown, however, that there's no clear line between the physiological and the emotional reasons for eating. So asking someone to decide whether they have a real, physical need for food is asking for the impossible. If you're deprived of food for any reason, you're likely to have an increased need to eat. And the more you deny that need, the more food-obsessed you can become.

So what should you do if you crave food?

I think you should go right ahead and have some. Sometimes, that means you'll eat when you're not physically hungry, but that's okay. You really do want to eat. Just eat the healthiest and lowest-calorie foods that you find satisfying.

- **There are no bad foods.** Candy is okay. Desserts are okay. You're not "cheating" if you eat those foods, but you are making choices. Yes, there are times when only the high-fat, high-calorie food will do. But there are also many alternatives.

- **There are no "correct" portions.** Hunger varies from person to person. The need for food goes up and down. Even if you eat a whole pint of sorbet or a whole box of frozen fudge bars or a dozen hard candies, the diet isn't a failure. Sure, you've eaten a lot because you were hungry, for whatever reason, but you haven't blown your weight-loss plan. You're still in the driver's seat. You're not out of control. Don't worry about "getting back on track" because you're never off track.

- **An eating plan needs to suit your tastes and lifestyle.** Many of my patients travel and entertain. Frequently, they have business engagements where contacts are made and deals are done over drinks, appetizers, lunch, or dinner. Can they give up these appointments? Of course not. And neither can you if business meals are a necessary part of your professional life.

What you can do, however, is take control of these situations. You can continue your normal activities without interruption as you continue to work toward losing weight. Once you've lost weight, you can maintain that loss by continuing to make the best choices.

Even if you're not a power luncher, other challenges may be built into your lifestyle. For some people, the challenge is breakfast. They just grab something and go. I won't try to change that pattern. If you're used to grabbing breakfast on the run, so be it. What you can do is choose what you eat for that "quickie" breakfast so that you get the energy you need and don't feel deprived.

Consider the food challenges that face someone who's home all day, with the kitchen near at hand. You can't change the circumstances, but there are things you can do to ensure that you're making the right choices when you're living that lifestyle. Again, you can do it without depriving yourself.

- **You're never on a diet.** Instead of dieting, you're participating in an ongoing process of learning to make satisfying food choices.

On a typical deprivation diet, people often eat ravenously as soon as the diet is over. With Food Awareness Training, you never feel this kind of deprivation. You'll adopt new habits that are completely comfortable.

Food Awareness Training begins when you *see* your food choices. When patients come to my office, the nutritionist sets up actual food for visual demonstrations. These demonstrations help people take the first step toward developing a new relationship with food.

Want to see one of these demonstrations? Please turn the page.

Surprised?

Or maybe *shocked* is the right word.

As you can see, this food demonstration tells the whole story in the form of a simple equation. The muffin on the left has no added fat or sugar, but it has 720 calories. The calories come from flour, the muffin's main ingredient. What's more, since the flour has been refined, the muffin has little nutritional value.

To figure out what that muffin equals—in terms of calories—just think of all the foods on the right.

The equation states a simple fact: *All* the food on the facing page adds up to the same number of calories as the corn muffin on this page. Have a couple handfuls of grapes. If you're still hungry, how about two pears, half a papaya, and half a cantaloupe? Enjoy half a kiwifruit, too. If you want a couple of rolls, go ahead. Still hungry? Then slice up a whole fresh pineapple, add it to everything else you've eaten, and just keep on munching until you're full.

The choice is yours.

1 fat-free, sugar-free muffin (9 oz) 720 **calories**

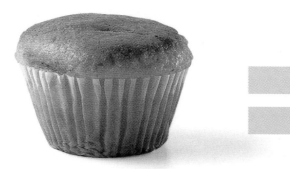

1 pineapple (2 lbs) 240 calories
½ cantaloupe (1 lb) 60 calories
½ kiwifruit (1½ oz) 10 calories
½ papaya (5 oz) 40 calories
grapes (5 oz) 70 calories
2 pears (6½ oz) 100 calories
2 whole wheat rolls (2½ oz) 200 calories

TOTAL 720 calories

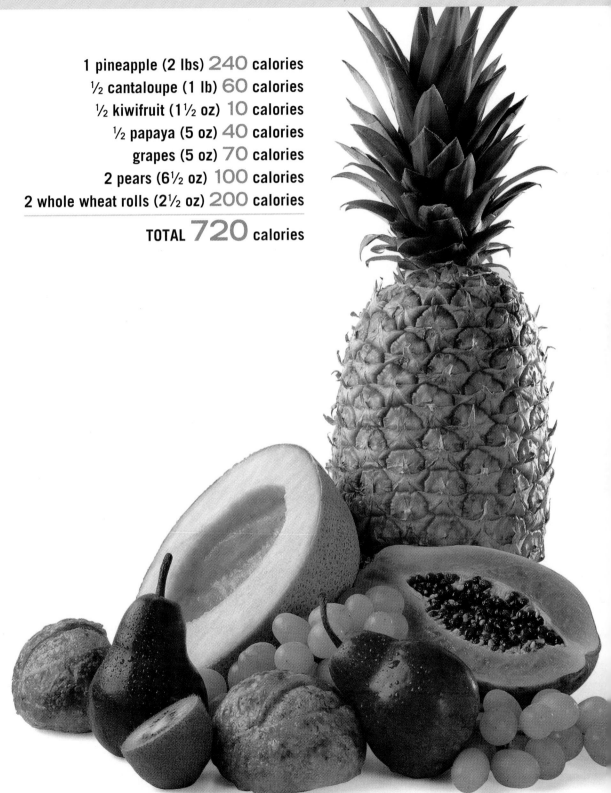

The simple equation sinks in quickly, doesn't it?

That's the first lesson in Food Awareness Training. It really doesn't take much to make us aware of what we're eating, but sometimes, you simply have to see it to believe it.

Now let's consider what happened when you looked at the visual equation on the preceding two pages.

Most of us have the impression that corn muffins are a healthful food. At least they might seem that way, compared with a Danish or a buttered croissant. So it might seem perfectly natural to have a corn muffin for breakfast or a snack. Even if you happen to know the number of calories in that muffin, why waste time counting calories when you're just plain hungry?

A View of Your Options

With Food Awareness Training, you don't have to count the calories. Instead, simply think of the picture you just saw. Then consider how much you can eat instead of that muffin. Even if you were starving, it's unlikely that you could eat all the food to the right of the equal sign.

I'm not saying that you can't eat the muffin. Of course you can. But you can also see what your options are. Very clearly.

If you're reading this book, you have probably dieted before and may consider yourself fairly knowledgeable about fat and calories. So you probably know the cold, hard mathematical facts about food, fat, and calories. Rationally, logically, you could get out a calorie guide and a calculator and work out how many calories you're getting from each food. But who has time for all that?

The reason why this food demonstration works so effectively is that the images appeal to a different part of your brain. Instead of calculating your choices, you can see your choices. Research shows that when visual images are stored in your memory, you retain them longer. And they have much greater impact on your behavior, so you can make the right food choices instinctively.

As a result of looking at the pictures in this book and reading the accompanying explanations, better food choices will become a matter of routine.

You won't feel hungry because you'll be eating a lot. You'll experience the pleasure that comes not only from having eaten but also from having eaten amply, wisely, and well.

Chapter 1

Seeing Is Believing: The Core of Food Awareness Training

Does it seem to you that everywhere you go, people are talking about their diets?

It's true. One-third of Americans are overweight, while another third struggle constantly not to be. In 150 million homes each day, clock radios go off and people get out of bed, go into the bathroom, look in the mirror, and think about a diet.

But only about 9.5 million people are actually dieting at any given time.

What happens to the 140 million other promises? They're broken as soon as the man in the too-tight vest reaches for that piece of Danish pastry in the bustle of the morning meeting. For the mom who's at home with the kids, the diet promise ends as soon as she takes a few more nibbles of the kids' snack foods because she needs energy. For the person who has been chained to a desk all day, trying hard not to think about food, the diet promise comes to a crashing end with a late-night bowl of ice cream.

Everyone knows that being overweight isn't good for you. The insurance companies certainly know it: To determine risk groups, they have gathered masses of statistics about what happens to people who are overweight. They've realized that if you're overweight, you're more prone to diseases such as heart disease, diabetes, stroke, and high blood pressure. People who are overweight are more likely to need surgery, and once they've had the surgery, they're more likely to develop complications. Being overweight even affects your buying power: Those who weigh more are likely to earn less money, especially if they're executives.

Enough Incentives?

Better health and more prosperity are fine motivators. But even with these incentives, the thought of going on a diet is difficult to contemplate.

A diet is rigid. A diet is boring. A diet means giving up all the foods you like. A diet means changing your lifestyle. A diet means feeling hungry. And many people have discovered something else that's incredibly discouraging about diets: Once they're over, you usually begin to gain back the weight.

Before you take the first steps toward Food Awareness Training, I want you to get rid of all those thoughts about dieting. This is not like any diet you may have known. Food Awareness Training is flexible, not boring. You do not have to give up the food you love or change your lifestyle. You will never feel hungry. You will change your entire relationship with food so you need never be on the same up-and-down weight cycle again.

This is not a "diet book" in any conventional sense. Start with the fact that it is not just for dieters. You won't have to rely on prescriptions, diet gurus, or prepared meals. While this book will help anyone who is trying to lose weight, either through an individualized or group program or with the help of a doctor, it is also meant to help people who are trying to maintain weight, eat in a healthier way, or make better choices for their children.

Who Are You?

To be sure, the way you approach Food Awareness Training is likely to be influenced by experiences that you've had with diet or weight-loss programs in the past. Fortunately, the program has worked for a wide range of people—from those who have never tried diets to those who have been through numerous plans and programs that were designed to help them lose weight. And there's a reason why Food Awareness Training is just as effective for men as it is for women, and just as effective for young

people as it is for those who are middle-age or older.

If you've never been concerned with weight loss, but you are now, Food Awareness Training can help you make food choices that assure you'll never have to go on a drastic weight-loss program. In fact, many people who come to see me are experiencing a weight problem for the first time.

Among the first-timers are women who notice small to moderate weight gain with the onset of menopause. The extra weight isn't a problem, and they want to make sure it doesn't become one. They feel like there are certain things that they can do now to lose some weight and avoid a lot of weight gain in the future. And they're right.

Some men meet their first challenge with weight gain just as they're reaching middle age. That's to be expected. Metabolism changes as we get older, and the food that we consume doesn't get burned up as quickly. Even if our eating habits don't change, it's easy to put on a few pounds—and much harder to take them off. In fact, by the time you're a mature adult, you need 100 fewer daily calories than you needed when you were growing up.

Some people who have never had weight problems in the past find that a new medication can have side effects. People often gain weight if they start taking drugs that contain steroids. And some people gain weight when they have hormone therapy or take psychotropic medications such as antidepressants.

Other factors that can cause weight gain? Maybe you've put on a few pounds because you've started traveling for business a lot more than you used to. Or perhaps you have young children who tie you to the home front and kitchen much more than you used to be. Working odd shifts, changing jobs, or going through a relocation can also initiate weight gain.

The Quick-Fix Lure

For anyone who starts to put on weight, a gimmick diet might appear to offer a quick fix. My advice: Stay away from those diets.

You need practical, easy-to-understand advice to make some healthful and easy adjustments in the way you choose food. With my program, you can continue to eat real food, and you don't have to follow a set routine of eating a certain amount at a particular time. Also, you don't have to deal with control and deprivation. While you're eating healthier food—for some people, the best food they've ever had in their lives—you'll also be controlling your weight, as long as you have Food Awareness Training to guide the hand that feeds you.

- If you have gone on diets many times during your life, you'll be relieved to discover that Food Awareness doesn't involve unusual regimes and extremes of deprivation.

  I know how extraordinary those programs can be, having met people who have tried everything from pills and injections to elaborate rituals that involve weighing each portion of food. Food Awareness Training will teach you how to make food choices for a lifetime. With this plan, you have the very best chance of losing weight and keeping it off—without ever feeling deprived.

  Most important, you won't have to go through the heartbreaking cycle of losing and gaining weight again. You will never again have to see a diet doctor or join a program. Why? Because you will be dealing with food in a totally different way than you ever have before.

- If you're particularly concerned about fitness and nutrition, Food Awareness Training will help guide you through the maze of information and apparent contradictions that relate to reduced-fat or low-calorie foods and beverages. Which of these foods really do make sense? Are there some low-fat or "light" foods that are nutritionally barren? With Food Awareness Training, you'll find out which of the diet foods are nutritional booby traps and learn to make other choices automatically. You'll also discover some of the nutritional superstars that can help you maintain a well-balanced, healthful diet even if you're trying to maintain or lose weight.

- If you're a teenager or college student, you may already think a lot about being overweight. But even if you know that certain foods should be avoided, you may not always find it convenient to sit down to a regular meal. Also, you may not be sure which foods are good choices for meals or snacking.

  With Food Awareness Training, you can pick up knowledge of your food choices with minimum effort. This book presents that kind of information in a memorable and easy-to-understand way. You can start to develop automatic eating habits that will help you for the rest of your life.

The Key to Weight Loss

When I was beginning my practice, I prescribed many different approaches to losing weight that were tailored to individual needs. I discovered that calorie reduction is the key.

On a long-term basis, there is only one safe, effective, foolproof way to get yourself down to a lower weight and keep off the extra pounds. That is to eat a healthy, reduced-calorie diet and get enough exercise.

But the really good news is that eating fewer calories does not necessarily mean eating less food. And it definitely doesn't mean that you have to walk around in a constant state of deprivation. After all, a feeling of deprivation is the surest way to make your weight-loss plan fail. Instead, you may be eating even *more* food. You will certainly feel satisfied.

I also found that most people don't enjoy counting calories. First-time dieters quickly discover that it's a time-consuming and complicated chore. Calorie counting almost always goes hand in hand with the feeling of being deprived that spells doom to a diet.

And that led to the next important step in my program: developing food demonstrations.

The Look of Knowledge

You've already seen one food demonstration on page 4. Coming up in this book are scores of others.

These are exactly the kinds of food demonstrations I use in my practice. The "demos" are a powerful, effective tool for teaching people to look at food in a different way.

We see so much information about fat and calories that this information may seem like first-grade stuff to most of us. But it's not always easy to judge the information given to you.

For instance, if you read a package label, you may register the fact that a food is "high in fat" or "low in fat," but you're less likely to pay much attention to serving size.

Just for fun, you might want to test some of the assumptions you have about different types of food. The food quiz on page 12 will help you do that.

One thing is certain about taking this quiz: Once you've *seen* the answers, you're unlikely to forget them. Seeing the actual food—and understanding how many calories are in that food—is a far more powerful message than reading a list of words and numbers.

These demonstrations—like the many in chapter 6 of this book—are likely to challenge many of your assumptions. Looking at their choices, people often say, "That can't be true! How can one little fat-free muffin have as many calories as all that fruit?"

But there's no trick to these demonstrations. Before preparing any visual display of food, my staff nutritionist checks food values with statistical tables provided by the USDA. If we're using packaged foods, we use the nutritional information on the packages, paying special attention to the serving sizes. And for some of the prepared dishes in the food demonstrations, we calculated the calories for the recipes using the USDA handbooks.

Each food demonstration has been carefully checked, using all the information that we have about calorie counts, nutritional values, and serving sizes, to make sure that the portions and amounts are accurate. Since you're always making choices about what foods you eat and don't eat, I want to make sure that what you see is what you get.

Help from the Demos .

The food demonstrations not only help you choose wisely but also help you interpret nutritional information correctly. Here, too, the advice of dietitians and nutritionists is extremely valuable. We find, for example, that many people have mistaken beliefs about what they should and should not eat.

Take the term *fat-free*. Thinking that fats should be avoided, many people believe that they can lose weight if they simply eliminate butter and oil from their diets.

What happens if you eat fat-free cakes and cookies instead of the conventional fat-filled kind? What if you eat bagels instead of croissants? What if you have jelly beans for a sweet instead of a chocolate bar, or pasta instead of a burger? Isn't weight loss guaranteed for people who adopt these fat-cutting strategies?

If that's what you've heard, and you've moved over to a low-fat or fat-free diet, then you may wonder why the scale isn't moving downward. Where's the flaw in the low-fat reasoning?

Here's the problem: A fat-free cake, as advertised, is probably free of fat, but it is high in refined carbohydrates. And the carbohydrates that it contains can easily turn to body fat.

Carbohydrate calories are very real calories. Like fat calories, they can either turn into energy when you exercise, or they can go to the fat cells in your body, where they're stored away. That's why food products that are advertised as "fat-free" do not by themselves help you get thin.

When I speak with people who have had lifelong struggles with weight control, I tell them that the program they will begin is not a short-term effort but the beginning of a journey during which their relationship with food will change. Even experienced dieters are surprised to discover that they don't have to stick with the foods that they thought were "good" for them—foods they might not even like—but that they can eat a wide array of foods that they really enjoy. Nothing I can say, however, drives home these points as powerfully as the food demonstrations.

A Male Message, Too

In the past, the overwhelming majority of people who came to see me about weight control were women. Their number one concern was appearance. Many women just didn't like how they looked in jeans or bathing suits, and they wanted to change that.

Few men seemed to share the same concerns. But that's starting to change.

Several years back, most of the men who came to see me were concerned about some health problem associated with weight. Some had heart problems, and their doctors had told them that they absolutely had to lose weight to help prevent future heart attacks. Others were threatened by what they found out about their family histories, which suggested that they might be in line for future health problems such as atherosclerosis (hardening of the arteries), diabetes, or other weight-related

(continued on page 16)

The Food Quiz: Testing Your Calorie IQ

Are you ready to face the challenge?

It's quite easy, actually. Just look at the pairs of "food comparisons" in the pictures below and guess which food in each pair is *lower* in calories.

The calories are based on the amount of food you see in the photographs.

Just from this short quiz, you'll get a better idea about which choices you're making the next time you see these foods. Even if you get 100 percent correct on the quiz, the images will remind you of things that you already know about these foods. You'll discover even more, and expand your choices, as you continue reading this book.

After you try, you can check your answers on page 14.

1.

assorted olives or fat-free pretzel

2.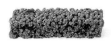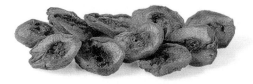

low-fat granola bar or dried peach halves

3.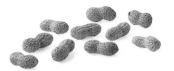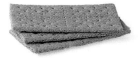

peanuts or graham crackers

4.

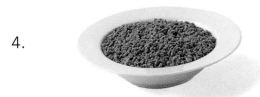

Grape-Nuts or **Frosted Flakes**

5.

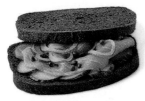

smoked salmon on pumpernickel or **roast beef on country white**

6.

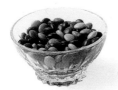 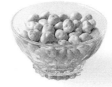

M & M's or **yogurt raisins**

7.

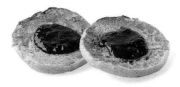 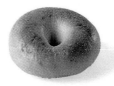

English muffin with jam or **dry bagel**

8.

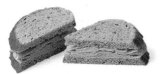 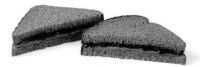

turkey on rye or **peanut butter and jam on whole wheat bread**

The Food Quiz: Testing Your Calorie IQ *(answers)*

1.

15 assorted olives 60 calories
1 fat-free pretzel 80 calories

Did you assume that the olives had the higher calorie count?

True, the fat-free pretzel looks bare, dry, and downright plain. Naturally, we're likely to assume that it must be low in calories. By contrast, we tend to think of olives as "fattening" foods, and their lush appearance and rich taste only add to that image.

It's accurate to say that olives contain fat, but many people don't realize they have the "good" kind of fat—the heart-healthy monounsaturated fats, not the saturated kind that raises artery-clogging cholesterol.

As for calories, this dish of olives has only 60 calories—versus 80 calories for the bare, dry, plain, fat-free pretzel.

2.

1 low-fat granola bar 150 calories
10 dried peach halves 150 calories

What we're looking at here is a tie as far as calories go. While there's plenty of nutrition in the granola bar, it comes at a fairly high caloric price. Look at all the dried peach halves you could eat for the same amount of calories. And there's an interesting twist here. Despite all the nutritional claims for that granola bar, you get *even more* fiber, vitamins, and minerals from the dried peach halves.

3.

10 peanuts 80 calories
3 graham crackers 180 calories

Graham crackers versus peanuts? Seems like an easy choice, doesn't it?

It's hard to believe—but absolutely true—that these three puny graham crackers, the least cookielike cookies around, have over twice as many calories as 10 peanuts, notorious for their fat content. And if this weren't enough, the graham crackers are virtually nutrition-free, while the fats in the peanuts are the essential fatty acids our bodies need.

4.

1½ cups Grape-Nuts 600 calories
1½ cups Frosted Flakes 220 calories

At first glance, you probably thought this question was a dead giveaway: What could be higher in calories than a cereal that has been sweetened like crazy—frosted with sugar!—to make it more palatable to children? Against a healthy, grown-up offering like Grape-Nuts, the kid cereal, Frosted Flakes, probably seems like a non-contender.

In this case, however, the kid's "junk" food is the better caloric bargain: 220 calories versus 600 calories for an equivalent portion of Grape-Nuts.

The fact is that almost all cereals have about 110 calories per ounce. The denser the cereal, the higher the calorie content per cup. Grape-Nuts is a particularly dense cereal. Just eat ¼ cup of Grape-Nuts, and you'll be consuming a full ounce.

5.

2 oz salmon 90 calories
2 slices of pumpernickel 140 calories
cucumbers and capers 5 calories
TOTAL 235 calories

3 oz roast beef 210 calories
2 slices of country white 150 calories
TOTAL 360 calories

Smoked salmon is a treat—a fancy, fatty fish we reserve for special occasions. Lean roast beef—hold the dressing—is what we eat for lunch when we're trying to drop a few pounds. Right?

Well, if that has been your thinking, you might want to take a second look. In this comparison, the roast beef sandwich is *not* the lower-calorie item. In fact, the salmon on pumpernickel "wins": Its 235 calories compare favorably to the roast beef sandwich's 360.

6.

5 oz M & M's 675 calories
5 oz yogurt raisins 675 calories

Let's face it: Yogurt raisins are pretty much everybody's idea of a "virtuous" snack. They're what you would eat if you were trying *not* to eat M & M's.

If you did so, however, you would achieve absolutely nothing in the weight-loss department. This bowl of yogurt raisins has exactly as many calories as the bowl of M & M's. Eat yogurt raisins if you want to, but not to save calories; that's a virtue they simply don't possess.

7.

English muffin with jam 170 calories
Dry bagel 400 calories

If it's calories you want to save, you're far better off with the English muffin and jam than with the plain bagel, chaste though it appears. But both of these snacks are, in the words of staff nutritionist Phyllis Roxland, "nutritional wastelands." In other words, the vitamins, minerals, and fiber you get from these typical breakfast foods are so minimal that there's really no difference between them. Only the calories are much different. If they are the only snacks around, you might as well go for the sweet taste of the muffin and jam rather than the dry, unadorned bagel.

8.

5 oz turkey 250 calories
2 slices of rye 160 calories
TOTAL 410 calories

1½ Tbsp peanut butter 150 calories
1½ Tbsp jam 75 calories
2 slices of whole wheat 140 calories
TOTAL 365 calories

Surprise! A sandwich of skinless white-meat turkey—hold the mayo—looks like the perfect "diet" lunch. By contrast, good old peanut-butter-and-jelly—the notorious PB&J of our reckless youth—seems an obvious no-no. But in this case, looks are deceiving; the truth is in the numbers. If you choose the PB&J, you'll be getting fewer calories.

problems. Again, their doctors' warnings gave them an urgent nudge toward my office.

These days, more men are concerned with appearance. Yes, health concerns are still the dominant issues, but I am seeing many more men than I used to, and they have other issues. Some top executives, for instance, now make room in their crowded calendars to visit my office to deal with their weight.

The Costs of Being Overweight

Why are more men visiting me than before? Well, for one thing, there's been a change in our society, and men are no longer embarrassed to admit that they care about how they look. I see a lot more men working out, going to spas, coloring their hair, having cosmetic surgery—and coming to me to deal with their bodies.

The appearance factor is more than skin deep. Many male professionals have learned—sometimes the hard way—that no one has a lifetime guarantee of employment. It is not unusual for a top executive and even a CEO to be let go. If you are in the position of having to present yourself as a job candidate in competition with young people in good shape, you want to look as youthful, fit, and healthy as possible.

Fair or not, in many competitive business environments, people who are trim and in good shape are perceived as being disciplined. Being overweight is more often seen as having a lack of willpower.

I've seen many men and women who were extremely talented, well-paid, and pro-

motable. But they understood that they could go even farther in their careers if they were more "presentable." Many of my patients—both men and women—tell me that once they lost weight, they were suddenly treated differently at work.

One woman who holds a very high position at a global firm estimates that being severely overweight has probably cost her several million dollars in lost compensation. Men are beginning to realize that the same may be true for them—but having been less sensitive about weight, some have been slower to understand the professional and economic cost of being overweight. When they come to the door of my office, however, they're prepared to make some weight-loss choices that they feel will keep their options open.

As you begin using the information here, you may be facing similar issues in your professional life.

Meet Your Challenges

Over the course of my career, having interviewed thousands of people who are concerned with weight loss, I have discovered that each individual faces different challenges. But many are in similar situations in terms of their lifestyles and schedules. Here are the four lifestyle situations that seem to pose the most problems.

1. Tied to a desk. Let's face it: Many people who spend a lot of time in the office have fairly sedentary lifestyles. Lunch may be catch-as-catch-can from a vending machine, the office cafeteria, the local sandwich shop, or some other source. Often, food choices are limited, and snacks are all too available—no farther away than the desk drawer or office refrigerator.

If you're in this situation, you may find that you have a low-energy period in the late afternoon. The temptation is to remedy the problem with a "sugar fix." And, of course, if you're in an office all day, your responsibilities don't end there. Pressured by family demands or other obligations, you may be tempted to pick up convenience foods for breakfast or dinner. Again, your options may be limited because you need to act fast to get food on the table.

2. Home with the family. Stay-at-home moms (and dads) often have big snacking problems. When kids leave food on their plates, parents naturally hate to see it go to waste. So they take a bite here, a bite there, and it all adds up.

Also, in many families with children, it's likely there will be more junk food around. Chips and cookies find their way in, and when you have easy access, that's another problem. When you're spending a lot of time near "kid food," it's all too easy to grab a handful while you're taking care of the family.

3. Eating on the run. Young, single students are typical on-the-run eaters. But you may have the same eating pattern if you're so busy that you rarely cook. If you have little time to eat, you may be picking up practically all your meals. You get breakfast from a deli or coffee shop. Lunch may be fast food or whatever the nearest street vendor has to offer. Dinner ends up being takeout. It's not un-common to skip a meal or two, then eat as much as necessary to fill yourself up.

Often, this eating style is driven by necessity, and in some professions, nearly everyone eats this way. Police officers, for instance, rarely have time for sit-down meals, except when they're off duty. Department store clerks and other retail personnel have irregular breaks, so they can't count on fixed schedules. In fact, anyone who has to eat out most of the week is likely to have an eating-on-the-run lifestyle.

4. Wined and dined around the clock. Executives who spend a lot of time doing business in social situations are likely to eat well but rarely on the same schedule. They may start their days with a "power breakfast," hold a meeting at lunch, and go to a social event for dinner. If your lifestyle is like this, you're probably traveling a great deal, often grabbing a bite while you're on the road, in an airport, on a plane, or in a hotel.

Each one of these lifestyle situations makes different kinds of demands on us, and in each case, your food choices vary. That's why I do food demonstrations with so many different kinds of foods—not just things that you'll find in the cupboard or refrigerator but also with fast foods, street-vendor foods, takeout and restaurant foods, and common snacks.

In other words, I understand that you can't change your lifestyle just because you've decided to lose weight. Your lifestyle depends on such a wide range of factors—family, location, profession—that you need food choices that fit your lifestyle, rather than the other way around.

The idea is to help you *see* your choices, no matter what circumstances you're in or what lifestyle you follow. The right solution is the one that helps you eat healthfully, lose weight, and not feel deprived.

The Stress Connection

Do you eat more or more erratically when you're feeling a lot of stress?

For so many people, food is a stress reliever. And from what I have seen, people these days are under a lot more stress than they were in the past.

More women are juggling jobs and families. Men and women are spending more hours on the job. Of course, it's true that my office is located in New York City, one of the stress capitals of the world. But I think that what I see is replicated in many other places in this country.

Americans as a whole tend to be workaholics. Many people work two jobs to maintain the high standard of living to which they aspire. And in many two-career families, time is at a premium.

Not long ago, I began working with a group of police officers who were just starting Food Awareness Training as part of a health-improvement program.

We all know about big-city cops. Can you imagine a higher-stress job? But I was interested to learn that on-the-job stress wasn't necessarily their biggest concern. For many of them, the stress that they reported came from being so busy.

Many have spouses who also work. So a typical off-duty police officer has to take on a large share of household responsibilities. After they get home, they have to look after home maintenance, cleaning, cooking, and child care. For them—as for so many of us—these are the stresses that really add up.

The result? To many of these cops, food was a comfort and a reward. One officer told me that his biggest problem was snacking after 11:00 P.M. Not until then—after his workday was over and the domestic duties were taken care of—could he kick back and relax. And that's when he reached for snack foods.

I could not only sympathize but also empathize. For me, too, that's a time of day when I can wind down and when I am most tempted by food.

So what can we do?

In my view, late-night snacking is not necessarily bad. If that's the only time of day when you can get a break, why not enjoy it? But I helped the policeman by showing him that there are a number of satisfying and delicious snacks lower in calories than what he was eating. When he felt like sitting down for a snack, he could eat foods like pretzel rods, fruit, low-calorie frozen fudge bars, or Creamsicles.

I didn't tell him not to eat. I didn't tell him that he was eating for the wrong reasons. I just helped him make some different choices—equally satisfying and enjoyable, but for just a fraction of the calories.

Why You Gain Weight

As your own tastebuds will tell you again and again, food is not a villain.

Most of us love it. And that's a good thing because we need food for growth and repair of tissues. We need all that pent-up nutritional power to help meet our energy needs.

It's not the food itself but the storage process that makes us unhappy. If we eat more than we need for immediate use, our bodies put it into cozy, comfortable storage cells. Where are those cells located? You already know the answer. Most of the plump fat cells are located in the trouble spots that we know about—bellies, hips, thighs, buttocks, and all the other areas that have fat-holding cells.

People who tend to be overweight have bodies that scientists would describe as efficient. At first blush, efficiency might sound like a good thing, but in the modern world, it's a liability. If your body uses food efficiently, you get the energy you need immediately, and then store the excess.

For some people, that's fine. Their bodies, almost mysteriously, don't store much of the food they eat. You know who I'm talking about—those few people who seem to be able to eat anything and still stay thin.

For the vast majority of us, however, the fat that we store just keeps hanging around. If only there were some way to reset the controls on our bodies. If we could do that, maybe we could turn the storage function from high to low.

Of course, as you know, scientists have not quite figured out a way. Until they do, some people will be more likely to gain weight than others. The reasons have to do with body chemistry.

On the other hand, that doesn't mean your body is going to fight you all the way. Many people can maintain a significant degree of weight loss, but that's easiest to do when you don't feel deprived.

Bon Hunger

For many years, we were fed the myth that there was a difference between genuine hunger and mere appetite. Hunger was supposed to be a good or normal sensation that came after prolonged periods without food.

For years, we believed the myth that you could actually tell the difference between appetite and hunger. Experts said that if you hadn't eaten food for hours and were genuinely hungry, you would know it. Dizziness, weakness, or acid stomach are the symptoms of real hunger.

Appetite, they claimed, was something different. Appetite was the result of out-of-control impulse. Your appetite, not hunger, made you head for a box of cookies despite the fact that you had just finished dinner. If you polished off a whole bowl of peanuts while chatting with your friend at the bar, that was the fault of your appetite again.

By this reasoning, the hunger-versus-appetite dichotomy was black and white. If you were legitimately hungry, that was okay. But if your appetite was making you eat, well, that was deemed less okay, even shameful.

Appetite, we were told, was an emotional response rather than a biological one. Appetite led you to eat out of boredom or frustration or anger. Eating for emotional reasons sounds like a wrong reason to eat.

But as scientists have begun to unlock the secrets of weight gain and weight loss, they have learned that people's reasons for eating can't be labeled in such neat and precise ways. The difference between hunger and appetite is hazy. Researchers have discovered that there are several hormones and neurochemicals in the body that have a profound effect on your life.

Listening to Your Chemicals

There are at least six body chemicals that have a profound effect on your life—and your weight. Their names are strange, and there's no reason to memorize them. But as weight-loss research continues, it's likely that you'll see these chemicals mentioned again and again. They are cholecystokinin, cortisol, dopamine, leptin, neuropeptide Y, and serotonin.

At the moment, there are no adequate explanations about how each of these affects your weight individually. What researchers do know, however, is that these substances relay messages to your fat cells, blood, brain, and intestines. They play a role in regulating body weight, appetite, eating behaviors, and even the way we think about food.

This is not to say that we are automatons programmed by chemicals. Our eating is also affected by other factors, from psyche to circumstances. Since the whole issue of eating is so complex, no researcher can tell you with absolute certainty why someone can resist the temptation of the bread basket one day but lust helplessly after chocolate cake the next day.

While it's nearly impossible to know the reasons why you need to eat a particular food at a particular time, it's very important to be in touch with that desire. You can't understand all the ways in which chemicals work, but you must listen when they talk to you. Most dieters have not learned to do this.

The urge to eat is a need that must be filled.

If we don't respond to that urge, the need-to-eat feelings—call them hunger, appetite, or anything else—will get the upper hand. And here's the irony: As a result of trying *not* to respond to the need to eat, there's a good chance that you won't be able to lose weight or maintain weight loss.

Beyond Good and Bad

Most dieters have built-in defenses. A statement as simple as "I'm hungry!" is unacceptable. Before acknowledging something that simple, dieters are already worrying about how that hungry feeling can lead them into going astray, going out of control, or messing up. People who have been on diets tell me that they constantly feel either good or bad, in control or out of control.

But you can't repress a feeling that says, quite simply, "I want to eat that." You might try to keep that chemically driven impulse in check, but it's sure to get the upper hand.

Overweight individuals typically have so much anxiety about the urge to eat that their bodies operate defensively. They don't even allow the hunger to come to consciousness. They find all kinds of rationalizations.

A person may come home from the supermarket with a cake. She says, "I bought it to serve to company." But lying just below the surface of that statement is the real reason, which is simply the desire to eat cake. The chemicals are talking. But what happens when we don't allow the chemicals to be heard?

What I'm telling you is something that

In Command of Appetite

Deep in the command center of your brain, a protein with a funny name may play a role in telling you whether you're feeling full.

The newly discovered protein, GLP-1, is made in the hypothalamus, the body's control center. When you eat, GLP-1 tells the intestines and pancreas to slow down digestion.

In animal studies, rats injected with GLP-1 showed signs that they were full before they finished their normal rations of food. When an inhibitor of GLP-1 was injected, the rats ate *more* than usual and grew fatter. More research is needed, however, before scientists can establish the role of GLP-1 in humans.

you may have always suspected if you've struggled repeatedly with your weight. That struggle is caused by something other than lack of determination. It's not being caused by a deficit in willpower. By identifying the chemicals that play a role in your hunger, we're beginning to get to the real causes. Soon we should have the information that proves your suspicions are true: Gaining and losing weight are *not* matters of self-control, determination, or other intangible factors.

In the meantime, that doesn't mean that your only choice is to throw up your hands and say, "Well, it's fate. I was born to be overweight." That is definitely not the case. You can reshape (literally) your destiny—or at least you can achieve a more modest goal of just taking a few pounds off.

I like to think of a person's underlying body chemistry as a kind of metabolic hand of cards that he is dealt at birth. Maybe, when it comes to weight issues, you weren't dealt the genetic equivalent of four aces, but I can tell you that if you play your cards right, you can still come up a winner.

Why Deprivation Diets Don't Work

To lose weight successfully, you either have to decrease your caloric intake or increase the number of calories expended through exercise—preferably both. To lose weight successfully and keep it off, you have to accomplish calorie reduction without feeling deprived. This is a key concept, and it is the heart of my program. Feeling deprived comes around and kicks you in the rear end—right in the direction of the nearest hot-fudge sundae or the local bakery.

I have been working with dieters for many years, and I know that they do not have a problem with willpower. Quite the contrary. People who can cling to a rigid diet, despite everything else that's going on in their lives, often have unusual discipline in many areas. Some have managed to stick with extremely rigorous programs for an amazingly long time to reach their goal weights.

I have had people who stayed on a liquid protein fast without a morsel of real food for as long as 4 months. Don't tell me this demonstrates a lack of willpower!

I have also seen, however, many people who have worked unbelievably hard to reach a certain weight-loss goal, only to gain all the weight back again. The feelings of deprivation were just too much for them, and once they had reached the numbers on the scale that they longed for, they resumed their old eating patterns. Yet, all the time they were dieting, they were not aware of feeling deprived.

People who are attempting to lose weight typically do not report feelings of deprivation; they bury them instead. They say that they had a bad week or that they ate because they weren't focused. They will say things like, "I had plenty. I didn't need to eat the brownie"; "I wasn't hungry"; or "I don't know why I did it."

If those phrases sound familiar, I can assure you that people who are deprived of food do need to eat. If you eat, it's because you're hungry.

What Diets Can Do to You

Dieters don't eat unconsciously. They don't have blackouts. They know when they're eating the whole box of cookies. What they lack is an awareness of the feeling of being hungry or craving the food. They've blocked the feeling because they thought it was bad. They tried to protect themselves from those urges.

I suggest that people in the Food Awareness Training program get comfortable with these urges. I tell them that it's okay to eat, but to do it mindfully. In fact, you *have* to learn to work with those urges. If you don't, the inevitable result is a binge.

A woman once came into my office reporting that she'd had a terrible week. She went to a birthday party that featured a lavish buffet. Smelling the food, she was tempted, but what really called out to her was a piece of cheesecake. She resisted it because she thought it was bad.

Instead of having the buffet food or the cheesecake, she had a cupcake that she thought was a little less bad. The cupcake didn't satisfy her, so she had another cupcake. After that, she just continued eating, having far more food than she was comfortable with. She ate so quickly, and with such feelings of guilt, that she didn't enjoy any of it.

What was the alternative?

My message to her was that giving in to her urge and eating the cheesecake would not have been a problem. Where she had a problem was with her attitude. Instead of saying, "This cheesecake looks good to me," she said to herself, "How can I avoid this cheesecake?"

To lose weight successfully, you have to figure out a way to have that occasional piece of cake and still feel like you're in the driver's seat.

Some people have the cake and tell me, "Okay, I decided I would have the piece of cake and get it over with."

Now, why should anyone want to get it over with? Do you plan not to have a piece of cake for another 6 weeks or 4 months or a year?

It is a mistake to put eating on hold, to think that you can turn off your desire to eat as if you were turning off a switch. That would be sad. You will have the urge to eat cake or whatever else tempts you from time to time. That urge is not an evil thing. You don't have to view a piece of cake, or whatever you desire, as an unfortunate or disastrous lapse of self-control.

Having Your Cake and Your Waistline, Too

As you're looking at your wide range of food choices, I urge you to figure out a way to recognize the foods that you enjoy and then work them into your eating plan. Yes, that includes food like cakes and cookies.

It doesn't mean that you should have a piece of cake every day for the sole purpose of teaching yourself to work cake into a weight-loss program. It does mean that if, on a particular day, you feel like having cake, you figure out a way to work it in or find a suitable substitute with which you're comfortable.

I ask people to try to become aware of the times when they experience the feeling of wanting to eat. By the way, it's perfectly okay to want food because you feel bored, frustrated, or anxious.

You don't need to distinguish between hunger and appetite or figure out whether the impulse is coming from the stomach, the brain, the elbow, or the television set. It doesn't matter. I don't want you to try so hard to put a label on it. Just being aware that you want to eat and knowing that it's okay helps put you in charge.

Remember: There is no wrong reason to eat.

Once you have recognized the impulse to eat, you can learn how to respond to it. You'll realize that there's no reason to feel guilty about having an appetite.

You're Choosing, Not Cheating

There's a good reason why I wage war on the concept of cheating. I simply don't believe that people cheat when they're hungry.

If someone decides she has to have a brownie, I say, "Go ahead, if you really want it. But make it a choice, not a cheat."

"That brownie is 400 calories!" she replies. "What's the difference whether you call it a 'cheat' or a 'choice'?"

The difference, I maintain, is logic. When you use logic to make the decision to eat some especially tempting, high-calorie food, you have the upper hand.

"I didn't have a good week," Andrea told me during an office visit. When she'd gone out to dinner, she told herself she wasn't going to dip into the bread basket. Andrea considers bread her weakness. But the bread came, and she couldn't resist. She broke off a chunk of sourdough bread.

She would have felt okay if it had stopped there. But after that first bite of sourdough bread, she broke off another chunk. And then, perhaps because she was hungry or stressed, she had a third.

Somewhere between the second and third chunks of bread, she made the transition from feeling like she was in control to feeling that she'd blown her diet for that day. She told herself that she'd cheated, and she believed it. So she no longer felt good about herself. Since she felt like a failure anyway, she decided to have breaded veal cutlet followed by the Death by Chocolate cake for dessert. On the way home, she picked up some ice cream and pretzels to snack on.

Eating with Awareness

Susan's evening started out like Andrea's, but the ending was quite different. Susan knows that she loves freshly baked breads and rolls. She, too, went to a restaurant. When she saw the fresh, warm bread in the bread basket, she decided that she really wanted to have some, so she took a roll and enjoyed it.

I'm very familiar with Susan's history as a dieter. I know that in the past, taking that roll would have created a cascade effect. Instead of seeing the roll and deciding to eat and enjoy it, she would have picked at it—taking as little as possible, then taking some more, then finishing it. To someone with the mentality of a dieter, the roll is a trigger, and Susan would have finished the roll, then worked her way through the rest of the bread basket. She would have felt guilty the whole time because she was cheating.

Instead, Susan ordered fish and vegetables while she finished her roll. She enjoyed the whole meal—the high-calorie roll as well as the low-calorie meal—and came away from the table feeling good about herself.

With another few weeks of Food Awareness Training, I'm confident that Andrea will arrive at the level of decision-making where Susan is now. But Andrea's not quite there yet.

Notice that Andrea didn't tell me about the bread problem right away. Instead, she began by saying that she hadn't had a good week.

We worked our way back to the point when she'd dipped into the bread basket. That was the point where she lost focus, but not because of the bread itself. A good-size chunk of sourdough is only about 30 calories. What sabotaged her, instead, was the feeling of failure—that she had somehow given in.

With Susan, on the other hand, the decision was just that: a decision. She wanted to treat herself to a roll, so she did. As it happens, that roll was about 150 calories—a lot more than the sourdough bread that Andrea ate—but it didn't trigger any feelings of failure. So the woman who had a 30-calorie chunk of bread ended up having a "bad week" as a result of all the bad feelings that it triggered, while the woman who had a 150-calorie roll enjoyed the treat and felt okay.

What's the Difference?

The woman who *chose* the roll was listening to her feelings. Susan worked the roll into her "diet"—if we use "diet" to mean the standards that you set for yourself. Andrea, by contrast, didn't allow herself the awareness of what she was feeling. She tried to suppress the desire for bread. So when she finally gave in and ate the bread, not only did she mess up her eating plan but also she didn't feel good about herself.

The problem? An impossible standard. If you love bread, there will be times when you want to decide to have some. It's that simple.

Right or wrong, self-image and self-worth for many people are very much related to what they're eating and how well they are sticking to their diets. With Food Awareness Training, you're always choosing, never cheating. So you never have to feel like you're falling off the wagon. And you never have to live up to impossible standards.

Making Your Decision

Obviously, you can't have every dessert in the world and still lose weight. But you do have some choices. You can pass up dessert, you can eat it, or you can choose one of many lower-calorie alternatives that may be just as satisfying. I recommend that you substitute the lower-calorie foods when possible, but have the brownie or the roll every now and then.

But please, whatever you do, recognize that the decision is up to you. I encourage you to recognize each urge that you feel. Ask yourself, "What am I really in the mood for? Is it chocolate? Will a frozen fudge bar or a Tootsie Pop do?" If not, have the brownie and know that you're still on track. By definition, the brownie should be considered a choice if none of those lower-calorie options can possibly satisfy your desire for the flavor and texture of a brownie.

Making a conscious decision to enjoy something is very different from eating it and feeling like a failure. In the latter case, people often go on to an all-out binge, having decided that it doesn't matter since they've already blown the diet.

Your attitude about what you're eating is as important a factor in how successful you'll be in weight loss as the calorie count of the food.

Written Permission from the Doctor

If you've been on diets before, you're probably wondering how I can be telling you

that it is possible to eat until you feel satisfied—even to have a whole box of frozen fudge bars when you feel you have to—and still lose weight.

I won't ask you to weigh yourself daily, measure each portion, stick to elaborate menus, or buy certain endorsed weight-loss food products. Instead, I'll help you make choices by giving you exactly the same food demos that my patients get to see.

Many people find that they learn one thing immediately from these visual demonstrations: They can eat a whole lot more than they do now and still take in fewer calories.

And it's delicious food. The pictures in this book speak to the urges that you may have tried to suppress. Yes, I'm giving you permission to eat, and the pictures show you why. They show large portions of foods that look and taste great. And they start to influence your relationship with food because these pictures will convince you that *it's okay to eat*, even when you have a goal of losing weight.

What's a Lot and What's Not

Unfortunately, most veteran dieters expect the acceptable foods to be something like lettuce leaves and celery stalks. But if you page ahead, you'll see many pictures of foods like bread and corn on the cob, hot-and-sour soup, scallops with black bean sauce, lollipops, pretzel sticks, and butterscotch candy. We're suggesting foods that you may decide to substitute for higher-calorie foods while getting the same satisfying taste.

Let's run a quick test right now. Do you like chocolate ice cream? Okay, you can have the richest chocolate ice cream available—for about 1,350 calories a pint. But you have some other choices. Instead, you can have chocolate frozen yogurt or sorbet—those have 450 calories a pint or less. If you think that a frozen fudge bar or two would be just as satisfying, you're really in luck, since a low-calorie fudge bar has only 30 calories. In other words, you'd have to eat 45 frozen fudge bars to consume the same number of calories that you'd get from one pint of rich ice cream. And if you have only one or two frozen fudge bars, which is likely to be enough to meet your chocolate craving, you will have satisfied your hunger for a lot fewer calories.

Now, how can anyone possibly expect to remember all that?

You'll find a picture on page 97 that will show you what I'm talking about. And I guarantee, with that picture firmly planted in the part of your brain that records visual images, you'll think very differently about the choices that you're making when you have a chocolate craving.

Some Is Yummier, Too

Call me biased, but some of the foods that I recommend taste even better than foods that you're already eating.

Bruce had been eating a turkey sandwich for lunch almost every day—not because he enjoyed it but because he thought that it was a healthy, low-calorie choice. He also loved soup, but he always assumed that a thick, hearty soup was much higher in fat or calories.

Time for a food demonstration. Our dietitian showed Bruce the trade-offs. He was thrilled to learn that a big bowl of lentil, black bean, or split-pea soup was a much better option than a turkey sandwich. He also found that when he started ordering those soups for lunch, he was looking forward to lunchtimes with considerably more anticipation than he used to.

Diane used to eat fat-free, sugar-free cookies as afternoon snacks. Her preference would have been dried fruit, but that was on her taboo list because it was full of sugar.

Five minutes with our dietitian and a quick food demonstration was all it took.

Now Diane readily passes up the cookies in favor of her snack of dried pears and apricots. Why? Because she discovered that she saves a couple hundred calories with that choice and, by the way, gets a good dose of minerals, vitamins, and fiber that she'd never get from the diet cookies.

Here's the point: In addition to discovering better-tasting alternatives, you may find that you can easily replace some kinds of foods with others that you prefer and, in so doing, save thousands of calories that you've been consuming unnecessarily.

That's why people come into my office and say that they don't feel like they're dieting. They're eating foods they enjoy, new foods they never before tasted, foods they stayed away from that they discovered were fine. Many times, the lower-calorie choice is a delicious food that they didn't even realize was an option.

Chapter 2

CALORIES AND WHERE THEY COME FROM

Nutrition is boring. Even nutritionists admit that. Fortunately, you don't need a course in nutrition to make Food Awareness Training work for you. We've taken a lot of the recent findings about nutrition and incorporated them in the food descriptions that are in this book. So while you're making your food choices, you can take note of the health benefits as well.

As you're making food choices, you will naturally lean toward foods that have lower calorie counts, since it's reasonable to assume that you want to lose weight. But in addition to this, I'd like to steer you toward foods that are high in nutritional value. It's another way to ensure that your needs are met when you're hungry. And, of course, it's a good way to make sure you're getting all the vitamins, minerals, fiber, and protein that your body needs.

While I'm not going to give you a mini-course here, I'd like to add a few notes to what you may have learned in high-school nutrition class or picked up from your own reading—just enough to make nutrition awareness part of food awareness.

The Big Picture— And What It Means to You

Nutrients are divided into two basic categories, macronutrients and micronutrients. Macronutrients are food substances like protein, fat, and carbohydrates that end up supplying us with calories.

I say "end up," because calories are actually a measurement of how much energy is produced. Throw a bunch of dry sticks in a pile and what do you have? Just a pile of sticks. But if you light them, they burst into flame—which is a kind of energy. For food to turn into energy, it has to be "ignited" by the chemical processes in your body.

A macronutrient has the potential to supply energy, and the actual production of energy is measured in calories. Calories are calculated by measuring the amount of heat a food gives off when it is "burned."

If you've ever used an exercise bike that shows a digital readout of the calories you're burning, you've seen how those macronutrient calories can go up in smoke when you're pedaling hard. Every action from breathing to scribbling a message on a post-card burns *some* calories. But, obviously, if you're pedaling an exercise bike, you are burning a lot more than you do when you scratch your chin.

Micronutrients are food components like vitamins and minerals. These supply no calories, but they help release energy from food. So they're the sparks that help light the fire.

This might surprise you, if you have always thought that vitamins give you energy. They don't. Certain vitamins do give you better *access* to the macronutrients that supply the energy, but the vitamins themselves are not the fuel that feeds the fire. They're simply the sparks that help to ignite the energy-burning process.

What about water? Technically, it doesn't fit in either category. It's not a macronutrient, because it has no calories. And it's not a micronutrient, because it's neither a vitamin nor a mineral.

But we all know we need water to live. It's absolutely essential for digestion as well as many other bodily processes.

Protein Sources

The nutrients—along with water—work like instruments in an orchestra. Each one has a specific task, but they work together to get the overall job done.

Proteins, among the macronutrients, are needed for growth and repair of tissues. The average person needs 40 to 100 grams of protein a day. This requirement can be met with a bowl of bean soup and a seafood entrée along with a good variety of vegetables and grains.

Each gram of protein—less than $\frac{1}{28}$th of an ounce—has 4 calories. Typical high-protein foods include meat, fish, legumes, cheese, and nuts, to mention just a few.

The reason that all protein foods don't have the same number of calories is because the fat and water content vary. That is why, say, most cheeses have 100 calories per ounce and most fish have about 30 calories per ounce.

Cheese is a good example of a protein-rich food that's also a high-fat food. Yes, you get a high dose of protein from your favorite Cheddar. But along with it, you get saturated fat, which is the kind that contributes to heart disease and other problems.

As a result, we often turn to other, healthier, lower-calorie sources when we're looking for protein. Among the prime candidates are seafood and legumes like peas, beans, and lentils.

The soybean is a legume that deserves special mention because of its health-promoting properties. That's why you'll see many soy products pictured in this book. Any time you opt for the soy products that are currently available in the form of burgers, franks, or deli slices, you're choosing a high-protein, low-calorie food. The products, which are sold under various brand names, are increasingly available in supermarkets as well as health food stores.

Counting Carbs

Carbohydrates usually provide about half of your body's energy needs when you're resting or performing a low-level activity. About half the energy you burned last night

Liquid Lunch

The phrase "liquid lunch" once conjured up visions of corporate vice presidents downing their third martinis before heading back to the office. Today, it's more likely to refer to the meal-in-a-can that serves as a lunch replacement—or breakfast or dinner replacement—for people on a diet.

Liquid meals are typically used by doctors to help sick patients gain nutrition. So it may seem logical to think that these meals are both healthy and convenient. Why not get our nutrition from a can?

There's a problem, however. While most of the weight-loss "shakes" contain a number of vitamins and minerals, they also contain substantial numbers of calories—as many as 250. Further, they contain plenty of fat—up to 9 grams in some cases. These numbers are identical to the calorie and fat content of an 8-ounce chocolate milkshake.

What's more, most meal replacements provide neither fiber nor phytochemicals, the kind of thing you get best from eating vegetables and fruit.

If it's a milkshake you want, have one. If it's lunch you're after, have a low-calorie, healthy lunch.

---

while sleeping came from carbohydrate sources. And probably 50 percent of the energy you're using right now, reading these words, comes from carbs.

Carbohydrates are considered the energy nutrient, because your body can break them down and use them very quickly.

How much carbohydrate do you really need in your daily diet?

For the average person, carbohydrate needs can be about 60 to 360 grams per day. That's roughly the equivalent of 2 to 13 ounces of pure carbohydrates.

You've probably heard of runners or triathletes who do "carb-loading" before a big race; that's because they're going to be tapping a huge amount of that particular energy reservoir when they exercise hard. The requirements are a lot less, of course, if you hardly exercise.

Sources of carbohydrates are all over the place. See that sugar bowl? Carbohydrates. Rice has carbohydrates. So do raisins, apples, spaghetti, popcorn, potatoes, and cookies. And in baked products labeled "fat-free," most of the fat content has been replaced with carbohydrates.

Simple and Complex

All carbs are not created equal. There are two basic types. The so-called simple carbohydrates are the sugars. Table sugar, any syrup, honey, and the sugar in fruits are all simple carbohydrates.

Then there are complex carbohydrates. Your mom and high-school nutrition teacher probably called these starches. Complex carbs include vegetables such as potatoes and corn and grain products such as bread, pasta, and cereals.

Among the complex carbohydrates, there's a further distinction. Refined grain products such as white rice and white breads tend to suffer from processing. While these foods are being spruced up for delivery to our plates, they lose a lot of their hearty nutrients. Often, the packager takes steps to remedy that by enriching the food with iron and some B vitamins that are lost in processing.

Whole grain products—also complex carbohydrates—retain more of Mother Nature's supply of nutrients. Whole wheat bread and brown rice, for instance, have more protein, fiber, vitamins, and minerals than their refined cousins. They also contain a whole category of beneficial nutrients that are often in short supply—the phytonutrients. These are health-promoting substances found in plants (aside from vitamins, minerals, and fiber).

Phyto Facts

In addition to the vitamins and minerals, there is another class of substances known as phytochemicals whose role in human nutrition is just becoming clear. Phytochemicals seem to have an important role in the prevention of diseases.

Phytochemical Family	Food Sources
Allyl sulfides	Onions, garlic, leeks, chives
Isoflavones	Soybeans (tofu, soy milk)
Isothiocyanates	Cruciferous vegetables
Phenolic acids (ellagic acid, ferulic acid)	Tomatoes, citrus fruits, carrots, whole grains, nuts
Polyphenols, flavonoids	Black, green, and oolong tea; apples; onions; citrus fruits; carrots; broccoli; cabbage; soy products; parsley; tomatoes; eggplant; peppers; berries
Saponins	Beans and legumes
Terpenes (perilyl alcohol, limonene)	Cherries, citrus fruit peel

While these phytochemicals have no direct effect on weight loss, a person who is eating the type of healthy diet I recommend—rich in fruits, vegetables, and beans—will be getting a good dose of phytochemicals to decrease the risk of heart disease, cancer, and other diseases.

Check the Index?

Apart from the simple/complex division of carbohydrates, there's another way of categorizing carbohydrate foods that you may have seen in some popular diet books: glycemic index, or GI.

The GI reflects the rate of entry of sugar into the bloodstream. In terms of weight loss, the slower the rate, the better. So the lower GI foods are considered better choices than the higher GI foods.

Many factors affect GI. Fiber, protein, and fat content as well as the degree of processing of a food have a big effect on the glycemic index. For example, whole wheat bread has a lower GI than white bread because of its fiber content. Sponge cake has a lower GI than plain, boiled rice because of its protein and fat content. And old-fashioned oats have a lower GI than instant oatmeal because of processing. Rice cakes happen to have a very high GI. Chocolate eclairs are relatively low!

You can see why discretion should be used when working with the GI. If you're encouraged to eat a wide range of fruits, vegetables, beans, and whole grains, that's fine. But if following the GI leads you to avoid potatoes, onions, or carrots (which are high GI foods), that's not fine. And, please, go easy on the eclairs!

Fats in the Fire

Every gram of fat has 9 calories.

Compare that to the 4 calories in every gram of carbohydrate or protein, and you can see where fats get their ugly reputation. If you eat 1 gram of fat—that is, any kind of vegetable oil or animal fat—you're getting more than twice the calories as you would get from 1 gram of carbohydrate or protein.

We need fats to survive. But researchers have had a hard time establishing how much fat we absolutely need in our diets.

The "good" or unsaturated fats are those that usually come from plants. They provide the essential fatty acids needed for good health. Unsaturated fats, studies have shown, have beneficial health effects: They help lower blood levels of low-density lipoproteins (LDLs), the "bad cholesterol" contributing to artery-clogging plaque that clings to blood vessels and helps induce heart disease.

Among the beneficial, unsaturated fats are soy oil, canola oil, olive oil, and all other nut and seed oils. And fish oil—especially the kind that comes from cold-water fish—is among the most beneficial of oils. Another "good" fat for preventing health problems is flaxseed oil, which is the highest natural source of omega-3 fatty acids.

The "bad" or saturated fats are usually of animal origin. (Fish, high in omega-3 fatty acids, is the significant exception.) Bad fats tend to raise levels of LDL cholesterol and may increase the risk of certain cancers. Examples are chicken fat, beef fat, lard, butterfat, and the fat found in eggs.

Another type of "bad" fat is trans fat. This is the kind found in many margarines, solid shortenings, and some fried food. It's formed when liquid oils are hydrogenated or hardened, or when they are heated to very high temperatures.

Dressing Down

Researchers report that salad dressing is a major source of fat in the American diet. This is especially the case for women under the age of 50, who eat a lot of salad—no doubt on the theory that it's good for them. So it is, as long as you watch the dressing.

A ladle full of salad bar dressing may contain as much as 48 grams of fat and 450 calories. Commercial dressings are pri-marily fat, with 85 percent of their calories from oil.

Try the fat-free or low-fat commercial dressings. Or, when you're at home or at the salad bar, make your own lower-fat vinegar-and-oil dressing, stretching it with lemon or tomato juice and a range of such condiments as ketchup, salsa, relish, and hot sauce. In restaurants, ask for low-fat dressing or for oil and vinegar "on the side."

You will probably meet your requirement for essential fatty acids—unless, that is, you become fanatical about removing every trace of fat from your diet. By fanatical, I mean picking the few olives out of a Greek salad, being afraid to order grilled vegetables in a restaurant because they might contain some oil, or eating sole instead of salmon even though you dislike sole.

Remember, though, that all fats, whether "good" or "bad," are a very concentrated source of calories—9 a gram. That's about 120 calories per tablespoon of any kind of oil. So even if a fat is called "good," like the fat in nuts, you *can* have too much of a good thing. At 900 calories per cup, nuts come at a high cost.

Multitasking

Why do we need fats?

Like carbohydrates, fats are used for energy. But our need for fats goes beyond that. For instance, we require small amounts of essential fatty acids for functioning of the immune system. Your nervous system also needs fats.

And fats have been hired as ushers in the great theater of our bodies. Many nutrients mix well with fat but not with water. If we're going to absorb these nutrients in our bodies—and get the benefits we need—fats have to help them make their way into our cells. We also need fat to help our bodies absorb some fat-soluble nutrients such as vitamins A, D, E, and K.

And then there's the ice-cream effect. Fat contributes to a sense of satiety—that "feeling full" sensation at the end of a meal. If you've cleaned your plate of the 23-vegetable special and you're still picking away at your dining partner's leftovers, maybe it's because you don't feel full. You want the gourmet ice cream at the end to achieve the "Done!" feeling that you're after.

Why Calories Do Count

When you consume more calories than you burn up, your body converts the unused carbohydrates, proteins, or fats into body fat. This is why excess calories from any source can add interesting dimensions to your fat-absorbing belly, hips, and thighs.

If we could just find a high-calorie, delicious food that would take 12 hours to eat, it wouldn't be such a threat to the waistline. The real "problem foods" are the high-calorie gang that are quickly and easily consumed—such as candy bars, cake, chips, and cookies. Not coincidentally, these are the villains that are usually considered "fattening."

But they're not *necessarily* fattening. They're just easy to eat—and extraordinarily high in calories.

Regardless of how high they are in calories, you *can* have candy, cake, chips, or cookies. But when you make the choice to eat these types of foods, you also need to figure out how you can eat low-calorie, filling foods as well.

Where Does the Low-Fat Diet Go Wrong?

Zero-fat diets are unhealthy.

Why? Quite simply, because you need some fat in your diet if you want your brain, nerves, and body to work.

But many people have heard that fat is the main culprit in weight gain. I have had patients who scrupulously followed a diet that prescribed "No fat!" They conscientiously checked the fat grams on every food product they purchased.

So . . . if they *still* gained weight, what went wrong?

Ardent dieters often make the mistaken assumption that only fat calories can make them gain weight. Fat-free food is not the answer, however.

Consider fat-free cakes, cookies, and muffins. You might assume that you can eat all you want. However, the refined carbohydrates in these foods can have more potential for weight gain than fat does.

I do not mean to suggest that people should necessarily avoid all low-fat products. Some low-fat dressings, sauces, and frozen desserts make weight loss a lot easier than it used to be. It's the baked goods that are the culprits.

Getting the Nutrients You Need

For a quick review of your vitamin and mineral needs, take a look at the chart on page 34, which comes from The Food and Nutrition Board of the National Academy of Sciences. This chart shows the Recommended Dietary Allowances for the vitamins and minerals needed by healthy people in the United States. As you can see, the recommended amounts are different for women and for men. In addition, you'll notice that our requirements change as we get older.

Do you meet these minimum requirements, given your daily diet?

While you may eat a wide range of vegetables, fruit, beans, and grains, I would recommend that you also take a multivitamin supplement with minerals each day.

A "multi" provides an extra margin of
(continued on page 36)

Recommended Dietary Allowances

Age (Years) or Condition	Weight (lb)	Weight (kg)	Height (in)	Height (cm)	Protein (g)	Vitamin A (micrograms RE)	Vitamin D (mcg)	Vitamin E (milligrams Tocopherol Equivalents)	Vitamin K (mcg)
Infants									
Up to 6 months	13	6	24	60	13	375	7.5	3	5
6 months–1	20	9	28	71	14	375	10	4	10
Children									
1–3	29	13	35	90	16	400	10	6	15
4–6	44	20	44	112	24	500	10	7	20
7–10	62	28	52	132	28	700	10	7	30
Males									
11–14	99	45	62	157	45	1,000	10	10	45
15–18	145	66	69	176	59	1,000	10	10	65
19–24	160	72	70	177	58	1,000	10	10	70
25–50	174	79	70	176	63	1,000	5	10	80
51+	170	77	68	173	63	1,000	5	10	80
Females									
11–14	101	46	62	157	46	800	10	8	45
15–18	120	55	64	163	44	800	10	8	55
19–24	128	58	65	164	46	800	10	8	60
25–50	138	63	64	163	50	800	5	8	65
51+	143	65	63	160	50	800	5	8	65
Pregnant					60	800	10	10	65
Lactating									
1st 6 months					65	1,300	10	12	65
2nd 6 months					62	1,200	10	11	65

	Water-Soluble Vitamins							Minerals						
	Vitamin C (mg)	Thiamin (mg)	Riboflavin (mg)	Niacin (milligrams-Niacin Equivalent)	Vitamin B_6 (mg)	Folate (mcg)	Vitamin B_{12} (mcg)	Calcium (mg)	Phosphorus (mg)	Magnesium (mg)	Iron (mg)	Zinc (mg)	Iodine (mcg)	Selenium (mcg)
	30	0.3	0.4	5	0.3	25	0.3	400	300	40	6	5	40	10
	35	0.4	0.5	6	0.6	35	0.5	600	500	60	10	5	50	15
	40	0.7	0.8	9	1.0	50	0.7	800	800	80	10	10	70	20
	45	0.9	1.1	12	1.1	75	1.0	800	800	120	10	10	90	20
	45	1.0	1.2	13	1.4	100	1.4	800	800	170	10	10	120	30
	50	1.3	1.5	17	17	150	2.0	1,200	1,200	270	12	15	150	40
	60	1.5	1.8	20	2.0	200	2.0	1,200	1,200	400	12	15	150	50
	60	1.5	1.7	19	2.0	200	2.0	1,200	1,200	350	10	15	150	70
	60	1.5	1.7	19	2.0	200	2.0	800	800	350	10	15	150	70
	60	1.2	1.4	15	2.0	200	2.0	800	800	350	10	15	150	70
	50	1.1	1.3	15	1.4	150	2.0	1,200	1,200	280	15	12	150	45
	60	1.1	1.3	15	1.5	180	2.0	1,200	1,200	300	15	12	150	50
	60	1.1	1.3	15	1.6	180	2.0	1,200	1,200	280	15	12	150	55
	60	1.1	1.3	15	1.6	180	2.0	800	800	280	15	12	150	55
	60	1.0	1.2	13	1.6	180	2.0	800	800	280	10	12	150	55
	70	1.5	1.6	17	2.2	400	2.2	1,200	1,200	355	15	19	200	75
	95	1.6	1.8	20	2.1	280	2.6	1,200	1,200	355	15	19	200	75
	90	1.6	1.7	20	2.1	260	2.6	1,200	1,200	340	15	16	200	75

safety. It simply ensures that you get all the recommended micronutrients that you need.

If you have a basically healthful diet, that multivitamin is probably all you need—unless your doctor has a particular reason for prescribing something extra. (For instance, you might be prescribed folic acid before or during pregnancy, calcium for osteoporosis, or vitamin E for heart disease.)

I am opposed to megadoses of vitamins or minerals. If you're eating a healthful diet and taking an adequate multivitamin, it's a pretty safe bet that you're getting all the micronutrients you need.

What about Miracle Formulas?

Not only am I opposed to multidoses of certain vitamins, I am also opposed to some of the over-the-counter remedies for weight loss.

It's important for every consumer to realize that substances sold as natural food supplements are not subject to the same regulations as prescription drugs. But weight-loss supplements—sold under a host of inviting names—can be just as potent as prescription medications.

My objections to weight-loss medications are based on issues of safety and efficacy. Here are my views.

- There is no standardized means of extraction. The quantity of the *active* substance might vary widely from one product to the next, even though both labels bear the same description. Also, impurities may be present.
- Some remedies may be utterly useless, which defrauds the public.
- Some may have toxic effects either alone or in combination with other drugs that people may be using.
- There may be insufficient or no warnings about usage or dosage.

Overfilling on Fat-Free

Our brains communicate with our bellies in interesting ways.

If a label says "fat-free," studies show, there's a good chance you'll eat *more* of that food—just as if you were giving yourself permission.

This conclusion is supported by a study at Pennsylvania State University where students were fed yogurt products with a variety of fat content. When the students ate what they believed was a fat-free yogurt, they ate more than normal at their next meal. But if they were told they were eating a high-fat yogurt—and then followed it with a meal—they ended up eating *less* than usual.

Same for potato chips? It would seem so.

In another study, researchers compared people eating fat-free chips to those who ate regular chips. True, the people eating fat-free chips consumed less fat overall. But at the end of the day, they had consumed as many calories as the people who ate regular chips.

Functional Foods: Health Weapon or Marketing Fad?

Cholesterol-reducing candy bars? Mood-lightening pasta?

With the functional food industry growing at an estimated 8 to 10 percent a year, such fantasies are increasingly possible. Functional foods go beyond "fortified" foods—those containing extra vitamins or minerals—to add a range of putative nutrients to a variety of food products.

Because the manufacturers of functional foods assert only that their products affect body function rather than fight disease, the nutritional claims that appear on the labels of functional foods don't need government approval. And, since many of the ingredients are natural, functional foods strike consumers as being healthy.

Are they?

Not necessarily. Some functional foods may provoke allergic reactions. Some may not combine well with medications you might be taking. Some may have side effects. Besides, the food label won't tell you how much you should eat or for how long you should eat it—the kind of information that is required for "real" medicines.

Where "Natural" Is Not All

What is unfortunate is that people believe readily available herbs and herbal formulas are not medicines. Many people think, "They're just herbs," and because they are "natural," they are perceived as safe and healthful. This could not be farther from the truth.

Some of the most potent, toxic substances known to mankind are natural. Just because something is herbal or derived from a plant doesn't mean it's safe.

People are often drawn to these products because they get a feeling of control over their own health care. As a physician, I am concerned that a person's response to these substances is not monitored. Some of these natural remedies can have profound effects on body functions such as heart rate and blood pressure.

What a Friend in Fiber

You get fiber in your diet from fruit, vegetables, beans, and grains. Technically, fiber is a very complex carbohydrate. It is a structural component of plants. Since humans lack an enzyme to digest fiber, it passes through our systems without being absorbed.

Why is it important? We used to believe that fiber had one function only: to prevent constipation. Many people called it roughage—not a particularly appealing name for something that's traveling through the tender interior of your body.

Because of its somewhat unappealing rep-

(continued on page 40)

Fiber Feasts

Want to add fiber without any calorie penalty? From soup to snacks, the comparisons listed here show how you can fill up on fiber—and get lots of additional nutrients—without adding a single calorie. In fact, in most cases, you actually save calories when you go for the high-fiber choice. It's a win-win situation—and a feast of fiber.

Soups

1½ cups minestrone soup
110 calories
10 grams of fiber

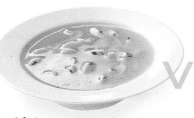

vs.

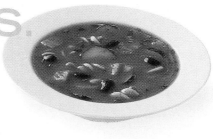

1½ cups chicken noodle soup
150 calories
No fiber

Entrées

1½ cups brown rice and beans
2 cups zucchini and tomatoes
6 slices grilled acorn squash
440 calories
19 grams of fiber

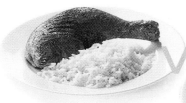

vs.

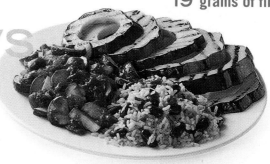

¼ chicken (leg and thigh)
1½ cups rice
720 calories
No fiber

Desserts

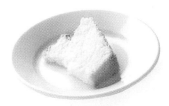

baked apple with raspberries
100 calories
8 grams of fiber

small slice angel food cake
100 calories
No fiber

VS.

Snacks

10 dried apricot halves
5 dried plums
6 dried apple rings
235 calories
9 grams of fiber

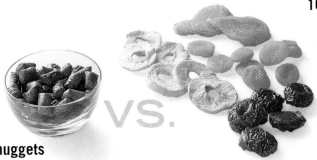

4 oz pretzel nuggets
480 calories
No fiber

VS.

Sandwiches

3 oz veggie lunchmeat on 5-grain bread
with lettuce, tomato, and coleslaw
240 calories
6 grams of fiber

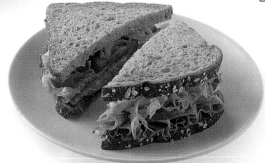

3 oz turkey on Italian bread
290 calories
No fiber

VS.

utation, if you say "fiber" to many of my new patients, they associate it with food that isn't tasty, like raw bran. But many tasty foods are also high in fiber, ranging in variety from minestrone soup and marinated artichokes to vegetarian chili, sweet potatoes, cherries, and dried apricots.

We now know that fiber is far more than a constipation fighter. People on high-fiber diets reduce their risks of a whole range of different health problems, from high blood pressure and heart disease to digestive disorders and cancer.

High-fiber foods are bulky. You can eat a large quantity and still consume very few calories. Most also take a long time to chew, so they slow down your eating. They contribute to a sense of fullness because they take up a lot of space in your digestive tract. Since they may take up to 24 hours to pass through it, they can take the edge off your appetite (and thus reduce your calorie count) for as much as a day.

High-fiber foods are also excellent sources of nutrients. If you're eating a diet high in fiber—including fruits, vegetables, and legumes—then you're eating a very healthy, low-calorie diet and not feeling hungry.

Chapter 3

SHARPEN THE FOCUS

Changing your relationship with food is the primary focus of the weight-loss program you're about to undertake, but that isn't the only thing that should change. You'll also want to alter or abandon a considerable number of misconceptions, misunderstandings, and plain myths that persistently surround the whole subject of losing weight. In fact, despite all the attention paid to it, weight loss is a subject that suffers from underexposure.

The subject goes back as much as half a century. That's when the diet game really seems to have gotten going in this country, and it marks the first of many phases that dieting has gone through since that time. Each phase of enthusiasm about new diets was driven by what dieters were told was a newly discovered truth, or a new-found system, or a newly invented magic bullet. This time, they were told, the new plan (or program or formula) was really going to make a difference!

In truth, as the fellow said long, long ago, there is nothing new under the sun. But that doesn't stop some people from spinning new fables, and it doesn't stop others from believing them.

When Counting Was the Rage

Back in the postwar period of the 1950s, the country was booming, suburban lifestyles were emerging as the norm, and thin was in. From then until the late 1970s, when I began my practice, the name of the game for weight loss was to count calories.

Calorie-counting devices were all the rage. All you had to do was spin a wheel or click a counter to see how many calories that apple or plate of spaghetti was costing you. Then you'd add up the calories for the meal or the day. And finally, you'd check your intake against a set formula that calculated exactly how much weight a person could expect to lose.

The formula was based on the "fact" that a pound of fat has 3,500 calories. Therefore, if you ate 500 fewer calories than normal, and you kept that up for 7 days (7 × 500), you would lose a pound. We now know this is too simplistic an assumption, but at the time, it was Holy Writ for calorie counters.

Fat Is the Enemy

The next big trend was fat restriction. By the early 1980s, the buzz was that all fats were bad, and the goal was to consume as few as possible. Carbohydrate calories, by contrast, were considered good—that is to say, it was assumed they wouldn't adversely impact weight loss.

People were encouraged to eat carbs to their hearts' desire, so long as they cut out fat. The result was a boom in the sale and consumption of pasta, bagels, breads, and fat-free cookies and cakes. Another result was that many people gained lots of weight.

By the late 1980s and early 1990s, the experts were taking a closer look at carbohydrates. Wasn't there a significant difference, they asked, between simple carbohydrates like sugar and the complex carbohydrates found in starchy foods?

According to the new thinking, complex carbohydrates were better for us than simple carbohydrates. Why? Because the complex carbs took longer to break down and were less likely to be stored as fat.

From Unrefined to Glycemic Index

About the middle of the 1990s, it became clear that the distinction between simple and complex carbohydrates wasn't so simple. You also had to know whether the carbohydrate was refined or unrefined. Down went dieters' consumption of such refined carbohydrates as white rice, most pasta, and white breads like bagels, semolina bread, and sourdough. Up went the intake of unrefined carbs. The stage was set for more whole grain pastas and breads along with lots of starchy vegetables.

And finally, in the late 1990s, the glycemic index became the rage. Foods with a high glycemic index included white rice, white potatoes, beets, and carrots. These were suddenly considered off-limits. Sweet potatoes and whole grains—foods with a low glycemic index—suddenly filled dieters' plates.

As we enter a new millennium, we find ourselves in a new phase of diet wisdom. Today, the prevailing trend is an emphasis on protein consumption. High-protein, low-carbohydrate diets now ride the crest of the popularity wave. (A review of these high-protein diets—and others—can be found in chapter 13 of this book.)

Gimmick Games

Everyone would like a formula that's guaranteed to work, and some folks have gone pretty far out on a limb to provide just that. Among the most creative and least credible of these formulas is "food combining."

The folks who promote food combining as a method of weight loss must have been absent the day the rest of us learned about nutrition in high school—or even grade school. Food combining is the theory—"notion" might be a better word—that because different nutrients are digested at different rates, the "wrong" combination of foods can lead to poor digestion and increased fat storage.

This is utter nonsense. Food that is not digested cannot be absorbed into the bloodstream and therefore cannot be deposited as body fat.

But people do lose weight on food combining programs. In fact, a number of people have told me that they met someone or talked to someone who actually lost several pounds on such a program.

No doubt. But the person lost weight because she probably took in less carbohydrate and/or fewer calories. Therefore, the weight loss didn't occur because she never mixed protein and carbs at the same meal.

"Fat-burning foods" are another cruel myth of the diet game.

There are those who maintain that grapefruit burns fat, or that vinegar or lemon juice melts it away. That's just so much applesauce.

No food burns fat.

Maybe it's the tart taste of these foods that inspires people to this wishful image of fat-burning, but it simply is not so. Exercise burns fat; food does not.

Gimmick Diets

Given all the people who mock gimmick diets, it's amazing how long many of these diets have been around. More amazing yet, it's likely that others will be created in the future.

Remember the cabbage soup diet? Cabbage shmabbage. It didn't stand a chance, but thousands of people tried it.

Then there was the watermelon diet. And the ice cream diet—yes, there was one.

All of these gimmick diets have a similar theme. They restrict your intake of total calories.

When your eating is restricted to one or two foods, you tend to eat less just because it's so boring to eat the same thing all the time. So naturally, for a week or two, you will be thrilled with what the scale tells you. But the large loss registered by that scale is not totally a loss of fat. Instead, it's mainly loss of fluid—in part because you've reduced your intake of sodium and/or carbohydrate—and it's temporary.

Advocates of gimmick diets typically recommend that you stay on them for 1 or 2 weeks only. They're not very healthy, and they probably won't continue to work after 2 weeks. The drop on the scale will taper off, the lost fluids will come back, and you'll regain the weight you lost.

Besides, by the second week, you'll be so

The Control Issue

Have you always associated weight loss with self-control?

I hope I can convince you otherwise.

Contrary to conventional wisdom, control is not the sure path to weight loss. In fact, control is the enemy. It suggests that someone *wants* to eat a particular food but refuses to do it with a mighty effort of will.

This kind of control goes hand in hand with deprivation, which ultimately spells trouble. There will be a breakdown of control sooner or later. When you lose weight by exercising control rather than by making choices, you're very likely to regain that weight again as soon as you "lose control."

bored with the dull sameness of what you're eating—not to mention with your low energy and generally blah feeling—that you won't follow the regime.

Pill Promises

Weight-loss products abound on the shelves of drugstores, health food stores, even supermarkets. They contain a range of ingredients—some of them utterly ineffective, some completely unsafe. Other ingredients do decrease appetite or increase fat loss, but their long-term safety has not been established.

What makes the products especially troublesome is that they are sold without prescription. Nor is it known if the weight that's taken off comes back, as is the case with most diets.

No weight-loss product is recommended in this book. As to the ingredients in these products, here's a partial rundown, starting with the "fat blockers."

How do they work?

Over-the-counter fat blockers prevent a certain amount of dietary fat from being absorbed from the intestine. In controlled studies, some people took chitosan, a fat blocker made from the exoskeletons of shellfish, while others received a placebo, a "blank" pill that looked exactly the same. The studies showed that the chitosan did seem to have some effect on weight loss. In other clinical studies, large doses of chitosan caused a sharp drop in the blood levels of vitamin E, intensified the loss of calcium from bones, and resulted in the loss of other minerals. So I'm reserving judgment on this one until more is known about its long-term effects.

Probably the most publicized of the pills with a promise is Fen-phen.

Fen-phen is the shorthand name for a combination of drugs that was first hailed as the solution for weight control, then banned because of health concerns. For popular consumption, however, prescription Fen-phen has been "replaced" by an herbal equivalent.

The so-called "herbal fen-phen" is a combination of ma huang (ephedra) and St. John's wort. This combination seems to be just as risky as the pharmaceutical version. Even though these herbs are available without a prescription, I believe they can be nearly as potent as prescription drugs and are potentially dangerous.

St. John's wort is a mood enhancer and antidepressant that affects brain chemicals—specifically, serotonin, which influences both mood and appetite. That is thought to be the source of its power to decrease appetite. As for ma huang, some studies indicate that it does increase fat loss. But a number of fatalities have been associated with its use, and I strongly caution against the use of herbal fen-phen products.

Here are some of the ingredients in other popular products that promise weight loss in a pill.

- **Cassia (senna) and garcinia (camboge).** These act as laxatives and can be dangerous. People who have a history of intestinal obstruction and/or inflammatory intestinal disease should not take them.
- **Cellasene.** A very expensive treatment for cellulite, cellasene is made of herbs, seed extracts, fish oil, and soy lecithin. In a controversial, limited, and subjective study that I

find highly suspect, researchers in Europe reported reduction in thigh size in some patients who took the pill. I don't credit it. And the cellasene itself is considered dangerous for women who are pregnant or lactating, people with thyroid conditions, and people on blood thinners.

- **Chromium picolinate.** Its biological role is not well understood, although it appears to play a role in insulin metabolism. Chromium is an essential nutrient only in trace amounts, but there is not enough information as of yet to determine its Recommended Dietary Allowance. What is known is that it can be toxic in large doses. Early studies that demonstrated fat loss and muscle building were flawed, and the follow-up studies were unable to duplicate the results. It is clear now that chromium picolinate does not appear to change body composition and may adversely affect the way iron is transported in the body.
- **Conjugated linoleic acid (CLA).** This is a mixture of polyunsaturated fatty acids that form in the intestines of cattle. In studies on growing animals, CLA increased the percentage of muscle and decreased the percentage of fat. In studies on overweight human adults, however, CLA had no effect. People who took CLA had no more fat loss than those who took placebos.
- **Hawthorn, ginseng, and ginkgo biloba.** According to studies, these have no effect on weight loss.
- **Hydroxycitric acid (HCA).** An extract of a tropical fruit, *Garcinia cambogia*, HCA can block the body's fat metabolism by in-

hibiting the enzyme that turns citric acid to fat. It also has a laxative effect and has been shown to be toxic in animal studies. As for weight loss in humans, HCA has no consistent effect.

- **L-arginine and L-ornithine.** These amino acids are said to help metabolize fat when taken with L-lysine before bedtime. No studies have proven that these amino acids have any measurable effect.
- **L-carnitine.** An amino acid, L-carnitine plays a role in fat metabolism at the cellular level. Some overweight people may have low levels of L-carnitine, but supplements have not been proven to affect weight loss.
- **Phenylpropanalomine (PPL).** This is the active ingredient in such weight-loss products as Dexatrim and Acutrim. It suppresses appetite by increasing the brain level of a chemical called dopamine, which is essential to the normal functioning of the central nervous system. In controlled studies, people taking PPL lost more weight than those in a placebo group, but the usual warnings apply. You should not take PPL if you have heart disease, thyroid disease, kidney disease, or high blood pressure, or if you're pregnant or nursing. With so many health cautions applied to PPL, I do not recommend taking it.
- **Pyruvate.** This is another expensive weight-loss product. Made in the body and found in some foods—large doses of which can cause a slight fat decrease and slight muscle increase—pyruvate has an insignificant effect on total weight loss. The impact of pyruvate in small doses is unknown, as is its long-term safety.

Accounting for Taste

Tastebuds, filled with nerve fibers, are on your tongue, on the roof of your mouth, inside your cheeks, even in your throat. Complex interactions take place within and among the tastebuds and brain both to evaluate flavors—sweet, sour, bitter, salty—and measure the level of savoriness. What's more, senses in your mouth and nasal system augment the tasting process, which is why you "can't taste a thing" when you have a head cold.

A nerve connecting the brain, nose, and mouth is another player in the taste game; it detects spicy irritants in such foods as hot chile peppers, the cool sensations of foods like mint, and the carbonation effect in certain beverages.

What's more, hot food is easier to taste than cold food—first, because it gives off more vapor, and second, because heat actually increases the intensity of sweet or bitter flavors, while cold diminishes it.

So keep these facts in mind when you're enjoying good food. Your tastebuds need looking after. And if they get what they want, your stomach may feel very satisfied.

● **Willow (*Salix*).** Willow contains salicin, a naturally occurring salicylate. (Aspirin is a commonly used synthetic salicylate.) In lab studies, salicylates doubled the effect of ephedra—ma huang—but had no effect on fat loss when administered alone. And ma huang, as I've noted, has been shown to be unsafe.

Correcting Our Course

Over the years, as we've moved through various diet fads and phases, I've noticed that many of the assumptions behind these diets do have merit. Consuming fewer calories will certainly help you lose weight. Restricting fats, within reason, is probably a good health move. Eating more protein-packed foods and fewer carbohydrate-heavy foods may lead to weight loss.

But if these pearls of diet wisdom aren't lies, they're not the whole truth, either. And around them have swirled a maelstrom of assumptions, assertions, and assurances that have been repeated so often they've been accepted into the dieter's canon of laws.

So before you eat another thing, let's cut through the fuzz and put the whole picture into sharp focus.

Let's look at food.

You can't stop eating, and you don't want to. So let's figure out how to make choices about the food you eat.

How Sweet It Is

Sweets are invariably the first thing people believe they must give up when they are trying to lose weight. Candy, cookies, and cakes are seen as obvious taboos. But the fact is, you don't have to give them up at all. In fact, it's unnatural to do so.

Liking sweets is a fundamental human instinct. It's basic, ingrained, almost organic. Deprive yourself of sweets for too long, and when you finally do allow yourself some, you tend to run amok. Then it's blow-out time, as you binge on your favorite dessert, and after the blow-out comes the guilt, the regret, the self-recrimination—and more sweets.

Instead of depriving yourself of sweets, turn to the lower-calorie sweets that are pictured in the food demonstrations and described in the Anytime List on page 222. There are plenty of low-calorie choices you can eat with enjoyment without undermining your weight-loss effort.

Fluid Facts

Our bodies are filled with enough liquid to fill a good-size puddle. If you've ever been stranded on sea or land without a drop to drink, you know how much you depend on a constant supply of fluids to keep you feeling hale and hearty.

But you don't have to be lost in the Mojave to suffer from dehydration. In general, you will lose 2 to 3 quarts of water every day through breathing, perspiring, even sneezing. You lose more when the air is dry or stale—as in an airplane—or when the air is very hot or cold. Hence, the often-quoted recommendation that you should drink the equivalent of eight 8-ounce glasses of water every day.

But does it really have to be water? And how do you keep count?

Here are some ways to measure your liquid assets without keeping a water meter running all the time.

Drink when you're thirsty. Some people believe they have to force themselves to drink those eight glasses of water if they're going to get enough liquids every day. Thirst is a fairly reliable indicator of the need for fluids. However, there are times when thirst may not be the best indicator—for example, when you're exercising strenuously.

Don't scorn soda. While pure water is the easiest, quickest, and probably the best way to get fluids into your body, you'd probably like to have a soda now and then. The fluid in beverages does count, especially if you're drinking a low-sodium, low-carbohydrate beverage such as a diet drink.

Gain from the garden. Fruits and vegetables definitely have fluids that contribute to your total daily consumption.

Count tea and coffee, too. It's a common misperception that the caffeine found in tea, coffee, or other caffeinated drinks actually "drains" fluids from your system. Though caffeine is a mild diuretic, when you drink a caffeinated beverage, your body still retains as much as half the fluid.

Is Alcohol Fattening?

You're more likely to put on weight if you drink alcoholic beverages.

In fact, drinking alcohol is a double whammy. Not only is booze high in calories, but it also evidently leads to increased appetite.

In a study, researchers alternated giving alcoholic and nonalcoholic aperitifs to a group of men and women lunchers over a 7-day period. On the days when the group drank alcohol, they ate faster, ate more, ate for a longer time, became "full" later, and kept on eating even after they had reached satiety.

Certainly, the alcohol prompted the people in the study to eat more and eat faster. Perhaps it also made them throw caution to the wind.

How 'bout a Drink?

What about my evening cocktail? What about my glass of wine with dinner? Sometimes, this is the first thing people ask me.

Well, awareness comes first when you're making this choice. The first thing to be aware of is that some recent studies have suggested that alcohol may actually increase appetite. What is almost certain is that it decreases resistance and can tend to muddle the decision-making process.

Since your food choices are the key to your weight loss, if alcohol tends to put you in a devil-may-care mood, that's something you ought to recognize. If you find that a bowl of peanuts at the bar disappears in the blink of an eye when you're meeting the gang for some pitchers of beer, you may want to order by the glass. Here's some overall advice for those times when drinks are being served.

- Choose seltzer or mineral water with a twist of lime or lemon for your first drink or two, as the first drink goes down so quickly. Only then move on to a glass of wine or a spritzer.

- Order a bottle of mineral water to come to the table when the bottle of wine is ordered. After that, alternate your glasses: first water, then wine. You'll pace your drinking.

Vegetables: Cooked versus Raw

Some people are under the impression that cooked vegetables have more calories than raw vegetables. In a sense, they're right: A cupful of raw spinach has fewer calories than a cupful of cooked spinach. That's because when spinach cooks, it shrinks, and you can therefore pack more into a cup.

But that's measuring by volume. By weight, the calories are the same whether you eat your spinach cooked or raw. And the same is true with broccoli, zucchini, carrots, and any other vegetable that can be eaten either way.

I am constantly telling my patients that it makes good sense to eat your vegetables cooked as well as raw. There's no calorie difference and no healthfulness gap, and cooking vegetables certainly extends the range and variety of tastes and textures you can enjoy.

Cooked vegetables seem more filling and satisfying, more like real food, especially if they're well-flavored. How about grilled portobello mushrooms, or baked eggplant, or curried pumpkin soup, just for openers? These foods seem like real meals.

What I'm saying, of course, is that I don't want you to think you have to eat the "rabbit food" that many people associate with dieting. Cold, raw vegetables—lettuce leaves, sprouts, celery, and carrot sticks—aren't for everyone. In fact, even people who love the rabbit-food veggies find there's only so much of them they can eat. So to the extent that cooked vegetables extend your vegetable options, they're a definite plus for weight loss.

Here's something I'm going to repeat a number of times throughout this book. If this advice becomes your mantra, so be it. Simply this: Eat as much as you want of vegetables, any way you want them.

Use vegetables in soups and stews. Marinate them—or choose the marinated vegetables at the salad bar. Puree your vegetables, sauté them, chop them into slaw, pickle them, grill them, or serve them with a range of low-calorie sauces, dressings, relishes, chutneys, condiments, spices, and herbs.

Salt and Weight Loss

I would guess that about 95 percent of my patients are concerned about their salt intakes. Chronic dieters—and that includes a lot of the people who come to me—tend to assume that anything they like should be restricted, so they take it for granted that salty foods like soy sauce, pickles, and soups are going to be bad for them.

But that's not necessarily so. Sodium, which plays a big role in the body's fluid balance, is a nonissue when it comes to losing fat. There may be a medical reason for you to restrict your salt intake, but that's a matter for your regular medical doctor.

In fact, for two very obvious reasons, salt can actually help the weight-loss process. First,

De Gustibus . . .

In matters of taste, the old saying goes, there's no point arguing. In fact, differences in people's perception of flavors are rooted in their genes. So is your threshold of perception—as measured in the number of tastebuds you have.

Research has shown that about a quarter of us—the super-tasters—possess a higher number of tastebuds and experience flavors more intensely. Another quarter of us have fewer tastebuds than average.

These people are known as non-tasters.

Super-tasters tend to be women—estrogen actually enhances taste perception—and have a particular genetic sensitivity to a compound found in some vegetables, such as broccoli, that makes them feel strongly, one way or the other, about these foods. Non-tasters can be absolutely blind to this taste as well as to the so-called bitter aftertaste of such foods as artificial sweeteners.

salt has no calories. Second, salt flavors food. All those sodium-packed dressings, sauces, and condiments are flavorful inducements to eat the vegetables, seafood, and soups that make such good, low-calorie choices.

Your scale may go up a pound or two if you choose such high-sodium foods as canned soup or tomato juice. But that's because sodium tends to make you retain water. You really haven't gained or regained fat.

Similarly, if you eat a very low salt diet for a while, especially if you're drinking a lot of fluid, you can trick your kidneys into sending out a lot of water. You'll urinate a lot, so it may seem that you've lost weight. But you really haven't lost fat.

In both these situations, by the way, the normal balance will restore itself. As for fat loss, that will come, with or without salt, through calorie reduction and exercise.

The Scale Is Your Enemy

You walked to the office this morning and were on the move all day at work. You showed up for an exercise class after work. As soon as you got home, you stepped on the scale to see how well you'd done.

Sure enough, you lost 5 pounds! You're thrilled to have this knowledge before you head out to your favorite restaurant. This calls for a bit of a binge.

Think again. That easy 5-pound weight loss isn't really a fat loss after all. What you lost was water—all the sweat from that exercise at the gym. And because it was water your body needs, you will eventually get it back—along with the "lost" 5 pounds on the scale.

Let's take another scenario, which might be just as likely to happen on another day.

Again, you walked to the office and stayed on the move all day. Again, you put in your time at exercise class. Feeling confident about your weight loss this day, you once again stepped on the scale as soon as you got home.

But . . . *what's this?*

Nothing lost! Not an ounce! The needle is right where it was this morning—maybe even a smidgen higher! All that effort for nothing.

Might as well give up and binge!

Again, the scales have lied. What really happened is that you drank a lot today. Or maybe it was that salty soup you had for lunch. Or both. What's registering as a slight weight gain is a water gain—and it's as temporary as water loss.

The moral is this: Let some time pass between weigh-ins. A stuck needle can be demoralizing, especially when it may be due to water retention. If you can't stay away from looking at the scales, check yourself no more than once a week. And be aware that a plateau or even a gain may be due to water, not calories from your food choices.

A better measure, if you want one, is to try on an article of clothing that either doesn't fit you at all or is very snug. Then, try it on again once every 10 days to see how it fits you differently. The clothing doesn't change size, so any difference in the way it fits is an indication that you're losing weight.

No Time Forbidden

Does any of this sound familiar?

"Eat your main meal at lunch, not dinner. . . . Eat a healthy breakfast whether you're hungry or not. . . . Eat several small

That Bedtime Snack

It's a Spanish tradition: Have your last meal late at night, at about 9:00 P.M., not long before you head for bed.

Eating right before bedtime? Isn't that an invitation to obesity?

Evidently not. There's now scientific evidence that you don't gain more weight if you eat late at night. Several studies confirm that when you eat has no connection with weight, and a survey by the Department of Agriculture has demonstrated that evening eating in particular has no more effect on your weight than morning eating.

It's the total number of calories consumed daily and expended in activity that makes—or breaks—weight gain. Apparently, the time of day when you consume those calories or burn them is really not an issue. The calories in your bedtime snack will be burned when they're needed. Even sleep burns about 50 calories an hour.

meals throughout the day rather than three meals at specific times. . . . Eat three meals a day at regular intervals and at the same time each day. . . . Eat nothing after 9:00 at night."

We're deluged with helpful hints, tips, prescriptions, schedules, instructions, injunctions, and formulas about when to eat and when not to eat.

Here's my advice: Forget it all.

As I tell my patients: Don't check the clock to see when to eat. Eat when you're hungry. Your body will tell you when it needs food. And while there may be some small benefit to be gained in terms of energy or weight loss or overall health from each of the decrees listed above, what really counts is the number of calories you consume in a 24-hour period.

I see no particular advantage to eating a big breakfast—or any breakfast at all—if you're not hungry. And if you are hungry and want to eat at 4:00 in the morning, be my guest.

At any time of day or night, food *choices*, not timing, will be the factor that makes the biggest difference.

Playing the Numbers

"How many calories should I eat in order to lose weight?"

It's the question everyone asks and no one can answer. I can't either. I won't give patients a specific number, and I certainly can't come up with a number for the readers of this book.

But this much I can promise: If you take in fewer calories than you need to maintain your present weight, you will lose pounds. That's why the weight-loss program in this book focuses on expanding your awareness. Once you know there are low-calorie alternatives to what you're currently eating and you go for those alternatives, you free yourself from the calorie-counting competition.

Needless to say, if you're curious about the calories in a specific food, it's easy to determine that. Just check the nutrition label. Comparable foods often do have slightly different calorie counts.

The Olestra Story

With all of America clamoring for low-fat and fat-free foods, the research people at food companies have been hard-pressed to come up with substitutes. And the one substitute that seems to fit the bill has been the source of a lot of controversy.

Still just a few years old, synthetically produced olestra is a fat substitute that is not absorbed by the digestive system. Since the body doesn't absorb it, it is free of calories. It is also free of cholesterol and can be used in deep frying. Best of all, it tastes good.

What a bonanza: olestra potato chips that taste like the real thing and have fewer calories than baked or fat-free chips. Sounds too good to be true.

And it just may be, because there's a painful downside to olestra. In many people, anything more than a very small amount of olestra-filled food may cause harsh stomach cramps and diarrhea. What's more, researchers still have not determined exactly how olestra may affect the body's absorption of the fat-soluble vitamins A, E, D, and K. Though the manufacturers have enriched their olestra products with additional amounts of these vitamins, they may leave the body along with the unabsorbed fat.

This means that eating large quantities of the good-tasting, reduced-calorie olestra foods may deplete your supply of fat-soluble vitamins. You may also lose carotenoids—like beta-carotene—that function as antioxidants and play a role in preventing such diseases as cancer and heart disease.

We just can't say for certain how much of the fat-soluble vitamins and carotenoids you're losing and what the effects are over time. Until we know more, I'd recommend small quantities of olestra food at infrequent intervals. Even better, have none at all.

But, frankly, a few calories one way or another, a few more calories one day than another, make little difference and are beside the point. The real goal is finding a way to eat that is comfortable for you—and a way of eating that you can continue over a lifetime. The point is to change your relationship with food in a positive way.

The Small-Portion Solution

Most of my patients instinctively assume that they are eating too much. They're pretty sure that if they could just "cut the portion in half," as the saying goes, they would lose weight.

But if you need X amount of food to feel satisfied, which is what you're eating now, half of X simply will not work. You'll end up feeling deprived, which inevitably will lead you to the place you don't want to be. Deprivation, in fact, is the enemy of the person trying to lose weight. It's a setup for regaining the weight you lose.

To me, portion cutting seems like an ill-advised exercise in a false kind of willpower. And it's not necessary.

The truth is that most weight-conscious people aren't eating enough. What they really need is larger quantities of lower-calorie food. They need to eat enough to satisfy both their senses and their psyches. They need to fulfill the craving for food and, at the same time, feel good about themselves.

Saboteur Foods

Saboteurs often travel in disguise. And "saboteur foods" are no exception.

Their disguise? Well, they pretend to be foods that help you lose weight.

But the fact is, those foods serve no purpose in weight control. They are the high-calorie/empty-calorie foods that we give ourselves permission to eat because they are lower in fat or sugar than their "regular" food counterparts.

All too typically, when we give ourselves permission to eat these foods, we can easily rationalize *overeating* them. That is why saboteur foods are the only foods I suggest you avoid in my weight-loss program. Quite simply, they will sabotage your weight-loss efforts and undermine the results.

High on the list of saboteurs are low-fat and fat-free baked goods. To read the advertising on these products, you'd think weight would vanish in an instant. The evidence—and there's lots of it—shows otherwise.

Ever since fat-free baked goods were introduced into the U.S. market, Americans have collectively gained weight. Why? Because everyone eating those products simply replaced fat calories with refined-carbohydrate calories.

If you've been eating these foods, you may have thought you were "saving calories." All you're really doing is exchanging one kind of calorie for another.

There are many other saboteurs besides these obviously misleading (and oh so tempting) baked goods. In fact, I divide saboteur foods into two main categories: the have-nots, and the haves.

The have-nots are all those snack foods with advertising that lists all the "bad" ingredients they do not contain. They are low-fat, reduced-fat, sugar-free, low-sodium, low-cholesterol, and so on. Examples of the have-nots are fat-free muffins, low-salt pretzels, and sugar-free cookies.

The no-cholesterol claim is the one that really gets my goat. Cholesterol-free foods can still be high in ingredients that really add weight. Potato chips and french fries, for example, have no cholesterol, but they are loaded with fats and are very high in calories.

The other category of saboteur foods—the ones I call haves—are the ones I refer to as "healthy naturals." We mistakenly perceive them as having some redeeming nutritional benefit.

Maybe the product is sweetened with fruit juice or honey instead of with refined sugar. Or the candy bar is made of carob instead of chocolate. Perhaps the pretzels are covered with yogurt instead of white chocolate, and the chips are made from vegetables other than potatoes.

The list goes on and on. The replacement item sounds healthy and natural, so we rationalize that it isn't as bad as an empty-calorie food.

But a cookie sweetened with honey is just

Reduced to What?

If you're a cheese lover who's also watching your weight by shopping for reduced-fat cheese, here's an eye-opener: This 2-ounce chunk of reduced-fat cheese has as much fat and as many calories as a 2-ounce chunk of salami. In fact, many reduced-fat cheeses have the same number of calories as the richest Brie or Camembert in the cheese shop. So . . . which would you rather eat?

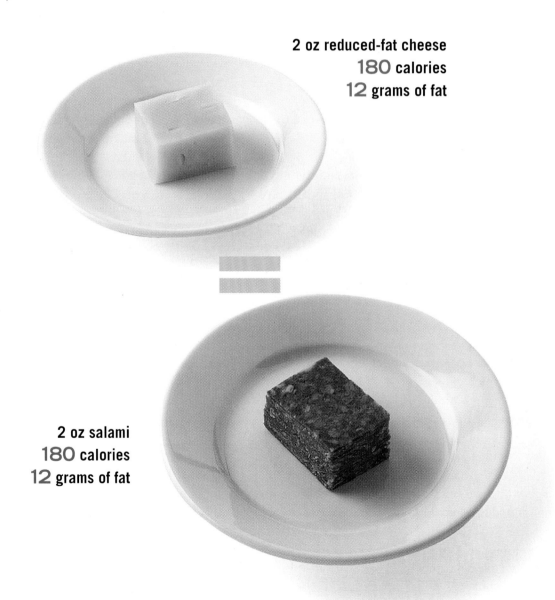

2 oz reduced-fat cheese
180 calories
12 grams of fat

2 oz salami
180 calories
12 grams of fat

Less Fat, Same Cals

Tufts University researchers compared some regular and reduced-fat products. The objective: to find out whether reduced-fat, low-fat, and even fat-free products also delivered fewer calories. The results go a long way toward explaining why, after the introduction of thousands of these "weight-loss" products on the market, Americans who eat them still gain weight.

½ cup Campbell's Vegetable Soup (with beef stock)	80 calories
½ cup Campbell's 98% Fat-Free Healthy Request Vegetable Soup (with beef stock)	80 calories
2 Drake's Yodels	280 calories
2 Drake's reduced-fat Yodels	290 calories
2 Tbsp Jif peanut butter	190 calories
2 Tbsp reduced-fat Jif peanut butter	190 calories
5 Nabisco saltine crackers	60 calories
5 Nabisco fat-free saltine crackers	60 calories
5 Wheat Thins	45 calories

as caloric as one sweetened with sugar. Yogurt-covered pretzels have the same fat and calorie count as pretzels covered in white chocolate. And chips made from sweet potatoes and beets instead of from regular white spuds differ from traditional potato chips only in content, not in calories.

How Saboteurs Snag You

Most of the time, you're better off eating "real" cookies, pretzels, or chips rather than one of the "have-nots" or "haves" that are such saboteurs.

Here's why. Even if a saboteur is lower in fat, sugar, or calories than the regular food, it's almost certain you'll give yourself permission to eat them more frequently—and probably in more generous quantities. Over time, then, they'll add more calories.

It's easy to find out whether these foods are high in calories. Just check the nutritional information on the label. But it's unlikely you'll do that. Instead, we tend to rationalize by saying, "Well, I really need to have a cookie—and since I'm going to have a cookie anyway, it might as well be low-fat." In other words, it's easy to fall into the habit of thinking the so-called diet cookie is "not as bad."

(continued on page 58)

Fruity Filler

Our staff nutritionist says she has seen more people gain weight on fat-free cookies than on any other food. This cookie is not only fat-free but also has fruit, so it's easy to rationalize that it's both healthy and low-calorie, especially if it takes half the package to make you feel full.

But maybe the photos below will leave a lasting impression. Can a whole cantaloupe really have the same calorie count as a single fat-free cookie?

It does. And not only that—the cantaloupe also has a generous helping of fiber, vitamins, and minerals.

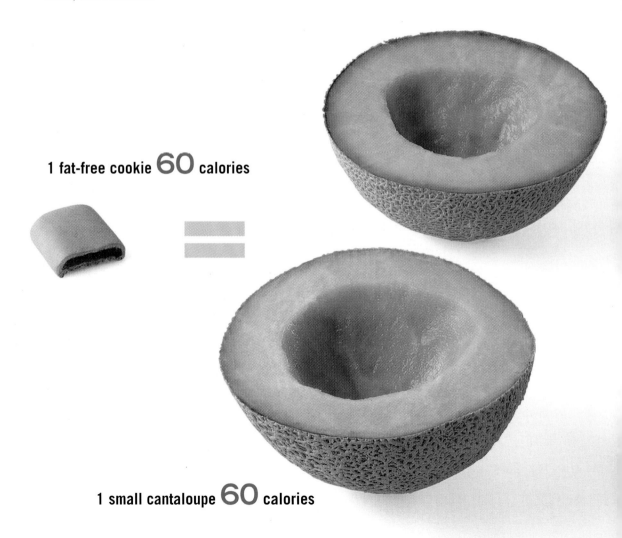

1 fat-free cookie 60 calories

1 small cantaloupe 60 calories

Carob: The Chocolate Saboteur

A carob bar like the one pictured here is the classic food saboteur. It seems nutritionally correct and bills itself as the low-fat answer to chocolate. But in fact, the bar is a substitute that has the same fat and calorie content as real chocolate—thanks to the processing that turned the carob into a candy bar.

If it's chocolate you want, eat chocolate. And if you're wondering how *much* chocolate you could eat (not that you'd want to), keep this mental image on file. For the same calories as the single carob bar, you could satisfy your craving with 10 scoops of chocolate Italian ices or 20 chocolate licorice sticks.

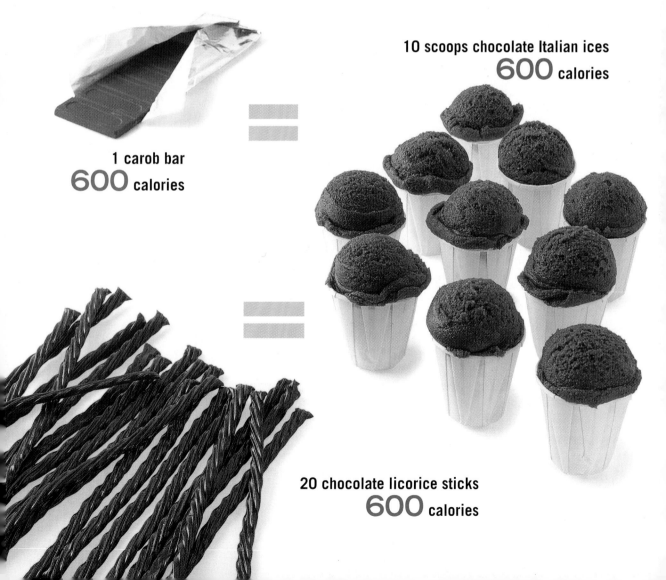

10 scoops chocolate Italian ices
600 calories

1 carob bar
600 calories

20 chocolate licorice sticks
600 calories

But then look what happens. Since the diet cookie isn't nearly as satisfying as what it's replacing, you eat more in an effort to satisfy the craving. See why I dub these foods saboteurs?

A recent patient was a classic case of this cookie confusion. She simply could not be convinced that fat-free cookies were her way of rationalizing eating cookies. She didn't believe that, in fact, she tended to eat many more cookies when they were fat-free.

Just the other day, she admitted to Phyllis, our staff nutritionist, that on a particularly stressful day at the office, she had bought low-fat cookies at the office vending machine.

"Would you have purchased a package of regular cookies?" Phyllis asked her.

"No," the patient replied without a pause. "I would never have considered it."

"That's my point," said Phyllis. "You would never have given yourself permission to eat real cookies, but the words 'low-fat' on the label are a green light to what is really a high-calorie food—and not a very satisfying high-calorie food at that."

Phyllis's solution is to ask yourself if you would have chosen the regular cookie—or muffin or cake or chips. If the answer is no, chances are you're using the fat-free substitute to rationalize your way into eating a food you believe to be inappropriate for you. It probably means you should find another alternative altogether.

To be sure, not all low-fat or sugar-free foods are useless. As you'll see in the pages that follow, I recommend many and include them on the Anytime List of foods on page 222 to keep on hand. And as the visual demonstrations throughout the book make clear, there is a range of low-fat, low-calorie foods you can eat in any quantity at any time.

But beware the food saboteurs!

Craving and Appetite: Is It All in Your Head?

We think of appetite as a generalized desire for something—for sweets, perhaps, or for "something salty." And we think of a craving as an extreme, almost obsessive requirement for a specific food—as when you absolutely have to have a hot fudge sundae.

The truth is that there is no known mech-

Hormones and Taste

Do your tastes change at different times of the month? For women, there's a hormonal reason why that happens.

Everybody knows that pregnant women are often seized by sudden tastes for salty or spicy food. The same thing happens premenstrually. Changing hormone levels affect the taste perception of salt, raising the salt taste threshold. Saltier, more savory, more highly flavored foods seem more appealing to women during these times.

Choosing Food
When You're Eating Out

Only dieters need to fret over where they eat, what they eat, and exactly how their food is prepared.

But making food choices is a process that will be ongoing throughout your life. Maybe you don't know where you're going to be eating dinner tonight. You can't refuse to eat—can you? With picture perfect weight loss, I want you to have the knowledge you need to make lower-calorie choices, whether you're cooking your own meal or ordering it from a menu.

Unless you've been invited to someone's home, where it would hurt a host's feelings to reject a food being served, there is really no occasion or location where you don't have some freedom of choice.

anism in the human body that translates a physiological need for a nutrient into a yearning for a food that is high in that nutrient. What's more, as everybody knows, the cravings that attack us are rarely for foods that are good for us. When was the last time you felt you just "had to have" a plate of broccoli? But how about a rich chocolate brownie? You can probably work up a good craving for that without too much trouble.

Cravings are born out of an interaction among a number of complex factors—neurochemical, nutritional, cultural, psychological—working together in ways we don't clearly understand. But that doesn't mean they're not real. They're very real—and quite powerful.

Searching for the mechanism that helps control appetite, researchers at the University of California at Irvine College of Medicine have discovered a receptor in the brain that is a major regulator of eating. The receptor binds to a nervous system chemical called melanin-concentrating hormone (MCH), which is known to regulate how often and how much we eat. A drug that blocks the receptor would probably control overeating, but experts don't expect such a drug to be available for at least 10 years.

From Deprivation
to Cravings

Clearly, some level of hunger works hand in hand with a multitude of learned factors to influence our eating. One hint about how it works is that a craving is usually for something we consider tasty and satisfying but that we don't allow ourselves to eat on a regular basis. Chronic dieters, for example, are seized by cravings much more frequently than nondieters. That's because food deprivation and/or loss of body fat can have a profound influence on the same brain chemicals that regulate appetite. The maddeningly skinny person who never diets, on the other hand, isn't deprived; she might want ice cream from time to time but won't obsess about it. The dieter will change her mind 15 times about the flavor, endlessly debate the use of sprinkles or a topping, and worry about the consequences of going off her diet.

Another factor that appears to work with the "appetite chemicals" is hormonal. Women are known to have more cravings than men.

The next time you feel a craving coming on, or even a mild appetite for a particular taste, ask yourself what you really want. Is it the hot fudge sundae? Will a chocolate frozen yogurt do just as well? A craving can often be satisfied by a lower-calorie food of similar flavor or texture. But sometimes, you just have to go for the sundae.

Planned Bingeing

I know that "planned bingeing" sounds like a contradiction in terms—and a pretty specious one at that. After all, bingeing implies something done wantonly, impulsively, with an out-of-control quality.

The image that comes to mind is of someone eating a whole box of cookies at one sitting, or scarfing down a huge bag of potato chips. It's something done hurriedly, almost furtively, as if consuming a large quantity of high-calorie food were an evil deed about which you should feel guilty.

By planning your binge, however—by preceding it with thought and executing it in the context of a decision—you can get all the enjoyment you deserve without remorse.

The demonstration on the right was designed in honor of a former—and highly suc-

cessful—patient. Call her Annie. Annie had always found that dipping into the bread basket at a restaurant would trigger an eating binge that would make her unhappy afterward.

After a minimal amount of Food Awareness Training, she came in to report a wonderful experience of the day before. I'll let Annie tell it in her own words:

"I met a friend for lunch and had a delightful time and a good low-calorie meal—a piece of fish and some grilled vegetables. On the way home, I passed my favorite Italian bakery. They were just setting out some freshly baked bread, and the smell was overwhelming. I went inside and bought a sesame-seed loaf, my absolute favorite bread. In the past, I would have eaten a few pieces and felt completely out of control—like I was cheating. But this time, I ate the bread by choice—half on the way home and the other half once I was there. I enjoyed every bite of it, and I didn't feel guilty because I didn't 'go off my diet.'"

The bread had 840 calories, and it certainly isn't a nutritionally adequate meal. But since Annie had eaten low-calorie, healthy food the rest of the day, her personal bread binge didn't produce either weight gain, nutritional deficiency, or self-recrimination. As Annie herself said, she felt good about herself. She felt she was in the driver's seat.

Unlike many dieters who make the mistake of eating something that doesn't really satisfy their urge, Annie had enjoyed her binge. She was in touch with her enjoyment, right down to the last, delicious morsel.

Whatever your binge trigger is—bread or

Annie's "Planned" Bread Binge

Annie chose to eat a whole loaf of fresh-baked semolina bread. That 820 calories was a splurge, for sure—but a far better calorie buy than the one tiny dish of Chex Mix that is hardly enough to whet the appetite.

5½ oz Chex Mix
820 calories

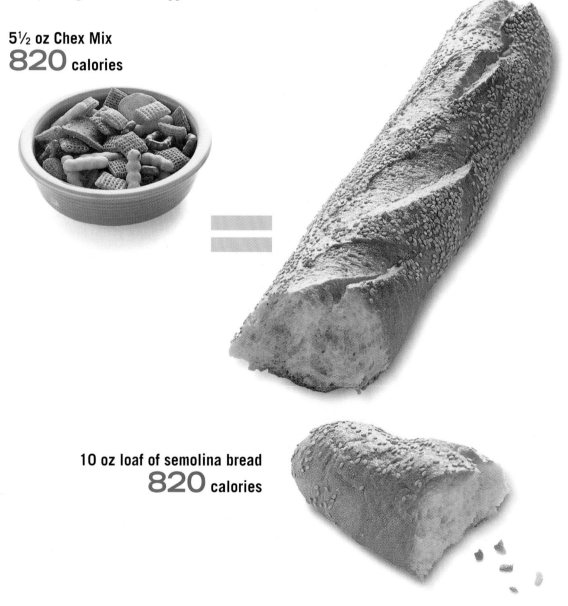

10 oz loaf of semolina bread
820 calories

chocolate or potato chips or Alsatian cassoulet, for that matter—when you make the decision to plug it into your eating equation, you'll gain enjoyment and a good feeling about yourself. And you can gain all that without gaining weight.

Boredom

Food is not boring. Diets are.

One reason diets never work is that people simply tire of eating the same food over and over. It's a great incentive to "cheat."

That won't happen on the picture perfect weight-loss program because no food is ruled out. You're not restricted to eating certain foods at certain times in certain quantities. Quite the contrary—I want to broaden the scope of your food choices.

For example, I am not telling you that you can never again eat a bagel with cream cheese. I'm simply asking you to be aware that when you do eat a bagel with cream cheese, you're choosing to eat 650 calories at once. You may decide that's exactly what you want.

On the other hand, you may look at the demonstration on page 108 and discover another choice that might be preferable—for the same or fewer calories.

The theory is simple: When people are bored by prescribed diets, they're propelled off of them. If you have a broad range of choices, you won't get bored. The weight-loss program in this book is all about choices.

No Failure Implied

When dieters "go off" a diet, they typically express the retreat as a failure. There's a moral undertone to it all: They've had a "bad" day or a "bad" week. A character flaw is implied. Feelings of self-worth can plummet; confidence takes a dive; the whole weight-loss effort suffers.

Patients usually adapt to my weight-loss program very quickly, not just because they're motivated but also because the choices offered in this program are very easy to live with. But many of my patients have days and sometimes even weeks in which they don't lose weight.

That's natural. It's human. It says nothing about your moral character. Expect it.

I get worried when people won't accept it. These people tend to be all-or-nothing inflexible types. They typically start with high and unrealistic expectations, and they stick to lower-calorie choices compulsively, failing to understand that this is a process in which, over time, they need to change their relationships with food. It's these people who are the most likely to blow it.

I feel much better about people who recognize they will have some days when they consume more calories than other days, and they keep moving on. They are the ones who understand that this is a process, and that what they are doing is changing their relationships with food.

Chapter 4

STARTING THE PICTURE PERFECT WEIGHT-LOSS PROGRAM

A journey of a thousand miles must begin with a single step, the saying goes.

That's the way to think of the weight-loss program in this book, too—not as a diet but as a first step on a journey into awareness that will continue forever, your opening stride into a life-changing experience.

For the most part, new patients making first-time appointments are referred to my office by other patients who are happy with their success. But I have one patient in particular who operates with an especially missionary-like zeal.

Her name is Karen. When a new patient is referred to me by Karen, I never know where they may have met. She may have had a conversation with a customer under the next hair dryer in the beauty salon. Or she was speaking to a fellow guest at a wedding. Or she just started talking to the guy sitting beside her on the commuter train. I don't know how these conversations get started, but as soon as the topic of weight comes up, pretty soon she has convinced whomever she's talking to that he or she should get involved with my program.

One day about a year ago, Karen showed up unannounced at midday. She had been lunching with a good friend and had managed to bring him directly to my office from the restaurant.

Definitely a first. Most people don't want to meet a weight-control expert right after a fancy lunch. Karen's friend was good-natured and gentlemanly about being "kidnapped," however, and I tried to allay what I was certain was his reluctance.

"I don't want to embarrass you," I told him. "You don't have to start this program because Karen is talking you into it. I'll explain the program to you, and you can go home and think about it before you make a decision."

I wasn't sure when or if I'd hear from him, but 5 days later, he called for an appointment. Now, 6 months later, he has lost 47 pounds and he can't thank me enough. I tell him it's not me he should thank, it's Karen. The truth is that thanks are owed to whatever internal force said to him, "Okay, today's the day. Today's the day I'm going to start changing the way I eat."

What Brings You Here?

The National Weight Control Registry, maintained by researchers at the University of

Pittsburgh School of Medicine and the University of Colorado Health Sciences Center in Denver, performed a study monitoring people who had lost at least 30 pounds and had kept the weight off for at least a year. Every one of those people said they could identify a particular "moment of truth"—a specific triggering incident or realization—that helped them get started on weight loss.

For one patient of mine, it was an inspiring article in a magazine. For another, it was seeing herself in a full-length mirror. Someone told me he couldn't play with his kid without wheezing. Another person was walking down the street and caught sight of her own reflection in a department store window. As she recalls it, that glimpse of herself "just blew me away."

Some come to see me because they have been advised by their doctors to lose weight for medical reasons—perhaps the threat of diabetes, or evidence of high blood pressure, or maybe a high cholesterol count. Other patients have been thin all their lives but are experiencing midlife weight gain.

Still others have gained weight in the wake of a traumatic experience—perhaps the end of a marriage or love affair, or maybe a professional crisis, or anxieties associated with the onset of middle age. And a great many of the people who come to see me have been dieting all their lives.

Sometimes, people tell me they've carried an article about my program for 2 years, and now here they are. I tell them how glad I am that they rushed right in.

Empowerment through Understanding

While every patient coming into my office in Manhattan has his or her own reason for being there, all share a similar need to change their relationship with food. The way we get them started on that change is not with a weigh-in. Once someone has made that all-important first move up the elevator and through the door of the office, he or she has an initial consultation with me, with my staff nutritionist, and with a staff psychologist. That's because all three disciplines—the medical, the nutritional, and the psychological—come into play in understanding the nature of each person's relationship with food.

If someone is going to be empowered to change that relationship, all three influences need to be brought into play. The change will show up on the scale. But that's not where the process of change begins—nor where it ends.

One thing I've come to understand over the years is that each person has an individual pattern in his or her relationship with food. I've seen those patterns emerge time and again over the years in literally thousands of people we've helped. Whatever the background, whatever the individual's dieting history, whatever the trigger that has propelled the person into my office, these patterns are most profoundly influenced by lifestyle.

In fact, just about everybody falls into one of four eating profiles. The "profiles" include not only a lifestyle but also the eating habits that go along with it. Before people begin to make changes, they need to recognize and clarify the most important aspects of their eating profile. It's an essential building block of the change they'll need to make.

The Four Classic Eating Profiles

The profiles are so real that I've named them after actual patients who best exemplified their classic characteristics.

- *Susan* was the classic example of the office worker tied to a desk.
- There's the business traveler, wined and dined round the clock—that was *Stan*.
- The mom stuck at home all day with the kids was *Diana*—to a T.
- The student or shift worker who always eats on the run is personified by *Doug*.

Now, I realize you might not be an office worker, a business executive, a mother with young children, or a student or shift worker. But I'm willing to bet my practice that you'll recognize your own eating profile in the scenarios of these four.

Here goes.

Classic Eating Profile #1: Susan—Tied to a Desk

"I've lost so many pounds in my life," Erma Bombeck once wrote, "that if you totaled up the net result you'd think I'd be hanging from a charm bracelet."

The words could serve as a slogan for the classic eating profile embodied by the tied-to-a-desk office worker. If you fit the profile, the rhythm of the day seems tied to food and thoughts of food.

Susan once told me that she believes she has thought about food for 45 of every 60 seconds of her life. Despite being on a diet "half the time," she always believes she's the fattest person in the room "and the only one who's starving."

Sound familiar? Chances are, you start every day with the conscious vow not to eat. You're filled with resolve—alert, alive, purposeful. You take your place in line at the breakfast counter, cafeteria, or coffee cart, determined to have only coffee this morning. But somehow, you hear yourself asking for the glazed cruller as well.

"Sometimes," says Susan, "I buy the diet doughnut instead—plain, hold the glaze, no sugar, no jelly. That has to be a few calories less, right?"

Stress makes you eat, and worry leads to stress, and I'll bet one of the things that worries you most is being overweight. Maybe, as with Susan, there's a family history of heart disease or diabetes or some other condition—and you know that weight loss could literally save your life. "But that doesn't seem to scare me enough into doing something about it," says Susan.

Anyway, most of us can find some way to avoid taking action. Susan stopped running because of a bad knee. And because she's an accountant, she's unbelievably busy and pressured from January through April, so she says she "really can't get anything going during those months." But that comment makes her pause. "Not that the rest of the year is easy," she finally adds.

You probably order out lunch and eat it

at your desk. And I wouldn't be surprised if you usually order from the same old place—and, often, order the same lunch you had yesterday and the day before that.

Or maybe you head for the company cafeteria. There, you try to keep it light. Susan's usual meal is "a chicken Caesar salad or, if I'm truly cutting back, chicken salad with just an oil and vinegar dressing and maybe a bread stick or two. Sometimes if I really, really want dessert, I get rice pudding."

Your work is hard—nobody says otherwise—and by late afternoon, your energy is flagging. Someone in the office always keeps candy or nuts on her desk. You certainly would never keep a supply on your own desk—you're too afraid your mouth would be full all the time—but you do occasionally dip into the bowl on a coworker's desk. And I wouldn't be surprised if you buy a replacement supply in bulk for that coworker every now and then, just so you don't feel too uncomfortable about helping yourself from time to time.

Of course, as Susan adds, "even if the company cafeteria is closed, there are vending machines if I want a snack. I get the low-fat cookies or a low-fat granola bar, which I figure is better than a chocolate bar."

When work is over, it's natural for a crowd of colleagues and coworkers to go out for a drink. "We go to one of those places that has a happy hour," says Susan, "but I usually try to resist the hors d'oeuvres. I figure the chicken wings and meatballs are the best choice. They're protein, at least."

Then it's off to home. You've had a long, hard day, some finger food you could have

done without, and a drink or two. The fact is, you're really hungry.

Susan says she usually has a couple of glasses of juice to take the edge off her appetite. "Then, if I'm feeling up to it, I'll make myself a grilled chicken breast. But then I'm still hungry. I'll have a bag of carrot sticks, but it's like eating medicine."

After medicine, of course, you deserve to have something you really want. Staying on the low-fat side, you might have low-fat cheese and crackers. Susan also eats low-fat pretzels. "I get the huge container from the wholesale club and go through it in 2 or 3 weeks. But then after the salty stuff, I want something sweet. Sometimes I have some low-fat ice cream. Or there's a 'lite' cake in the freezer and I dig into that. I don't care if it's frozen. I always feel that one of the best places for food to thaw is in my stomach."

When you look back over the day, it has been virtually defined by food. Does this ring a bell?

Classic Eating Profile #2: Stan—Wined and Dined around the Clock

Stan doesn't quite grasp the concept of moderation.

Ring a bell?

Well, if you're the type of person who works hard and plays hard, you probably eat whenever, wherever, and whatever is necessary to fuel your hard work and play.

To a person who travels a lot on business, eating is often an integral part of work. But certain parts of this eating equation—like when, where, or what you eat—don't seem to be entirely in your control. You eat because there are certain people you have to meet with, and doing business over meals just goes with the territory.

The fact is, if you're a business traveler, a lot of your most important meetings and conferences take place at mealtimes. The power breakfast, the working lunch, the dinner with customers: These are at the core of your professional life. You're expected to partake.

If you travel by plane, you can never really be sure what they'll be serving for the onboard meal or snack—if anything. Nor are you sure what the meal schedule will be where you're going. Or what the meal possibilities will consist of.

That's why a lot of business travelers eat on a kind of contingency basis. Stan finds he often eats in preparation for the possibility of not finding time to eat later. He'll pick up a muffin and coffee to eat in the car en route to the office, where he tries to squeeze in at least an hour of work before leaving on a business trip.

Later, at the airport, "I'll grab a sweet roll or something because I'm not sure what they will be serving on the plane. Or else I'll just wait, hope they serve something, and eat whatever they have on the plane."

Eat what's available when it's available: That seems to be the mantra. After all, you really may not know where or when you'll be having your next meal.

Then you arrive in a time zone that is 3 hours behind yours and guess what: They're serving breakfast—a lavish spread of eggs, bacon, ham, toast, and Danish. "My first assignment on the New York to California route," says Stan, "I gained 20 pounds. But now I try to eat lightly. If it's a breakfast buffet, I'll have just a bagel with some cream cheese."

If you're the typical business traveler, you no doubt feel you're at the mercy of a schedule set by others. And you want to be at your best at all times. That's why you need the fuel that food provides, and why you worry about exactly when you'll get the next chance to load up—and on what.

A weight-loss diet for someone like Stan? Forget about it.

"I don't want to skip meals when I'm traveling," Stan says, "because I need to keep up my energy. But I can't plan ahead when I'm on the road. I'm not in charge. I've tried following diet programs, but believe me, you can't carry your meals around in your attaché case or tell your colleagues that you can have only 6 ounces of lamb for dinner. It just doesn't work."

Much of the time, the business traveler is being entertained. It limits your choices. "When you're not in one of the bigger cities," says Stan, "even the 'best' restaurants don't offer very interesting lower-calorie choices. They're heavy on the steaks, roasts, chops, pasta—that kind of thing. So I eat whatever there is."

Conferences, seminars, and executive briefings are especially challenging. They're always putting food in front of you. At lunch, says Stan, "they just set out sandwiches and cookies, and I have no choice. The same with dinner at a conference: It's a set menu. Nothing I can do about it."

Or maybe you're staying in a hotel.

There's the hotel dining room, of course, but that's probably a routine meat-and-potatoes place. Anyway, you've arrived late and you're looking forward to tucking into something in the quiet of your room. But "the choices in room service tend to be really narrow," Stan says.

"I remember a 7- or 8-day stretch where I was staying in hotels that weren't great, eating terrible food night after night," Stan recalls. "Finally, one night I was so disgusted, I called back immediately after placing the order and told them I'd changed my mind, cancel everything. 'I'm so sorry, but we can't,' the kitchen staff person said. 'It's already in the grease.' That was my nightmare."

Your alternative to room service? A chocolate bar and a package of peanuts from the minibar.

Juggling time zones, coping with jet lag, and keeping your blood sugar at a semi-reasonable level is no picnic. Consider overseas travel. Did you sleep on the plane? If not, your body is confused about whether or not it's mealtime. Nothing's certain about the next meal, either. The only certainty is that you're due at another meeting.

"The tendency is to just go ahead and have something to eat," Stan says. "My energy is all the way down and I have to be 'on.' Since there's no downtime, I eat just to keep going."

At last the day or week of travel is finished. You're done with the meetings and on the plane, heading for home. All you want is to relax.

"I need those nuts and that glass of cham-

pagne," as Stan puts it. "As for the meal, sometimes I don't even like what they're serving, but I eat it anyway. It's just part of chilling out after the rigors of the day."

By the time you do get home, Stan complains, "it's too late to get a normal dinner since it's way past everyone else's dinnertime, so I scavenge whatever I can find in the cupboard or refrigerator."

Even at home on the weekends, the busy executive is frequently either entertaining or being entertained. Dinner out ritually begins with a drink or two. For Stan, "if I make the mistake of having a second drink, my guard goes down and I'm not very careful what I'm ordering for dinner. I always just figure I'll go to the gym—tomorrow."

Classic Eating Profile #3: Diana—At Home with Kids

The person who fits the home-with-the-kids profile rarely sits down to a meal, but she weighs more today than she ever has, and she can't quite figure out why.

How can you gain weight when you hardly get more than snacks all day long? Some scraps here, a few bites of this, some morsels of leftovers—what does it all add up to?

Well, snacking can add up to a lot if you do it all day long.

First thing in the morning, Diana makes breakfast for the kids. Even as she's pouring cereal into each bowl, she mindlessly pops a few handfuls of flakes into her mouth. The kids eat, she gets them packed up, sees them off on the school bus—the usual hectic morning in a family with young children. She comes home to a quiet house and a messy kitchen and finds the uneaten cereal left behind.

"Like Goldilocks," says Diana, "I polish it off. And then maybe I have a little piece of toast as a chaser."

Her day has begun. It is punctuated by almost unconscious snacking. As if driven by impulse, Diana will eat without thinking. Her eating will control her—instead of the other way around.

Diana cuts a tiny slice of the cinnamon apple coffee cake she bought for her husband, Joe, and nibbles at it as she picks up some of the kids' toys. When she does the laundry, she helps herself to another slice of cake.

A neighbor drops by. Diana takes a break from housework, brews some coffee, and spreads cream cheese on a couple of bagels. When the neighbor accepts Diana's offer of a slice of the coffee cake, Diana also cuts a sliver for herself.

Volunteer work at the school. Diana offers to help stuff envelopes. Without a job to go to anymore, Diana finds she is eager to help out at her children's school, and she likes the midday companionship as well. For the volunteers there are coffee and cookies. Taking some cookies from the edge of the platter, Diana instinctively rearranges the rest, so no one notices any cookies have been taken. In fact, people are constantly commenting that she hardly eats a thing, even though Diana knows that they're wondering why, then, she isn't thinner.

In fact, Diana says a lot of her eating is done "in hiding"—secretly, when she's at home alone. Diana realizes that without con-

sciously intending to, she has fallen into a pattern of hiding her eating from her husband, Joe.

Diana used to have a full-time job outside the home—and when she did, she was a lot thinner. "Weight was never a problem," she recalls. She assumes she'll get employed again after the kids are grown, and she certainly hopes the weight loss will be "automatic" then. But, rationally, that's beginning to seem more and more unlikely.

After the birth of her first baby, Brian, Diana gained 50 pounds. She lost most of that weight, but then came the second baby and more pounds. When she first came to see me, Diana was 60 pounds over her wedding-dress weight.

She tries to eat foods that are "not so bad," as she puts it. At lunch with an old friend shortly before she first came to see me, she ordered tuna salad, no bread. But the tuna salad came with potato salad. It wasn't her fault. She didn't ask for it. But she ate it just the same.

A package of crackers also came with the meal—so she ate them. For dessert, she ordered a corn muffin, toasted dry. It was a boring choice—so she figured it couldn't be too fattening. She really wanted the chocolate cake but didn't allow herself to have it.

"Brian learned the word 'diet' very early," Susan told me. "When he was 2½, I drove into the Carvel parking lot and he said, 'No, Mommy. Diet.' I looked at his beautiful little face and burst into tears. My kid is taking better care of me than I do of myself. I used to be able to do handstands. Now I can barely run around after the kids all day. I'm not that old, but I don't have that much energy.

"Joe isn't really a help. He'll say, 'Do you really want that?' and I'll say, 'Yes, I do,' and I'll eat it even if I don't really want it. If you asked him, he'd say he's being supportive. He thinks he's being supportive by offering at least once a week to pay for liposuction."

Daily life for Diana is driven by her kids' needs. It's a fact of life, but it's also influencing her eating. When she picks the children up from school and takes them for a treat, she has one, too. It's a time of day when she's tired anyway, so an ice cream bar serves as a picker-upper.

In the evening, she usually cooks two dinners, one for the kids and a second meal, later on, for Joe. She'll pick at what the kids are eating, then snack on wheat crackers or bread sticks because she gets hungry waiting for Joe. She eats a little something with him because he doesn't like to eat alone.

There's generally nothing for dessert. (What happened to that cinnamon apple coffee cake anyway?) So sometimes late at night, Diana will munch on some of the kids' peanut butter and jelly on crackers.

Classic Eating Profile #4: Doug—Eating on the Run

Maybe it started when you were in college—and doing part-time work as well. Your commitments kept you busy. When other people were sitting down to lunch or dinner, you were studying, working, or some combination of both.

Or maybe it's the nature of your job. When normal mealtimes roll around, your workday is just getting underway. Either you don't feel like eating, or you can't take a break right then.

Whatever the cause, the reality is that you eat on the run—when you can and where you can. On a nonschedule like this, whatever you see is probably going to be what you eat.

Doug is one of New York's Finest, a member of the New York Police Department. When he first came into my office, he certainly looked the part of the Mean Streets cop—big, burly, with a lot more in the midsection than he wanted to be there.

Doug says he was always generously proportioned. He was the big kid who moved on from neighborhood football to play in high school and college. By the time he got to college, however, he was "constantly snacking." Back then, he says, "I had a big beer-and-chips habit."

Today, however, Doug concedes he feels a certain amount of embarrassment about his kind of bulk. "It's fine out on the field, but when it comes to wearing great clothes and meeting people who don't know you're a football hero, I'd rather be slim," he says. "You don't get the cool clothes in my size, and most women seem to go more for a Brad Pitt kind of guy. It's a self-esteem issue."

But what's a cop to do if he works crazy hours like the noon-to-eight shift? He's working while others are having lunch and dinner, and he's sleeping while the rest of the world has breakfast.

Since Doug sleeps till 10:00 or 11:00 in the morning, he just skips breakfast. He usually goes out to lunch at 2:00 or 3:00 P.M. "because I'm really hungry by then. So I'll have something like a burger and fries, or steak and eggs and home fries, anything that comes along. Anyway, it's two meals in one—lunch and the breakfast I didn't have earlier."

Without a regular, "normal" schedule of meals to sit down to, dinner is usually something Doug orders in. "What usually happens is that someone will yell out, 'Does anyone want anything from the diner?' and I'll look at the clock and it's 7:00 or 8:00, so I'll yell back, 'Yeah, get me whatever you're having,' and that'll be meat loaf with gravy and mashed potatoes or whatever the special is."

For variation? "Maybe a few of us will go out to eat. We tend to look for a place that will give us the most food for the least money. It's kind of crazy—we'll go where the portions are biggest even if the food isn't that good. We just want more on the plate. We like the kind of places that give you soup, salad, bread, the main meal, and dessert. That's what I had yesterday, at an Italian place."

Then the shift ends, and what could be more natural than a couple of drinks with the guys—especially at the end of a high-stress workday when you're a big-city cop?

On the way home, Doug says, he'll usually stop at a McDonald's, especially if he hasn't eaten anything in a few hours. "It's a meal, I guess, but to me it's a snack: a big Mac, large fries, and a Coke and oh, yeah, why don't you throw in an apple pie while you're at it? I'll eat it all in the car."

The quantities may seem unusual, but the pattern is not. There are many, many people these days with unconventional schedules. And that means unconventional eating habits.

Eventually, of course, this kind of eating will catch up with you.

When Doug came to see me, he'd been through a fairly typical crash-diet experience. On a prepackaged plan, Doug had lost a lot of weight fast. Then the plan faded into the background, old habits took over, and Doug regained the weight just as fast—and put on a little extra.

Stubbornly, he tried again. " I went to another program, and that also worked for a while. I went to Weight Watchers and kept the weight off for a year and a half. Then all of a sudden I wasn't paying any attention, and because I had lost the weight, I was saying, 'Oh well, I'm not fat anymore, I can eat anything. I don't have to pay attention.'"

To Doug, "eating anything" means that he just grabs whatever tastes good. It has nothing to do with being hungry. "That's how I eat a lot of the time," he concedes. "There isn't a lot of planning. I just grab what I can and don't think much about it."

What's Your Profile?

Any of these profiles look familiar?

Again, I don't think any of us fits exactly into one category. These are individuals—and each of us has individual lifestyle challenges to deal with.

But I think it's important to recognize and respect the power of a lifestyle to influence our eating habits. Whether you're tied to an office job or you travel a lot on business, whether you're at home with the kids or working unorthodox hours, it's both impossible and unnecessary to completely change your lifestyle just because you want to lose weight.

But if your lifestyle won't change—what can?

This is where these profiles are useful. All four of these individuals were able to get the results they wanted with Food Awareness Training. Some lost more; some less. But all of them found a way to eat well, satisfy their appetites, keep their responsibilities going (just as before!), and, at the same time, develop the eating habits that enabled them to keep the weight off, once they lost it.

The truth is that all the people I've profiled were eating for different reasons but in the same way. They ate thoughtlessly—if not mindlessly. They really weren't paying attention to their eating or thinking about their food.

That's why they were not really *choosing* what they ate. Instead, they let the situation, their emotions, or somebody else's schedule choose for them.

Their relationships with food had a lot of interesting twists and turns—and those relationships are important to understand. But that's for the next chapter. Suffice it to say here, however, that their relationships with food were negative forces in their lives. Whether they knew it or not, that's why they had come to see me.

The Diary Revelations

After the initial consultation, I ask people to keep a food diary. I ask patients to record as accurately as possible the time they are eating, what they are eating, the situation in which they are eating, and the degree of hunger they feel at the time. Along with that, I ask them to jot down whatever comments they think are pertinent.

For it to be accurate and meaningful, there's really only one way to do this diary. You have to take notes in the diary as you're going through the day. It's simply impossible to re-create all the "eating events" of the day at the very end. Too many details can slip through the cracks.

Want a peek?

On the following pages you'll find the food diaries of Susan, Stan, Diana, and Doug—accurate representations of how they ate before starting my weight-loss program. I think their food diaries exemplify perfectly the four classic eating profiles.

The Food Diary: Getting Ready

Of course, there are lots of ways you can make low-calorie choices without keeping a diary. Just looking at the pictures in chapter 6 of this book will certainly help you.

But if you really want the *awareness* that comes with Food Awareness Training, keeping a diary—even for a short time—is absolutely the most helpful thing you can do for yourself.

The food diary will help you evaluate your own food choices and eating behavior, just as it helps my team of weight-loss experts analyze the food choices and eating behaviors of my patients. It's a spectacular awareness tool—which is why accuracy and attention to detail are so important.

As I well know, however, the mere thought of a food diary can provoke all sorts of reactions. One reaction is fear: Do I really want anyone (myself included) to know what it's like to be me, eating the food that I eat?

Then there's another reaction—well,

let's call it a tendency to stretch the truth a little bit. It's a lot easier to say, "I had a few snacks yesterday" than to recall and write down every snack you ate at different times of the day.

Plus, I can see how you might resist the requirement of having your diary handy and your pen ready through the day. Who wants to be bothered with writing this stuff down, meal after meal after snack after meal?

A small percentage of people—knowing they are about to "start a diet"—will eat everything under the sun. A kind of Last Supper mentality kicks in, as people binge on their favorite foods "one last time." Patients tell me they actually have Farewell to Food nights. Even before appearing in my office for the first time, they'll load up on all the high-calorie foods they love. These foods, they're certain, I'll be asking them to abandon forever.

Remember: No Deprivation Ahead

Before coming to see me, one patient planned a huge restaurant meal to be followed by a late-night snack of all his favorite junk foods, which he bought specially to have on hand in the house. The idea was to snack all he wanted, then throw out whatever he didn't finish and start fresh the next day. Imagine his

Profile #1: Tied to a Desk—Susan

Time	Food (Preparation, Serving Size)	Degree of Hunger (0–4)	Situation (Place, Activity)	Comments
9:00 A.M.	Dry bagel Unsweetened grapefruit juice	3	Working at desk	Starting good day of dieting
Noon	White-meat turkey on rye with mustard	3	Working at desk	Still on the diet
3:00 P.M.	Reduced-fat cookies (1 package)	3	Coffee break at vending machine	Feeling low; need a pickup
6:30 P.M.	Chinese takeout: Steamed veggies with beef Plain rice (1 pint) ½ egg roll	3	Watching TV at home	Tasteless diet meal; ate ½ egg roll, threw half away; had to have it
9:00 P.M.	Low-fat ice cream (¼ container) One slice low-fat cake, frozen	1	Talking on phone in kitchen	Wanted something sweet but didn't go out of control. Not a bad diet day.

Profile #2: Wined and Dined—Stan

Time	Food (Preparation, Serving Size)	Degree of Hunger (0–4)	Situation (Place, Activity)	Comments
8:00 A.M.	Bran muffin (6 oz)	2	Driving to work in car	On way to business presentation
9:00 A.M.	2 scrambled eggs 3 strips bacon Hashbrown potatoes Bagel (5 oz) with 1 Tbsp butter	1	Restaurant, breakfast meeting	Not very hungry
1:00 P.M.	Chicken Caesar salad, including 4 oz chicken Few bread sticks	2	Talking in restaurant	Business lunch
8:00 P.M.	Scotch on the rocks Mozzarella and sun-dried tomatoes Penne à la vodka Roll and butter 2 glasses of wine	4	Business dinner in restaurant	
11:00 P.M.	Large chocolate bar	2	Watching TV in hotel room; candy from minibar	Not really hungry, want something sweet

disappointment when he fell asleep after the huge dinner and didn't wake until 2:00 A.M. He faced quite a dilemma: Wasn't 2:00 in the morning technically "the next day," the day when his diet was to begin? Should he snack or not? (For the record, he did not.)

That Last Supper attitude is a tip-off to me that the individual is a chronic dieter who equates dieting with deprivation—and with failure. I try to impress on such a person that deprivation is not in his future, and that the food diary is not a weapon but a tool of his own empowerment.

More typically, my colleagues and I often find that the diaries of new patients don't quite match the information we gleaned in the intake interview. During the initial conversation, when we review a typical day's eating and try to understand the challenging times of day, people often overlook many of their snacks or impulsive buys.

It is human nature to try to look good, of

Profile #3: At Home with Kids—Diana

Time	Food (Preparation, Serving Size)	Degree of Hunger (0–4)	Situation (Place, Activity)	Comments
8:00 A.M.	Few handfuls low-fat granola	0	Kitchen, feeding kids	Busy
8:45 A.M.	Small slice coffee cake	1	Kitchen, folding laundry	Cake bought for husband
10:00 A.M.	Handful of cheese crackers	0	On way to get vacuum	Grabbed handful from box on counter
1:00 P.M.	Green salad with oil and vinegar 4 crackers Toasted corn muffin, dry	3	With friends in restaurant	In the who-can-eat-less competition; ordered muffin as better choice than cake
3:00 P.M.	Ice cream bar	0	At ice cream truck with kids after school	Not really hungry, want something sweet
6:00 P.M.	Leftover macaroni and cheese (½ cup)	3	Nibbled kids' leftovers	
8:00 P.M.	¼ chicken (6 oz.) Rice (1 cup) Vegetables (½ cup)	1	Dining room with husband	
10:00 P.M.	3 chocolate-chip cookies	1	Preparing kids' lunch boxes	Exhausted

course—and that could be one reason we don't get the whole story when we're asking people to work from memory. But I think there's something else involved, too. Before we can get a handle on our real relationships with food, we need to accurately record our eating habits. And that can't be done by memory alone. You need to have pen in hand and your diary ready—for at least a few days, and better, for a whole week.

The Diary: Your Mirror

I know I need the accurate record of a diary to help people. And I believe you need it, too, if you're going to help yourself.

In addition to accuracy, responsibility for

Why Writing It Down Works

"No need to write it down," you say to yourself. "I can keep my food diary in my head."

Yes, but keeping a diary in your head isn't nearly as effective as putting things down on paper, as researchers in health psychology have conclusively demonstrated. According to a study at the Center for Behavioral Medicine in Chicago, writing things down serves as "a focusing device." The requirement of keeping a food diary lends authority to the process itself and thus helps you pay closer attention to your eating.

Writing things down also increases your commitment by helping turn an abstract, long-term goal into short-term reminders. The food diary "helps create an internal dialogue," researchers say, in which you emphasize the importance of what you're doing.

Finally, writing down what you're eating lends an objective power to what you're doing: This is a problem you're solving, not a condition that makes you helpless.

The moral? Write it down—consistently, carefully, in black and white.

Profile #4: Eating on the Run—Doug

Time	Food (Preparation, Serving Size)	Degree of Hunger (0–4)	Situation (Place, Activity)	Comments
10:00 A.M.	McDonald's sausage and egg biscuit	2	Reading paper in restaurant	Not really hungry
2:00 P.M.	2 slices pepperoni pizza Coke	3	Lunchtime	Pizza was what everyone ordered
6:30 P.M.	2 pieces garlic bread Veal parmigiana Spaghetti Caesar salad Cannoli Cappuccino (sweetened)	3	Eating with friend in restaurant	Big portions
11:00 P.M.	Cheeseburger Fries Coke	1	In car	Feeling stuffed

keeping the diary faithfully is essential. The attitude that the diary is "just another chore—I'll catch up on it later" is a sure path to disaster. One busy executive wanted to hand over the assignment to his wife and secretary. Since the secretary typically ordered his lunch and his wife invariably dined with him, he believed they would remember what he ate better than he did. Besides, he contended, he was a busy man, an important executive, somebody used to delegating tasks he didn't have time for. "If you don't make the time to keep your food diary accurately and faithfully," I told him, "you're probably not ready to start a weight-loss program." He kept the diary religiously from that moment on.

For some people, the mere fact that they must answer to a piece of paper—the diary—is sufficient to raise their food awareness. The minute they know they have to write down what they're eating, forethought takes over—along with increased responsibility for the food choices they make.

And choice, of course, is what this program is about. It's about putting you in charge of your eating, changing your relationship with food without changing your lifestyle. The first step to that is mindfulness. That's what the food diary does and why its value is inestimable.

The Write Stuff: Your Own Food Diary

Now it's your turn. It's time to begin keeping your food diary. As you build awareness of your food habits and begin to see patterns in your eating, you will also begin to take more responsibility for your food choices.

Above all, you'll learn to be in touch with how you feel about food and about your eating habits. It's worth repeating: Hunger is caused by the interplay of internal and external triggers. We may not be completely aware of those triggers. We can't see the internal triggers, whether they're the physiological actions of hormones and neurochemicals or emotional states like anxiety, stress, depression, boredom, even loneliness. Even the external triggers may act upon us in obscure or unconscious ways: the clock telling us it's dinnertime, the family sitting down at the big table, the sight or smell of food—even a photograph in a magazine or a commercial on television.

By forcing you to pay attention to the feelings you have about food and eating, the food diary makes you aware of your own ability to make choices. That's why it's your first step toward better choices—choices that will help you lose weight and keep it off through your lifetime.

How to Start

Make seven copies of the diary template on page 78 and keep one copy with you at all times each day. For a week, record every bite and sip you take—with the exception of water and low-calorie beverages.

For the sake of accuracy, make certain you write down what you've had the minute you've eaten it—immediately. If you put off making the notation, you will almost certainly omit an important item in your diary entry.

The Food Diary

Time	Food (Preparation, Serving Size)	Degree of Hunger (0–4)	Situation (Place, Activity)	Comments

Here's how to fill out each entry on the diary template.

- **Time.** Record the exact time that you are eating.
- **Food.** Note what you have eaten—chicken, for example; how it was prepared, if applicable—broiled, fried, steamed, or roasted in the case of the chicken; and the size of the serving as best you can determine it. Describe as many ingredients in the dish as you think necessary—not just a roasted chicken but a roasted chicken stuffed with leeks and wild rice, or, in another example, not just a tuna sandwich but a tuna sandwich on whole wheat with lettuce, tomato, and mayonnaise.
- **Degree of Hunger.** For the purpose of this diary, I want you to define hunger as a desire to eat regardless of the reason. Rate the desire on a scale from 0 to 4, with zero indicating no hunger and 4 indicating extreme hunger.
- **Situation (Place/Activity).** Where were you—bedroom, restaurant, kitchen, taxicab, office—and in what situation—with a companion, reading a book, holding a meeting—when you had the food or drink? This information is helpful because I don't want you to change your lifestyle, just your relationship with food.
- **Comments.** Note anything you feel is relevant to your food choice or to the way you felt after eating. Some typical comments? "That piece of cake was worth it for the calories". . . "It was foolish to eat those cookies". . . "I was eating in someone's house and had no choice."

Chapter 5

THE PATH TO AWARENESS

*D*id you recognize yourself in any of the classic eating profiles in the previous chapter? Chances are there were characteristics in all four that resonated with you, parts of each that struck you with a shock of recognition—whether you identified with the exact lifestyle or not. Now it's time to get "down and dirty"—time to analyze your food diary to assess exactly what kind of relationship you have with food.

For context, I want to show you first the kind of analysis my staff and I do for the patients who come to my office. So that you have a point of reference, I would like to look back at the food diaries of our four classic profiles—Susan, Stan, Diana, and Doug—and reproduce my own notes for each.

Notes on Susan— Classic Eating Profile #1: Tied to a Desk

Susan consumes fruit juice—a bad caloric buy—probably in the mistaken view that because it tastes tart, it's low in sugar and calories. In fact, it's loaded with both.

She eats tasteless, bland "diet food" all day and doubtless consumes far more calories than she realizes. She's constantly hungry, too. Sug-gest more filling, tasty alternatives. Susan can be eating a larger quantity of enjoyable food for far fewer calories. Very low intake of fiber-rich fruits and vegetables.

Analysis: Susan is the typical "dieter." She goes for the low-fat choice in the mistaken assumption that it's the solution to her weight problem. She is unaware that low-fat does not necessarily mean low-calorie. Moreover, her food choices are now so boring that she needs the high-fat, high-calorie egg roll at dinner as compensation for the persistent tastelessness of her eating.

Notes on Stan— Classic Eating Profile #2: Wined and Dined

Stan eats in the car. Nothing wrong with this—there's no wrong place or time to eat. Obviously, he prizes convenience. But he needs to find an alternative to the muffin that is equally convenient and satisfying but lower in calories.

Stan is sometimes eating for social reasons when he isn't hungry. He can still sit down and eat in such situations, but when he is aware of what he is doing, he may be able to make lower-calorie choices—melon and an English muffin instead of eggs, bacon, potatoes, and a bagel.

Stan consumes several high-calorie, high-fat foods at the same meal. He should become aware of lower-calorie choices that are available—and that he would enjoy—in the types of restaurants in which he is dining.

Point out that alcohol lowers resistance to overeating. Suggest ordering club soda with a twist instead of the first alcoholic drink. The earlier in the day and the sooner in the meal Stan starts to drink alcohol, the more calories he is likely to consume. Suggest that a bottle of water be ordered simultaneously with a bottle of wine. Stan might alternate glasses of water and wine to cut wine consumption. Spritzer is also a possibility.

Stan experiences his most severe hunger at dinnertime. Suggest start-off food—soup or appetizer—to take the edge off his appetite early in the meal.

Note that he probably would not have consumed the chocolate bar if alcohol at dinner hadn't lowered resistance. He should be made aware of the possible interaction between alcohol intake and consumption of sweets. A good rule of thumb: Never insert the key into the minibar. There's nothing in there that is a good caloric buy.

Analysis: Stan needs nutrition education. At the moment, he has no concept of what he's eating, no idea about calories. The circumstances of his business and professional life are not going to change. We need to help him deal with each of these circumstances; they won't seem difficult to deal with when he is more mindful about eating, calories, and nutrition.

Notes on Diana— Classic Eating Profile #3: At Home with Kids

Diana nibbles all day long and never sits down to a real meal.

She is completely out of touch with whether she is really hungry or not and needs focus. She is taking in a tremendous number of calories. She also has a few misconceptions: perhaps that salad oil is less caloric than dressing, or that a muffin has fewer calories than the cake she really wants.

If Diana's lifestyle really requires eating little bits of food all day, I can help her make better choices. Suggest foods to keep on hand: hard candy, fruit, low-calorie popsicles. Refer her to the Anytime List.

Analysis: Classic mindless eating. Diana is simply not paying attention, not thinking about food. She is not focused on the fact that she is eating, not to mention of the eating choices she is making. In essence, the food is choosing her, not the other way around.

Notes on Doug— Classic Eating Profile #4: Eating on the Run

Doug eats when he's not hungry. He eats to be one of the gang, part of the crowd. There's no focus to his choices. He allows his odd schedule to be the excuse for eating as a social event.

Doug needs to be more assertive about the restaurants he goes to as much as he needs to be more knowledgeable about food choices. His crowd prizes quantity over quality. Quantity is not necessarily a problem, but Doug could eat the same quantity if his choices were better.

Analysis: Doug needs basic nutrition education and more focus. Put the two together and he could be making healthy, low-calorie food choices despite the odd schedule of his eating, the group choices of restaurant, and his desire for large quantities.

Evaluating Your Food Diary

After you have scrupulously kept your food diary for a week, sit down, look it over, and get ready to evaluate it.

The notes you see above—on Susan, Stan, Diana, and Doug—are just the kinds of notes you want to make about yourself and your own eating habits. You're looking for patterns—recurring situations in which you make food choices. The diary helps you see where you've chosen a high-calorie option or the less-healthful alternative.

Some situations may sound just like something you've seen in the four classic eating profiles. Some choices may leap out at you as unnecessary—even inappropriate. That's precisely what you're looking for.

Let's take a look, item by item.

● **Time.** Does the diary show that at certain times of the day you tend to eat more? Are other food choices available to you at those times?

If your diary shows that you have a late-afternoon craving for food pretty much every day, there are probably some foods you can keep on hand at home, in the office, even in your purse or briefcase. Eating those foods might make more sense than getting items from the vending machine or the coffee wagon or the ice cream parlor.

● **Food.** What kinds of choices do you usually make? Are you choosing mostly protein? Mostly starch? Or was it starch in the morning and protein in the afternoon?

Your food diary will show whether you eat lots of sweet foods or whether salt appeals to your taste. Once you know that, you can begin to think of lower-calorie options in the sweet or salty category.

● **Degree of Hunger.** Does the diary show that you ate when you didn't feel truly hungry? Sometimes? Often?

Many people eat in response to feelings of boredom or tension. Did you eat for those reasons? If so, were you in touch with that feeling when you made your food choice?

● **Situation (Place/Activity).** Can you find any connection between the situation in which you found yourself and the fact that you reached for food? Think about these entries a moment, and you may be able to see the connection between the situation and the kind of food you chose.

● **Comments.** Explore what you wrote. What do your comments tell you about your eating habits? What do they reveal about your hunger?

Be honest and candid as you evaluate your food diary. Remember: This is an exercise in awareness. Nobody is asking you—now or ever—to change your eating habits or patterns in terms of when, why, or how you eat. The aim will be to find healthier, lower-calorie ways of working with those patterns. To get there, you must start with awareness.

Your Personal Top 10 High-Calorie Favorites

People say, "Give me a specific plan, and I'll follow it. I've done it a million times before."

If you've "done it a million times before" and failed each time, isn't it time for something different? Isn't the need for something different what brought these people into my office in the first place?

I want to remind you again that there are no "absolute-must" or "absolute-must-not" foods in my weight-loss program. There's only food awareness—that "journey" I talked about that you will be able to stay on for the rest of your life.

Over the years, I have found that one of the best tools to help you along the way in that journey is what I call your Personal Top 10 List. These are the 10 highest-calorie foods that you allow into your life.

I'm sure you could tick them off right now, without any trouble: Would chocolate layer cake, chips, Brie, or french fries be on that list?

You fill in the blanks. I mean it. Right now. Jot down the 10 highest-calorie foods you regularly enjoy. And make sure they're the ultimate—every bit as calorie-filled as the foods I've just mentioned.

My Top 10 List

Take a hard look at this list. I'm not telling you *not* to eat these foods. I am simply asking you to put them in the forefront of your mind as you continue to read this book.

By the time you finish this book, you may find that the possibilities offered by the list have changed in your view. Some of the foods on the list might seem less "worth it" than they do now. You might identify foods that are just as satisfying and are lower in calories. Or you may end up confirming that these foods—some of them, anyway—are absolutely worth it and there's no low-calorie alternative.

Of course, it's your choice—always. I'm only asking you to write out this list so you have it on hand as a tool of awareness. What counts is how you decide to use this Top 10 List.

1. _____

2. _____

3. _____

4. _____

5. _____

6. _____

7. _____

8. _____

9. _____

10. _____

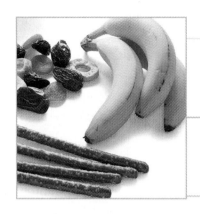

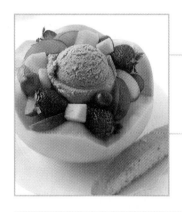

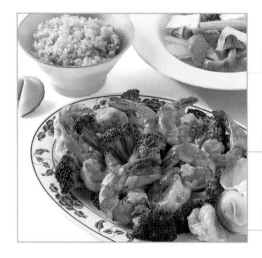

Chapter 6

GETTING THE PICTURE

"One picture is worth a thousand words," the ancient saying assures us.

You've read the words. Now here are the pictures.

One of the most useful discoveries I've made during the years of my practice—and one of the most important aspects of the weight-loss program I administer—is the importance of visual demonstration. A patient being treated for weight loss typically has weekly appointments, and each week, our nutritionist will prepare another demonstration for the patient. Maybe it's the bowl of black bean soup next to a chicken nugget that has the same number of calories. Or the small lemon tart and the seven scoops of lemon sorbet with an equivalent calorie count.

Whatever the specifics of the different demonstrations, one truth remains constant: The visual impact makes a difference. You can hear a message a million times, but when you see it demonstrated, it's really brought home.

That's why we're replicating the office demonstrations in the pages of this book, so you can see for yourself how wide-ranging your food options are, how easy it is to substitute one food for another, and how great a difference it can make.

The pictures that follow are not trick photography. No closely guarded secrets lurk here. But the food demonstrations you're about to see may seem to you to contain real insider information. Somewhere along the line, you'll be surprised. You'll see that a food you avoided because you thought it was "fattening" is really a good choice for weight loss. Or that a food you believed was a good "diet" choice is high in calories. Thirty-two butterscotch candies that have no more calories than a small serving of trail mix? Seeing is believing.

As you realize by now, these pictures are designed to do more than work up your appetite.

They show you exactly what your choices are and what the result will be when you decide to eat one food instead of another. Each of the portions shown is carefully measured. In each photograph, the food you're seeing has exactly the number of calories indicated. So you don't have to guess what someone means by 4 ounces, nor do you need to keep a measuring cup on hand. Just remember these photographs as you go through a normal day, and you can make your choices the way people *really* do—without measuring spoons or scales or calorie-counter books.

In this chapter you'll see a lot of what I call optical illusions. In some sections you'll see lots of food with relatively few calories. Other sections show the foods that would seem to be low-calorie but hide more calories than you can imagine. Throughout, we'll show you some of the many choices you can make when faced with decisions about what to eat.

Here's the way the food demonstrations are organized in the pages ahead.

- **Equal Calories, Different Portions.** You'll learn how much more you can eat—and discover healthier choices—when you see the food photographs on these pages.

- **Equal Portions, Different Calories.** Become an expert in making choices between the same quantities of the same types of foods. These photographs will help you select foods that may have one-half or one-third the calories of the alternative selections.

- **More for Less.** If you have a healthy appetite—and who doesn't?—you'll find that the foods in this section are worth learning by heart. Why? Because you can eat *more* of these foods and get *fewer* calories than you'd get from smaller amounts of higher-calorie choices.

- **Hidden Fat.** Prepare for a shocker. You probably know that some foods are exorbitantly high in fat—but wait till you see the equivalents measured by *pats of butter*. I predict these images will leave a lasting impression.

- **Looks like a Diet Meal.** You might assume that any salad is a good salad if you're watching your weight. Here's an image that will help you think twice—and choose some better calorie bargains.

- **Saboteurs.** A saboteur is sneaky, and this section will show you foods at their sneakiest. They may look healthy. They may even look low-calorie. But when you compare the saboteurs to your other choices, you may decide to avoid the calories that can sneak up on you.

- **Hazardous Situations.** Getting a snack from a street vendor? Stopping by the hot dog stand or grabbing some munchies to have with your drink at the bar? These are hazardous situations because you're making snap decisions. But with more food awareness—which you'll get quickly from this section—those decisions can be in your own best interest.

- **Holiday Meals.** Even when the table is groaning with holiday food, you don't have to back away. In this section, you'll find an easy visual guide to help you make lower-calorie selections.

- **Eating Out, International-Style.** Choose a cuisine—any cuisine—and you'll be faced with low-calorie versus high-calorie choices. This is the section that will help you decide. Have a look at some delicious international repasts that you can choose to satisfy your taste and appetite.

There's no right way to read these pictures. Whether they startle you or reinforce what you already knew—or both—let them be your guide to making mindful choices, and have fun with them. True, all you have to do is look at these demonstrations, and you're likely to have a lasting memory of what they show you about food. On the other hand, it won't hurt to return to this chapter a few days or a few weeks from now, just to make sure you remember what you've seen—and to reinforce the low-calorie choices you'll be making now and in the future. And if these pictures start to make you hungry, they also give you some very good ideas about low-calorie ways to satisfy your hunger. It's all part of the process of Food Awareness Training.

Elegant Eats

Want to start your meal with a touch of class? Well, before you make your high-class choices, consider what you're seeing here.

An ounce of liver pâté has 130 calories without the bread or toast points or crackers to spread it on. Or you can have 3 ounces of smoked salmon, touched up with the pungent flavor of capers and the cool taste of cucumber. It also has 130 calories.

1 oz liver pâté 130 calories

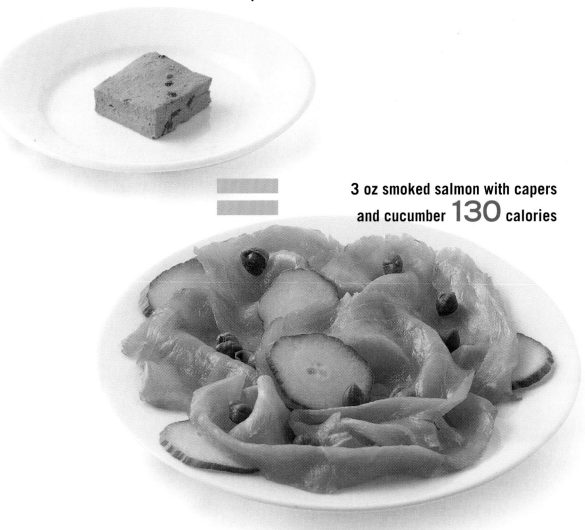

3 oz smoked salmon with capers and cucumber 130 calories

No More Waffling on Bagels

You know a bagel has a high calorie count, but what about half a bagel? Naked and unadorned, it has just 200 calories—the same calorie count as the light waffle breakfast pictured here. That's something to remember the next time you grab a bagel for your morning snack.

½ dry bagel (2½ oz) 200 **calories**

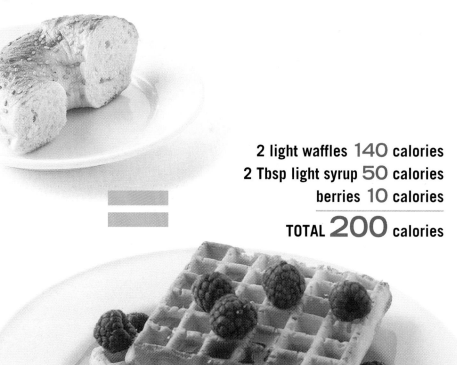

2 light waffles 140 **calories**
2 Tbsp light syrup 50 **calories**
berries 10 **calories**

TOTAL 200 **calories**

Snack Tricks

It isn't difficult to be deceived about snacks.

Consider the apple chips that you see below. If it's healthfulness and weight loss you're after, naturally you'll think of those chips as a good snack choice.

But not so fast. Those apple chips are not nearly the caloric bargain of a handful of pretzel rods. And for both nutrition and calorie-watching, nothing beats the real thing. Even if you ate four whole apples, you wouldn't be getting as many calories as you get from this 3-ounce serving of apple chips.

3 oz apple chips 460 calories

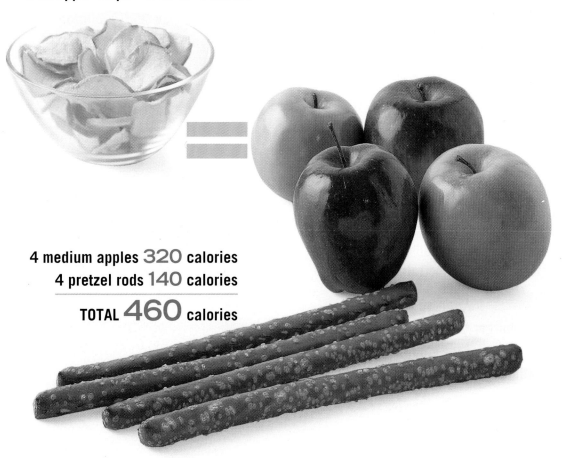

4 medium apples 320 calories
4 pretzel rods 140 calories
TOTAL 460 calories

Get the Picture?

Want a bite of bacon cheeseburger? Go ahead, but there's a cost. There are 210 calories in this bite. If you were to eat the whole burger, it would cost you 1,010 calories—not to mention saturated fats, cholesterol, and carcinogens.

The alternative is just as easy. Health food stores, supermarkets, and even fast-food chains now feature soy-based veggie burgers like Boca burger, the choice of the U.S. Air Force and an item that has been served at the White House. It has one-fifth the calories of the bacon cheeseburger without the health risk. In fact, the Boca burger is thoroughly good for you. And that goes for almost any other kind of veggie burger, too.

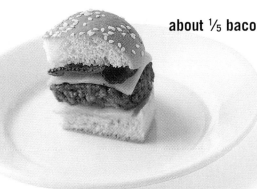

about ⅕ bacon cheeseburger 210 calories

4 oz burger 360 calories
2 oz cheese 220 calories
2 slices bacon 160 calories
bun 110 calories
2 Tbsp sauce 160 calories

TOTAL 1,010 calories
for the whole burger

=

veggie burger on bun with tomato,
onion, pickle, catsup, and relish
210 calories

Boca burger 85 calories
bun 110 calories
condiments 15 calories

TOTAL 210 calories
for the whole burger

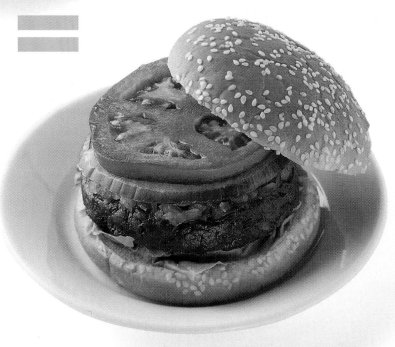

Sausage or Dill?

If you're in the mood for salty taste but not in the mood to waste a lot of calories, you can boost your food awareness by remembering the pictures below.

Consider that 32 large dill pickles have the same number of calories as one small sausage (1¾ ounces). Think about skipping the sausage and picking the pickles. They offer the salty taste you want—but without the saturated fats, cholesterol, and calories of the sausage.

As for the urge to satisfy your salt craving, you can probably go right ahead. Salt has no effect on fat loss.

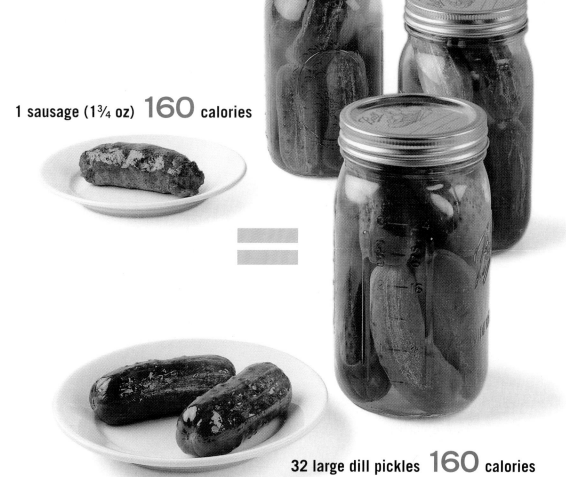

1 sausage (1¾ oz) 160 **calories**

=

32 large dill pickles 160 **calories**

The Color Orange

Love cheese? Who doesn't? But its calorie content can make it a costly snack. So here's a little imagery to keep in your memory bank. The two bites of Cheddar that you see on the left? While they're barely enough to satisfy a cheese craving, they contain as many calories as 30 dried apricot halves. And the apricots offer fiber—along with vitamin benefits too numerous to count.

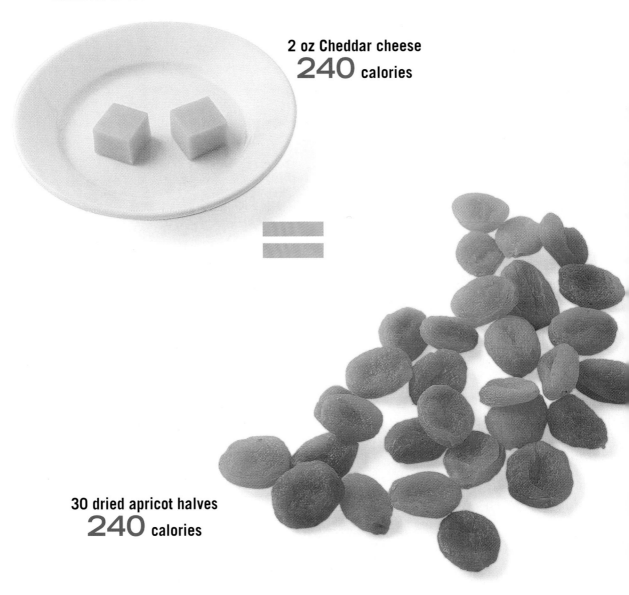

2 oz Cheddar cheese
240 calories

30 dried apricot halves
240 calories

Roll It

Even without the butter and/or jam you love to spread on top or inside, this croissant costs 320 calories. Now picture what you can have instead, if you happen to be hungry for a lot of breadstuff—both the bialy and the kaiser roll.

1 croissant (3 oz)
320 calories

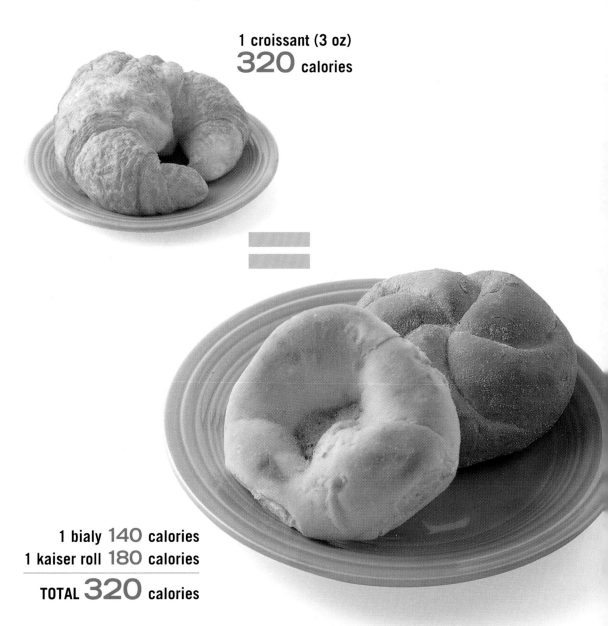

1 bialy 140 calories
1 kaiser roll 180 calories
TOTAL 320 calories

Equal Calories, Different Portions

Sweet Tooth Bargain-Hunting

If it's sweet taste you crave, keep your options in mind—as pictured below. The sorbet bars and dried figs on the right are equivalent in calorie count to the single chocolate-covered ice cream bar on the left. It makes any one of the items on the right—even any two—a caloric bargain.

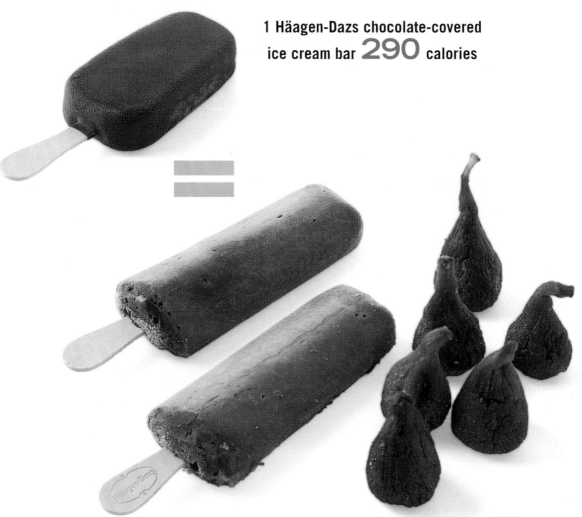

1 Häagen-Dazs chocolate-covered ice cream bar 290 calories

2 Häagen-Dazs chocolate sorbet bars 160 calories
6 small dried figs 130 calories

TOTAL 290 calories

Hot Dog!

If you love hot dogs, this one isolated chicken frank probably isn't enough for you. But look—and remember—what you can have instead.

If you try the platter of three veggie hot dogs, you'll get the equivalent number of calories that you find in the chicken frank. And since the veggie dogs' protein is from a vegetable rather than an animal source, they're also far healthier.

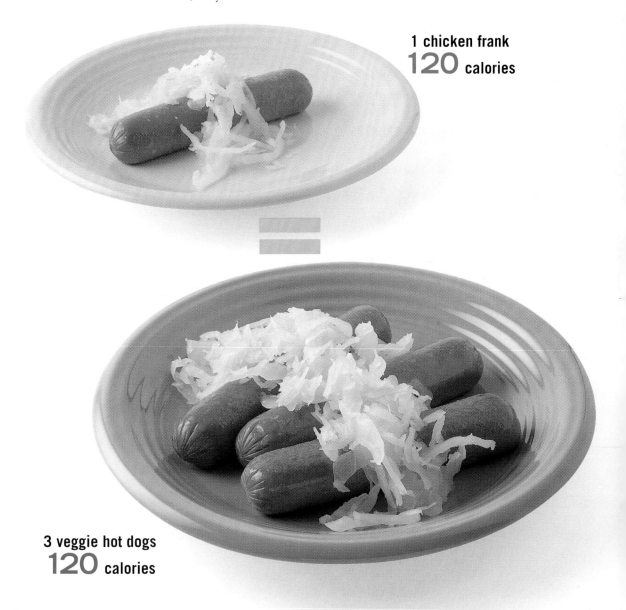

1 chicken frank
120 calories

3 veggie hot dogs
120 calories

Stacked Snack

In the mood for a rich snack? This scone—spread with a tablespoon of butter—will cost you 930 calories.

Now, to increase your food awareness, look at everything to the right of the equal sign. You can have one, or two, or even more slices out of this stack of raisin bread generously slathered with low-sugar fruit spread. Even if you could eat the whole stack shown here (an unlikely possibility), you'd just get the total number of calories that are contained in a single buttered scone.

1 scone (9 oz) 810 calories
1 Tbsp butter 120 calories

TOTAL 930 calories

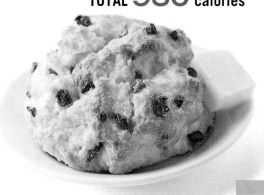

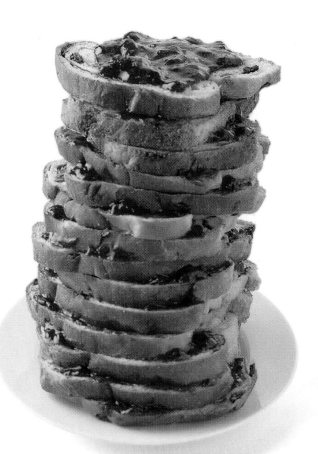

14 slices raisin bread 840 calories
4 Tbsp low-sugar fruit spread 90 calories

TOTAL 930 calories

Crowded Out

If you think this one lonely scoop of rich chocolate chocolate-chip ice cream doesn't look like much, you're right. It isn't. So the choices on the right should give you something to consider. For the same number of calories, you could eat 10 Tofutti chocolate fudge treats (not that you'd *want* to eat that many) or 15 fresh, succulent plums.

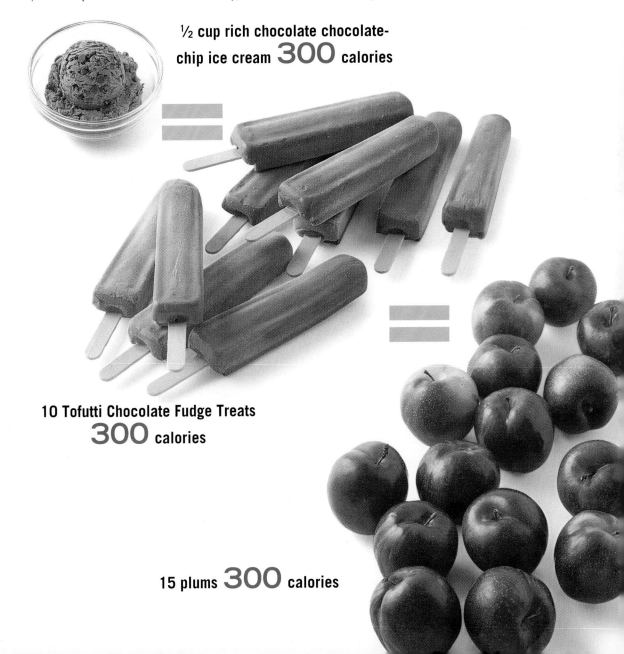

½ cup rich chocolate chocolate-chip ice cream 300 calories

10 Tofutti Chocolate Fudge Treats 300 calories

15 plums 300 calories

Equal Calories, Different Portions

Trade Deficit

A bagel is low-cal if I don't put any spread on it, you think to yourself. And it's filling, too. But contrast a bite of bagel with this vegetarian ham sandwich—a healthy entire meal. And next time you reach for a bagel, consider whether that's what you really want.

On light bread, with lettuce, tomato, mustard, and pickle, the vegi-ham sandwich offers protein, fiber, vitamins, and minerals for 140 calories. A third of a dry bagel, also 140 calories, offers virtually no nutrition whatsoever.

⅓ dry bagel (1½ oz) 140 calories

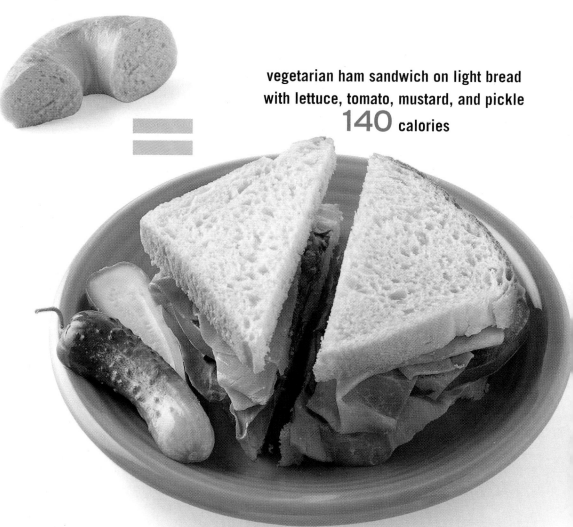

**vegetarian ham sandwich on light bread
with lettuce, tomato, mustard, and pickle
140 calories**

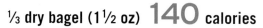

Lemon Aids

Sometimes, only the tart taste of lemon will do. But you'll want to remember what you see on this page before you automatically reach for a lemon tart for dessert.

One lemon tart can cost you as many calories as seven scoops of lemon sorbet or 14 lemon lollipops. Now you see why sorbets and lollipops are on the Anytime List of foods to keep handy: They're low-calorie options for the taste you crave.

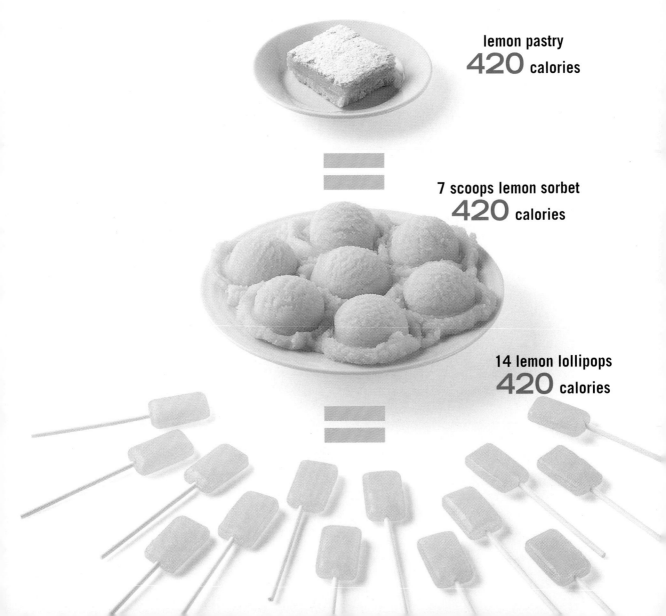

lemon pastry
420 calories

7 scoops lemon sorbet
420 calories

14 lemon lollipops
420 calories

Spuds 'n Nuts

Both potatoes and nuts are nutritious, healthy foods. The difference is in how we eat them.

Have a look at the comparison below. This single cup of cashew nuts costs 880 calories—the equivalent of eight baked potatoes with salsa! The next time you find yourself mindlessly snacking on nuts, remember this picture. If you're trying to lose pounds, the image of that tiny cup of cashews compared to all those lush baked potatoes may jolt you into thinking of an alternative.

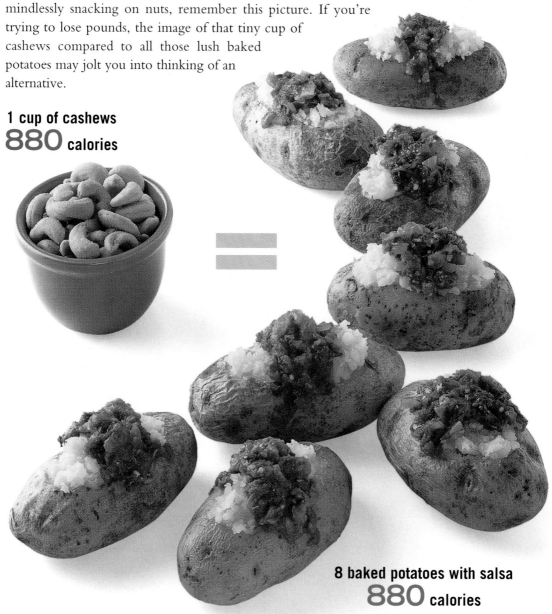

1 cup of cashews
880 calories

8 baked potatoes with salsa
880 calories

Measly Muesli

Muesli—the high-fiber, whole-grain, crunchy, nutritious cereal that has allegedly built the body strength of every Swiss mountaineer.

But what if you aren't climbing mountains?

A mental image of what you see here will come in handy the next time you have to make a decision about this particular health food. The tiny portion of muesli plus the three low-fat fruit slice candies have 310 calories. For the same 310 calories, you could eat a lot of food—four wedges of honeydew and four fruit leathers.

½ cup muesli 160 calories
1½ oz low-fat fruit slice candy 150 calories
TOTAL 310 calories

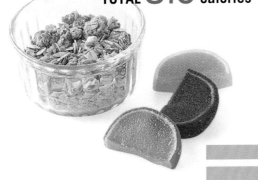

4 fruit leathers 180 calories
4 honeydew wedges 130 calories
TOTAL 310 calories

Sundae, Sundae

Who doesn't love a sundae? But alas! Its three scoops of ice cream, lathered with chocolate syrup and topped with nuts, whipped cream, and a cherry, will cost you 1,360 calories. Look again.

Each of those four sundaes shown on the right has one-quarter the calories of that whopper sundae on the left. The difference? Those four sundaes are made with nonfat ice milk or frozen yogurt or nondairy substitute. They're covered with just a little chocolate syrup and a lot of mixed fruit. All are topped with whipped cream and a cherry—but the sundaes you see on the right have no nuts. You'd never eat four sundaes, of course. But if you eat just one—made the way I've just described—it will cost you only 340 calories.

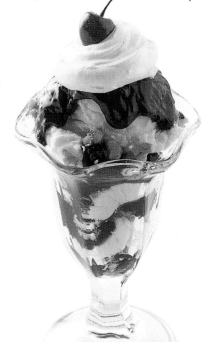

3 scoops rich ice cream (12 fl oz) 900 calories
6 Tbsp chocolate syrup 240 calories
2 Tbsp chopped nuts 190 calories
2 Tbsp whipped cream 20 calories
1 maraschino cherry 10 calories

TOTAL 1,360 calories

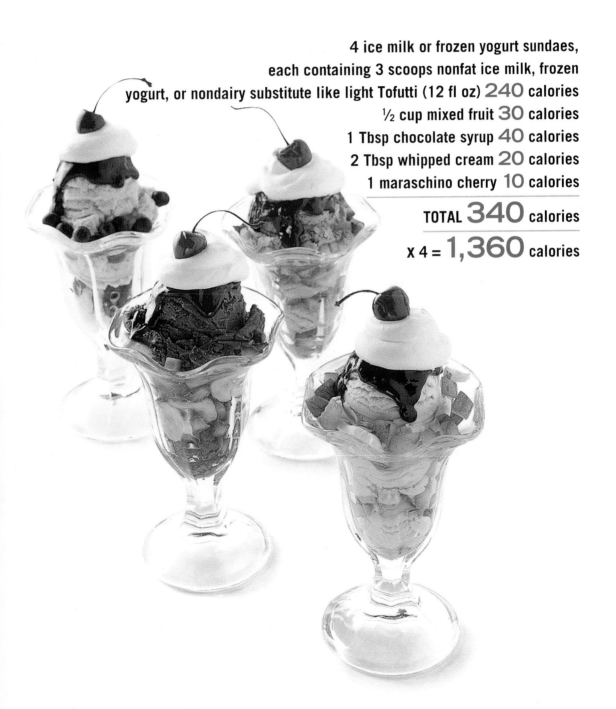

4 ice milk or frozen yogurt sundaes,
each containing 3 scoops nonfat ice milk, frozen
yogurt, or nondairy substitute like light Tofutti (12 fl oz) 240 calories
½ cup mixed fruit 30 calories
1 Tbsp chocolate syrup 40 calories
2 Tbsp whipped cream 20 calories
1 maraschino cherry 10 calories

TOTAL 340 calories
x 4 = 1,360 calories

Phony "Baloney"/Real Soy

The solo sandwich—naked bologna on naked pumpernickel—makes for a 520-calorie lunch or snack. Compare that to a sandwich made with vegetable bologna instead of the meat version. With the vegetable bologna option, you reduce the calorie count so much that you can go ahead and have a full-size meal. In fact, you would have to add soup and dessert to the vegetable bologna sandwich to match the calorie equivalent of the meat bologna sandwich. As for nutrition, the real bologna sandwich can't hold a candle to the meal that replaces it—with its soy protein and vitamins, minerals, and fiber from both vegetables and fruits.

4 oz bologna 360 calories
2 slices pumpernickel 160 calories

TOTAL 520 calories

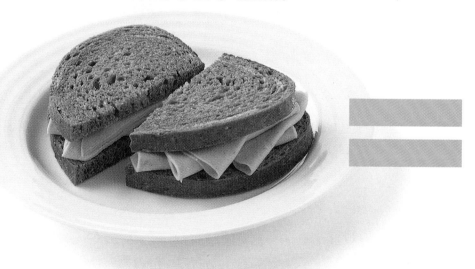

Equal Calories, Different Portions

4 oz vegetable bologna 120 calories
2 slices pumpernickel 160 calories
1½ cups tomato vegetable soup 90 calories
3 cups mixed fruit 150 calories

TOTAL 520 calories

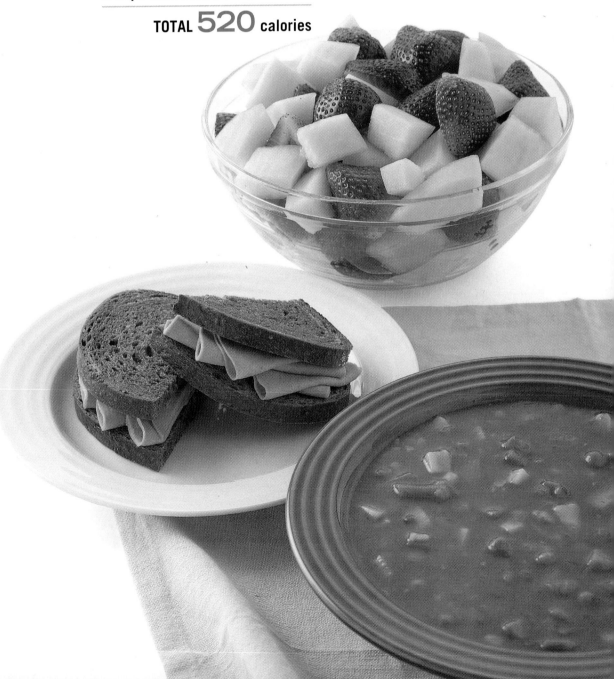

Nosh News

These pretzel nuggets are low-fat, salt-free, and contain oat bran. With all those advertising attributes, you might be lulled into thinking they're a good "diet nosh." But the picture below shows there's more to the equation—so it's worth keeping in mind.

The fact is, even a little bowl of pretzel nuggets contains 800 calories. That's the exact number of calories represented by all the noshes in the foreground—dried fruit, bananas, and four pretzel rods. What's more, the nuggets are not big on nutrition, whereas the bananas and dried fruit are packed with fiber, vitamins, and minerals.

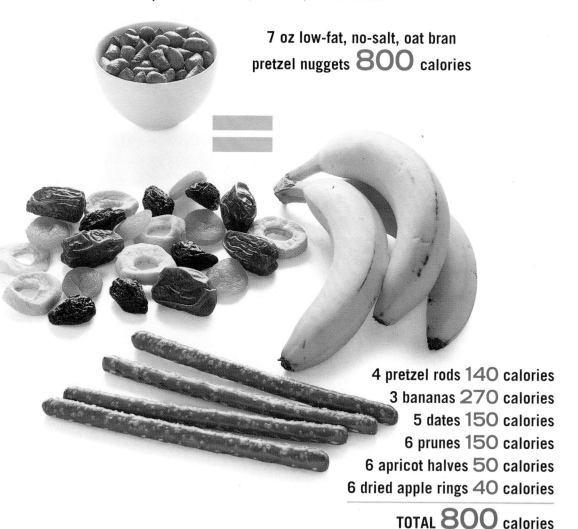

7 oz low-fat, no-salt, oat bran pretzel nuggets 800 calories

4 pretzel rods 140 calories
3 bananas 270 calories
5 dates 150 calories
6 prunes 150 calories
6 apricot halves 50 calories
6 dried apple rings 40 calories

TOTAL 800 calories

Eat the Starch, Hold the Fat

Any fried food is high in fat. In fact, there's so much fat in these fries that you'll probably consume more calories from the frying fat than from the potato.

How about four ears of fresh corn on the cob instead? The calories are equivalent. And if you eat just one or two ears—which is much more likely than four—you're choosing to cut your calorie intake by one-half to three-quarters. Plus, eating corn is a lot more fun.

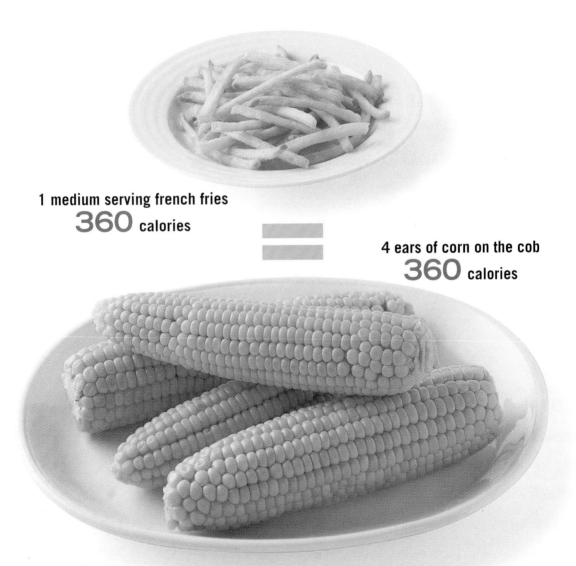

1 medium serving french fries
360 calories

=

4 ears of corn on the cob
360 calories

Equal Calories, Different Portions

Breakfast Bounty

Ah, breakfast! Time to fuel up for the full day ahead. How will you do it?

Before you answer that question, take a look at the calorie cost of a traditional bagel and cream cheese—and compare that to the breakfast on the right. While you might choose the bagel, it's a pretty big trade-off. For the same calorie count, you can have a bounteous feast of light pancakes, syrup, and veggie sausages plus vitamin-packed, fiber-rich fruit selections.

1 bagel (5 oz) 400 calories
2½ oz cream cheese 250 calories
TOTAL 650 calories

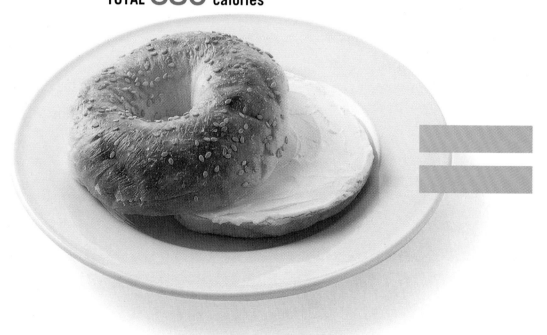

4 light pancakes 280 **calories**
4 vegetarian links 130 **calories**
2 Tbsp light syrup 50 **calories**
sliced starfruit and persimmon 190 **calories**

TOTAL 650 **calories**

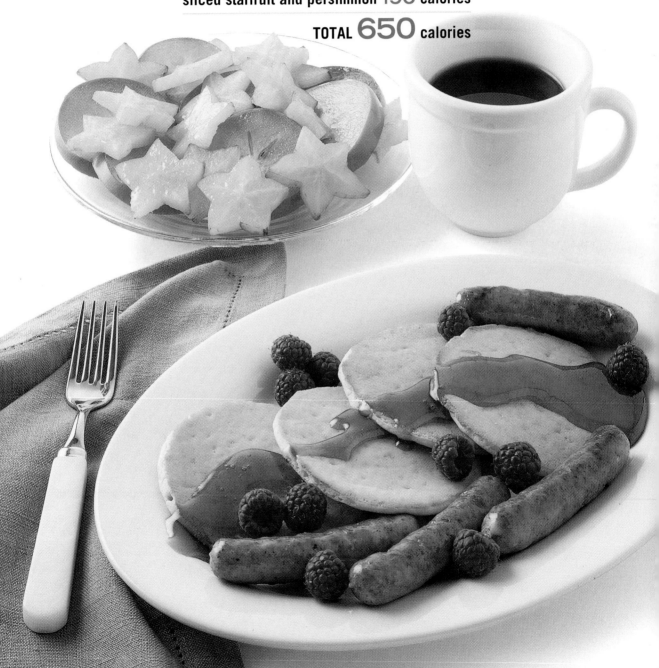

Lunch Package

A cheese-filled croissant is a bundle of calories, topped off with saturated fat and cholesterol.

Here's one of those images that says more than words or numbers could ever express. The number of calories in that whole platter of five sandwiches made with low-calorie cheese is equivalent to the calories in a single croissant sandwich. And with lettuce, tomato, and salsa on top of the cheese, these sandwiches are an excellent snack or lunch.

1 croissant with 3 oz cheese
650 calories

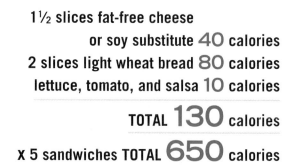

1½ slices fat-free cheese
or soy substitute **40** calories
2 slices light wheat bread **80** calories
lettuce, tomato, and salsa **10** calories

TOTAL **130** calories

x 5 sandwiches TOTAL **650** calories

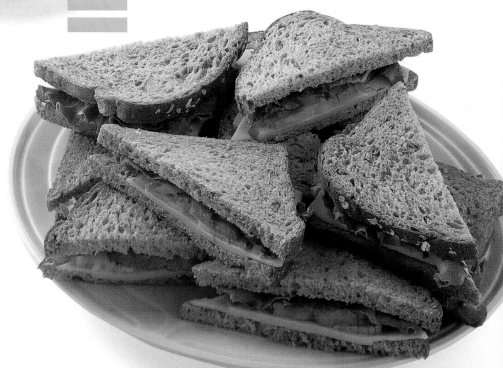

Mini Muffin, Maxi Impact

This tiny mini muffin has "only" 90 calories. But my guess is that you'll never see this mini muffin standing alone—nor eat just one, either.

These muffins usually come in packs of a dozen or 20. And they go down pretty fast.

Next time you think mini muffin, think yogurt cone instead. This frozen yogurt cone is a 90-calorie treat, the same as each muffin. But you can enjoy it for a good long while, rather than popping it into your mouth right away. So the cone lasts longer than a whole pack of mini muffins.

1 cone 20 calories
3½ oz frozen yogurt 70 calories

TOTAL 90 calories

1 mini muffin (1 oz)
90 calories

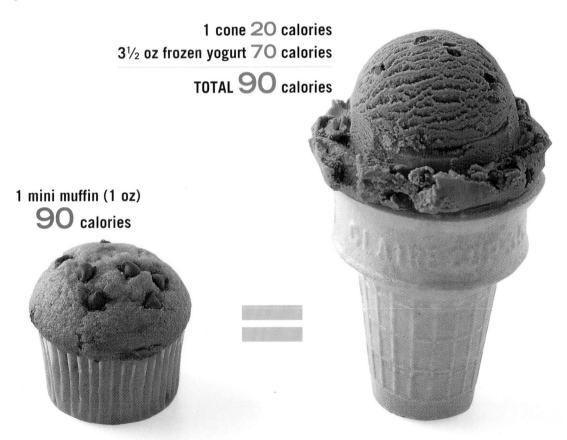

A Little White Lie

We all know rice is good for us. It's the world's "basic food," after all. We can feel virtuous eating the food that's the staple of the Asian diet. Right?

Unfortunately, that's a deceptive impression. We underestimate the calories in plain steamed white rice more than any other starch—probably because it has no color and little taste and is typically a side dish.

The next time you reach for white rice, think of the other white choice that's shown on the right. Consider that 1 cup of almost zero nutrition white rice has 220 calories—which is the same calorie count as these *10* cups of high-nutrition cauliflower.

1 cup white rice 220 calories

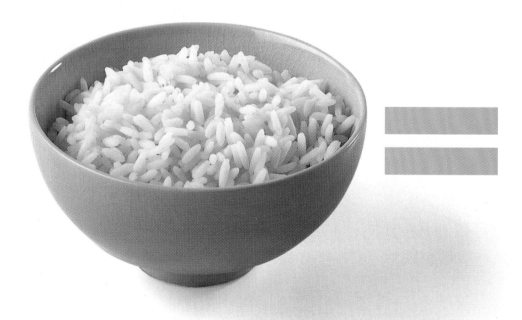

10 cups cauliflower seasoned with herbs and grated Parmesan cheese

220 calories

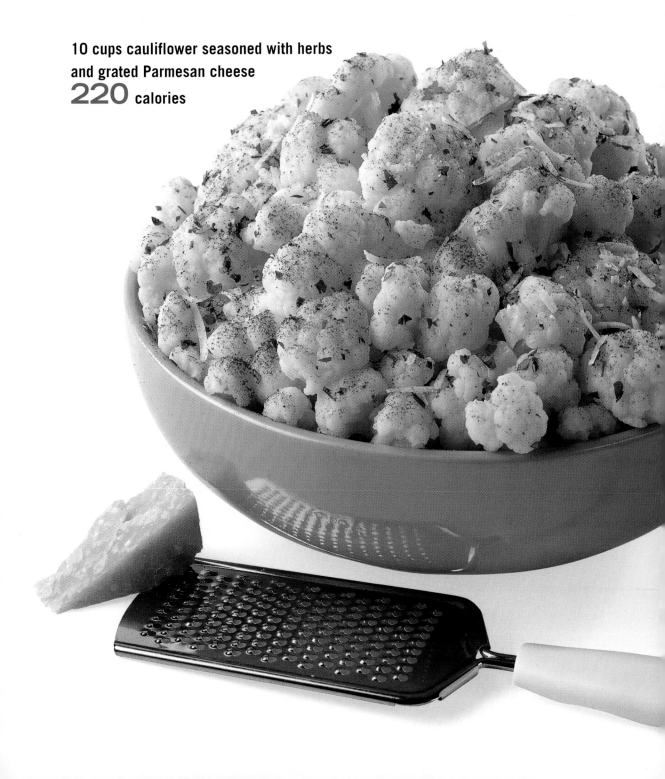

Deli with a Protein Punch

It's vegetable deli meat, but it looks and tastes like the real thing, especially when you slather it with spicy deli mustard. Contrast this plate of deli "meats" with the meager meat supply on these two small chicken wings.

Surely, these pictures tell the story. For the same caloric cost, you can have a lot of vegetable deli meat or very little chicken-wing meat. (If you dip the wings in sauce, the calorie cost will be even higher.)

And there's another notable difference—the health benefits you get from the vegetable protein versus the animal protein.

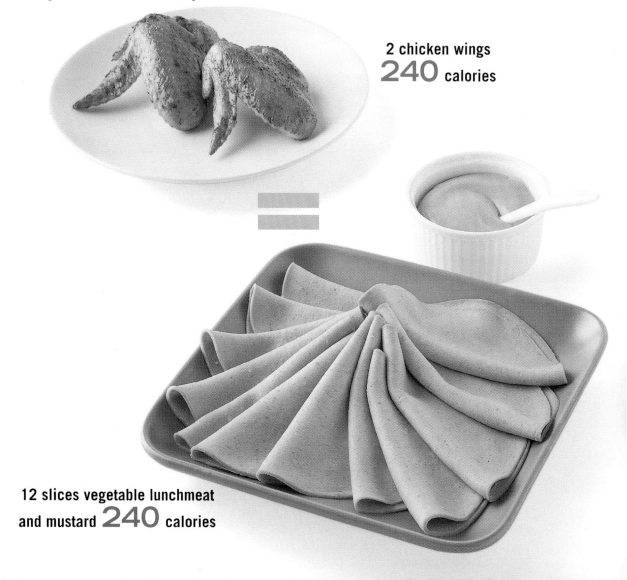

2 chicken wings
240 calories

12 slices vegetable lunchmeat
and mustard 240 calories

Juice or Fruit?

Oranges are good for you, right? And unsweetened orange juice must be just the ticket if you're concerned about weight loss, right?

Wrong. Think about what you see here the next time you reach for that glass of unsweetened orange juice. As you'll observe, the calories in one glass are equal to what you get from a whole pitcher of no-calorie orange beverage plus six oranges!

The lesson? Don't waste calories on beverage consumption. There's a far better choice—for instance, whole oranges with their abundance of goodness. If you eat the fruit, you get the pleasure and "full" feeling of a chewable food, and you also get the filling benefit of fiber.

1 glass (12 fl oz)
unsweetened orange juice
160 calories

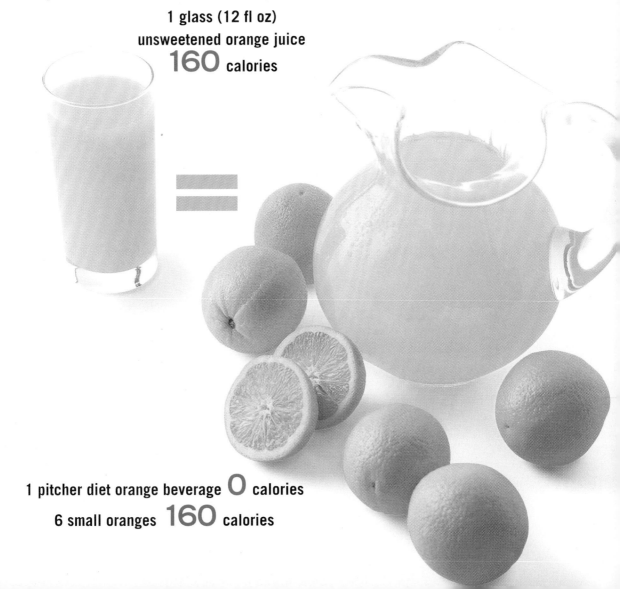

1 pitcher diet orange beverage O calories
6 small oranges 160 calories

Ice Cream in the Freezer

If you're accustomed to keeping some light ice cream in your freezer, you might want to study the picture below. One pint, which a lot of people can consume in one sitting, has as many calories as 32 low-cal Creamsicles. Put another way, if you had one of these Creamsicles every day for an entire month, you'd just about consume the same number of calories found in that single pint of ice cream.

1 pint light ice cream 800 calories

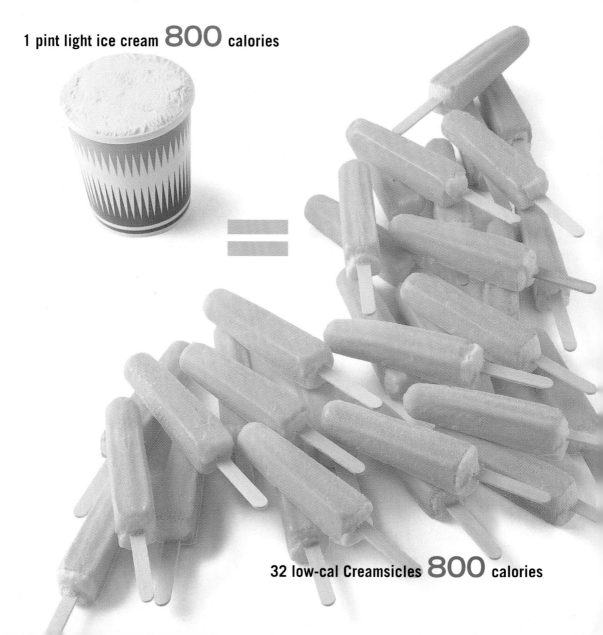

32 low-cal Creamsicles 800 calories

A Little Fruit

Want dessert? You'll pay 320 calories for a hint of the taste of apple in this small piece of apple crumb cake. But look at your choices. You can have the melon, mixed fruit, sorbet, and pastry taste of a biscotto for the same total calorie count. Plus, as soon as you dig into the real fruit, you're getting much more fiber and many more vitamins than the crumb cake can provide.

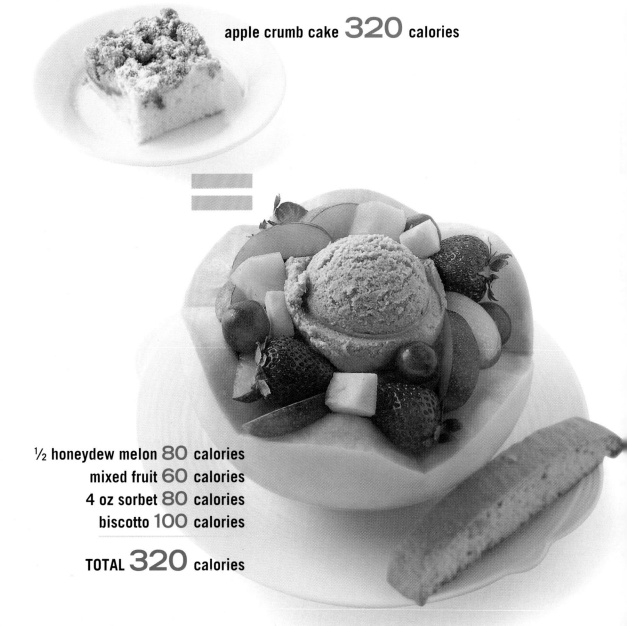

apple crumb cake 320 calories

½ honeydew melon 80 calories
mixed fruit 60 calories
4 oz sorbet 80 calories
biscotto 100 calories

TOTAL 320 calories

Plate Tectonics

It's lovely to precede a meal with a little something up front. But what will it be: three bites, or a bite for three people? Before you decide, consider what you're seeing on this page.

Yes, you can have two small bites of cheese and a sliver of pâté. But that doesn't go a long way. Instead, how about a platter of food that has a whole range of tastes—salty, smooth, pungent, and oily? The full platter that you see on the right will last quite a while—and might feed a few. As you can see, that platter of food has the same calorie count as the three-bite plate of cheese and pâté.

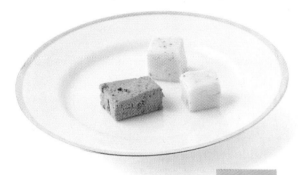

1½ oz cheese 170 calories
1 oz pâté 120 calories

TOTAL 290 calories

2 oz smoked sable 80 calories
3 blini 90 calories
1 oz caviar 90 calories
1 Tbsp sour cream 30 calories

TOTAL 290 calories

Dig In . . .

Help yourself to this heaping platter of vegetable pepperoni or this generous serving of shrimp. But before you reach for regular meat pepperoni, recall what you're seeing here.

Either the vegetable pepperoni or the shrimp has the caloric equivalent of one minute portion of regular meat pepperoni. But there's even more to be said for the vegetable pepperoni and the shrimp, because both add nutrition benefits that you don't get from regular pepperoni.

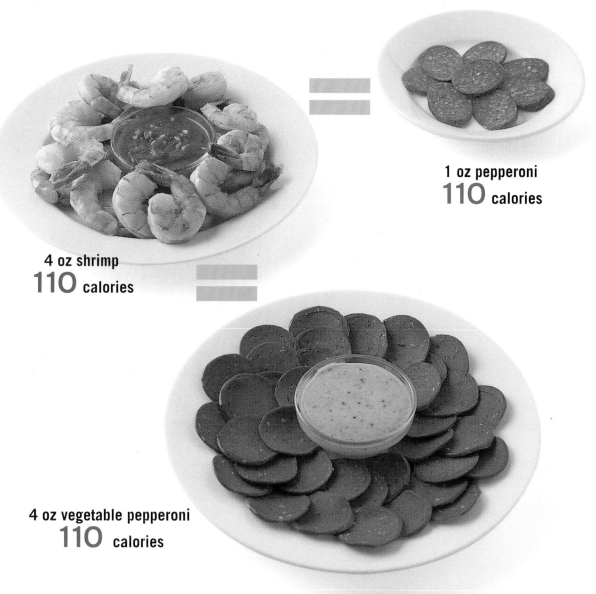

1 oz pepperoni
110 calories

4 oz shrimp
110 calories

4 oz vegetable pepperoni
110 calories

Equal Calories, Different Portions

Bites and Bowls

Each of these single bites of food is the caloric equivalent of the bowl of soup next to it.
Honest. And in each case, the bowl of soup offers a treasury of nutrition.

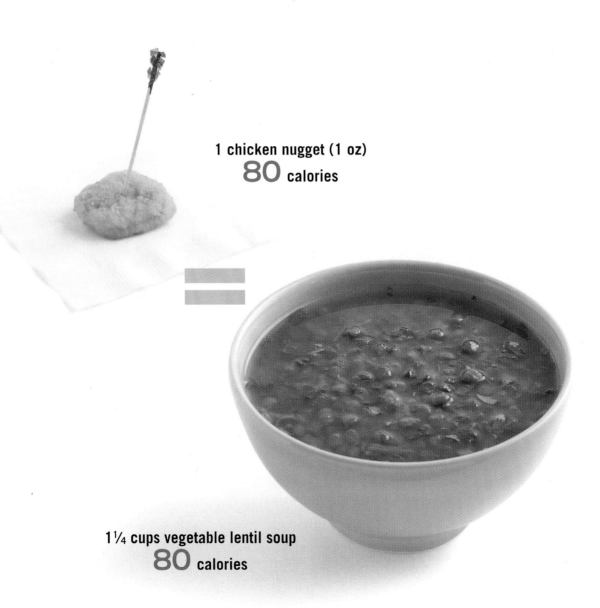

1 chicken nugget (1 oz)
80 calories

1¼ cups vegetable lentil soup
80 calories

1 ¼ cups black bean soup
100 calories

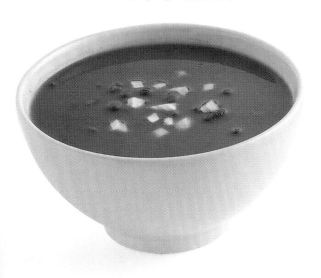

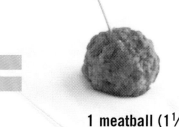

1 meatball (1 ¼ oz)
100 calories

¾ oz Cheddar cheese
90 calories

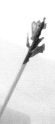

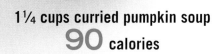

1 ¼ cups curried pumpkin soup
90 calories

An Apple a Day

If you're getting your apple intake in pie, it's costing you about 480 calories a wedge, the caloric equivalent of five baked apples. So before you make an apple pie—or buy one—consider what this picture is telling you.

1 wedge apple pie 480 calories

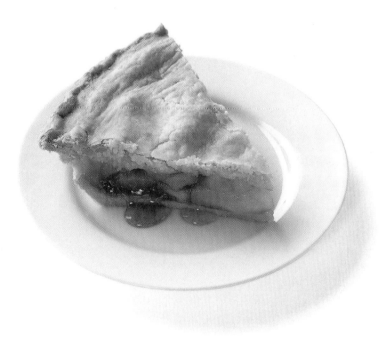
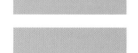

Equal Calories, Different Portions

5 baked apples (made with cinnamon, ginger, and low-calorie sweetener) 480 calories

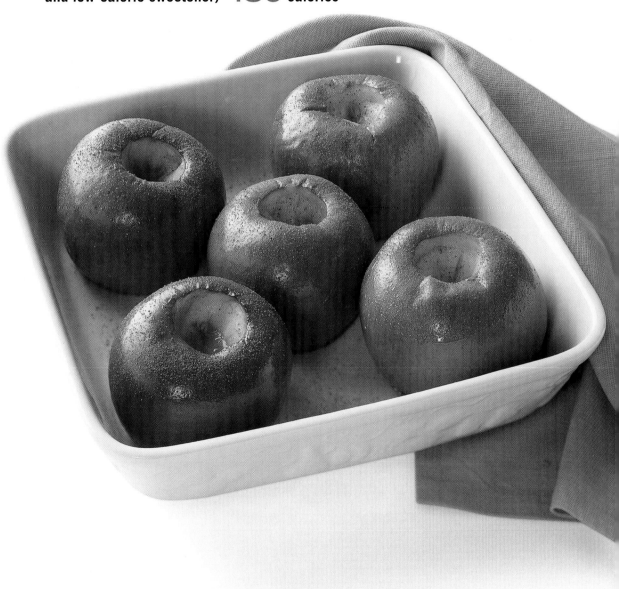

The Pastry Difference

Fruit tarts seem innocuous compared to desserts like cheesecake or chocolate layer cake. But if that's your view, it might be time for a tart reassessment.

If the images below tell you one thing, it's that you can eat a whole lot of raspberries for the same calorie cost as one little tart.

In fact, that fruit tart is made with a pastry that's so high in fat and sugar that it takes 8 cups of fresh raspberries with whipped topping to equal a single raspberry tart. If you want the tart, by all means have it—but not because it's a low-calorie dessert. For a low-calorie raspberry taste, feast on raspberries—the real thing!

1 raspberry tart 440 calories

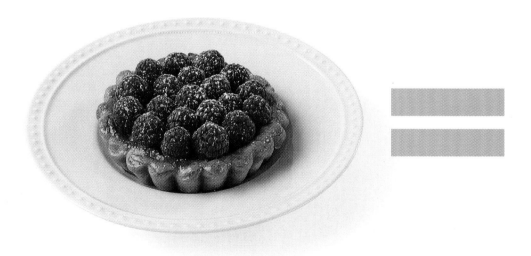

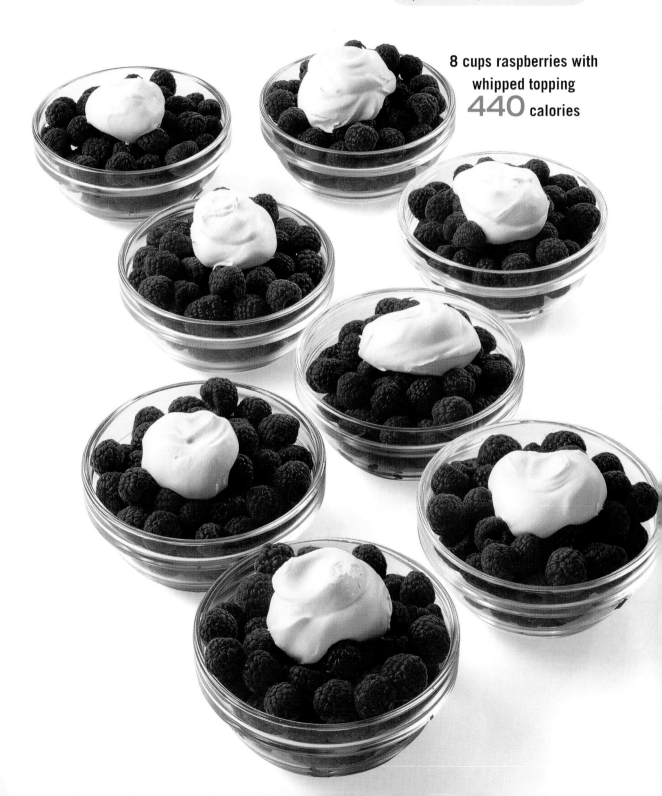

8 cups raspberries with whipped topping
440 calories

Equal Calories, Different Portions

Good Bread

Do you like bread? If so, you might want to spend a short time contemplating the pictures below. And remember what you see.

Each of these units of bread items has 530 calories. As you can see, that means one corn muffin has as many calories as 13 slices of light oatmeal bread. And it has just as many calories as five dinner rolls. Take your choice. But don't forget this visual advice on how to get the most bread for the fewest calories.

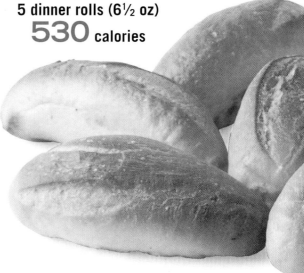

5 dinner rolls (6½ oz)
530 calories

OR

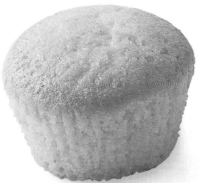

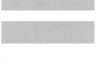

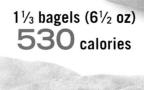

1 corn muffin (6 oz)
530 calories

1⅓ bagels (6½ oz)
530 calories

Equal Calories, Different Portions

13 slices light oatmeal bread
530 calories

OR

4 English muffins
530 calories

OR

4 pitas 530 calories

OR

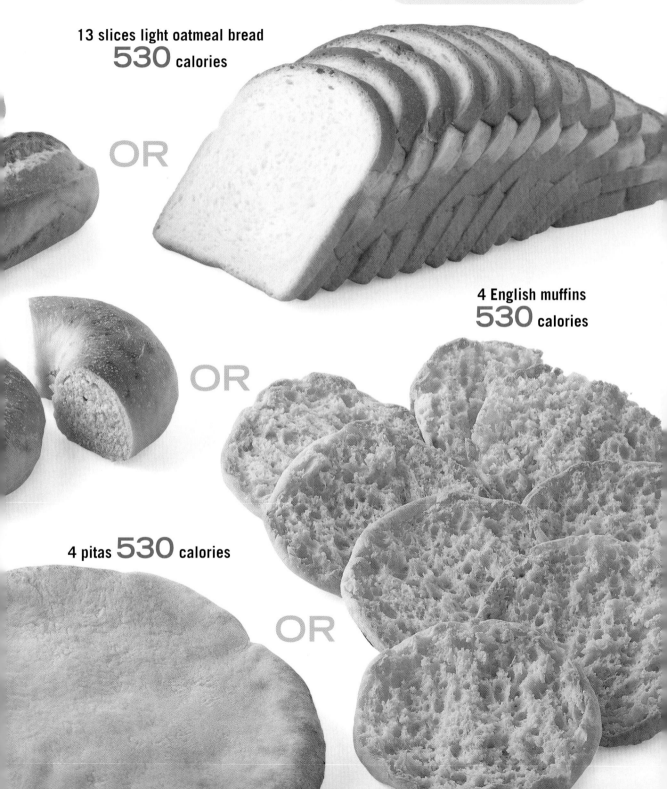

Cookie Monster

Love cookies? How much? The dessert bonanza pictured here—totaling up every last bite of fruit, frozen yogurt, and candy—has the same number of calories as this single, lonely black-and-white cookie. And the fruit provides nutritional benefits, too.

1 black-and-white cookie (4½ oz) 640 calories

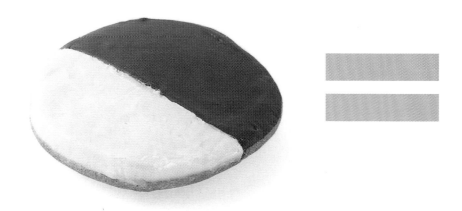

Equal Calories, Different Portions

2 frozen yogurt cones 200 calories
large plate of fruit 200 calories
6 hard candies 120 calories
8 chocolate mint sticks 120 calories

TOTAL 640 calories

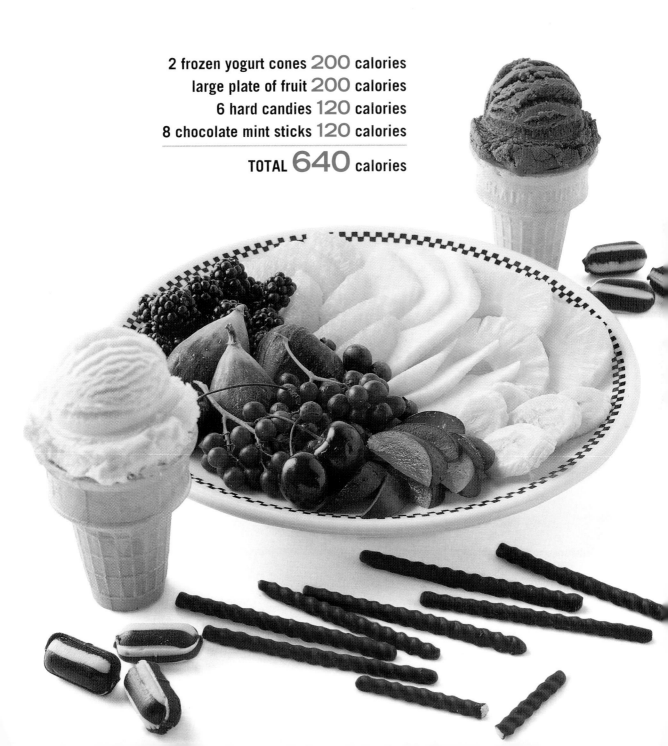

Well-Fed

Scones have become pervasively popular breakfast treats. But did you ever consider their breakfast calories?

The pictures below tell the story—and it's not one you're likely to forget. A scone is no bargain. At 700 calories, the single scone you see here is the caloric equivalent of everything else in the photo. So your trade-off is one scone or . . . an English muffin spread with jam, a dish of cherries, a bowl of corn flakes with banana, two slices of light toast with marmalade, the stem dish filled with sliced orange and pineapple, and a bowl of oatmeal with sliced peaches.

You decide. But if you need help deciding, don't forget the picture you see here.

1 scone (7¾ oz) 700 calories

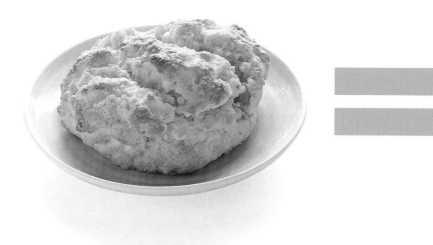

1½ oz (dry weight) oatmeal with peaches 170 calories
English muffin with jam 150 calories
cherries 80 calories
corn flakes with banana 160 calories
2 slices light toast with marmalade 100 calories
orange and pineapple 40 calories

TOTAL 700 calories

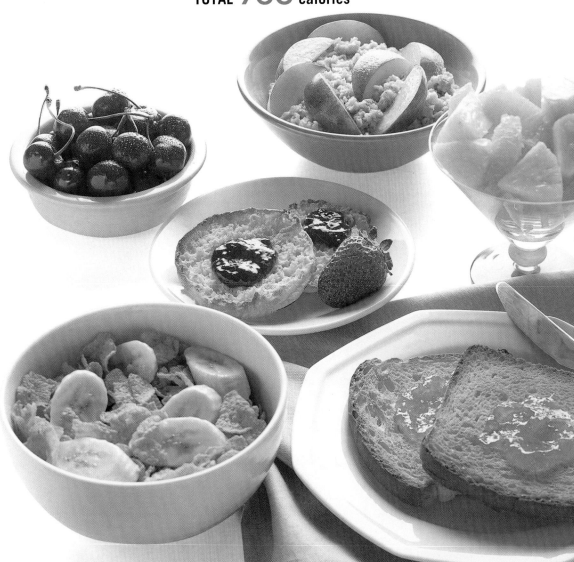

Fruit or Fruit Candy?

Consider what the photos on this page are telling you. Each of the fruits shown here has the calorie equivalent of the very small handful of low-fat candies beside it. But that's the only way the fruit and candy are anywhere near equivalent.

Keep in mind that the candies go down in a split second. But these portions of fruit can last a long time. The candies offer nothing in the way of nutrients. But each of these fruits is a treasure chest of vitamins, minerals, and fiber. And where the candies have many artificial flavorings that strive to give you fruit taste, at best it's only an imitation. The pineapple and melons are the real thing.

That's a lot to remember. But you won't have to, if you just allow these pictures to leave a lasting impression.

2 oz gummy bears 200 calories

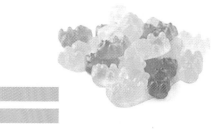

1 pineapple (2 lb) 200 calories

Equal Calories, Different Portions

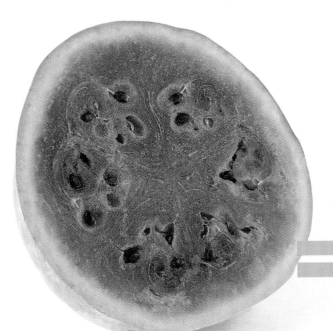

½ watermelon (4 lb)
200 calories

2 oz fruit slice candy
200 calories

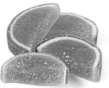

2 oz jelly beans
200 calories

1 canary melon (3 lb)
200 calories

Starch Binge

When you really crave starch—but want to keep calories in mind—choose carefully. There are lots of options including fresh corn, potatoes, and various kinds of bread. But calorie counts vary incredibly.

Actually, there's not a whole lot you have to remember. Just the picture you see here.

The single square of corn bread with butter goes for 820 calories. Want some other choices instead? Look at all the items pictured on the right. Their total calorie count is the same. So the trade-off is this: that square of corn bread with butter *or* two ears of corn on the cob, a roll with jam, a baked potato topped with salsa, a sweet potato, and two slices of raisin bread. It adds up: on your right, a binge; on the left, a bite.

1 square of corn bread (7 oz) 700 calories
1 Tbsp butter 120 calories

TOTAL 820 calories

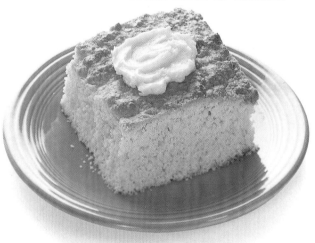

Equal Calories, Different Portions

2 ears of corn on the cob 170 calories
roll with jam 200 calories
baked potato with salsa 150 calories
sweet potato 160 calories
2 slices raisin bread 140 calories

TOTAL 820 calories

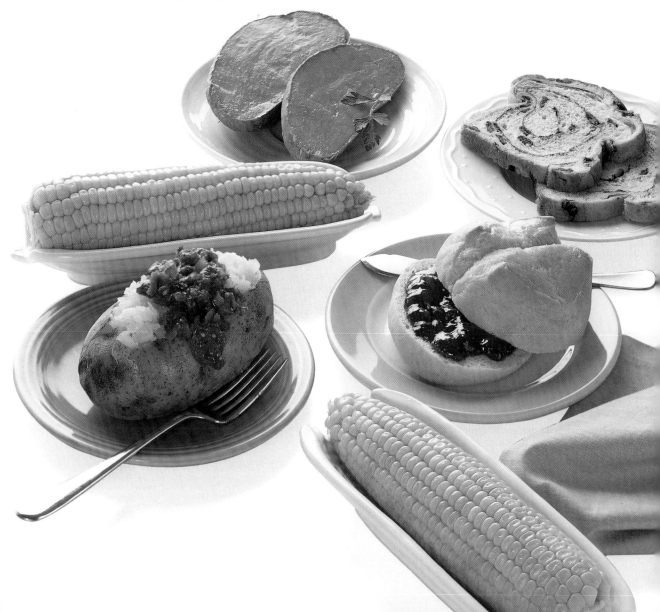

Pop Goes the Corn

Here's a mental image that will probably stick—*all* that popcorn, compared to those meager portions of nuts, chips, or vegetable crisps.

How high in calories could a tiny handful of mixed nuts be? Or even a few potato chips? And vegetable crisps, especially a number as small as pictured here, are surely a good bet for weight loss.

Think again. Ten whole cups of popcorn are equivalent to one handful of the nuts, chips, or vegetable crisps.

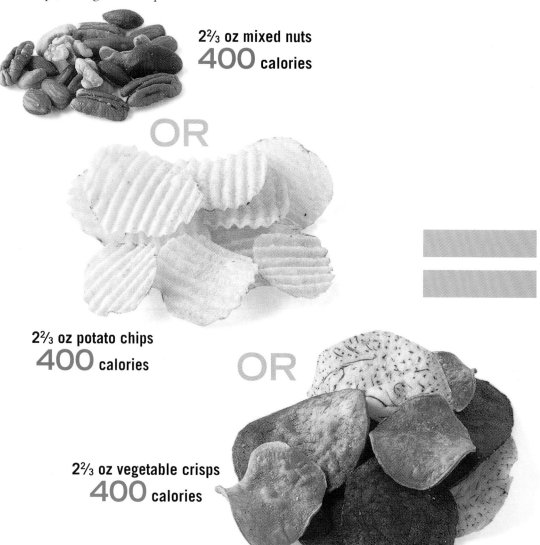

2⅔ oz mixed nuts
400 calories

OR

2⅔ oz potato chips
400 calories

OR

2⅔ oz vegetable crisps
400 calories

10 cups popcorn
400 calories

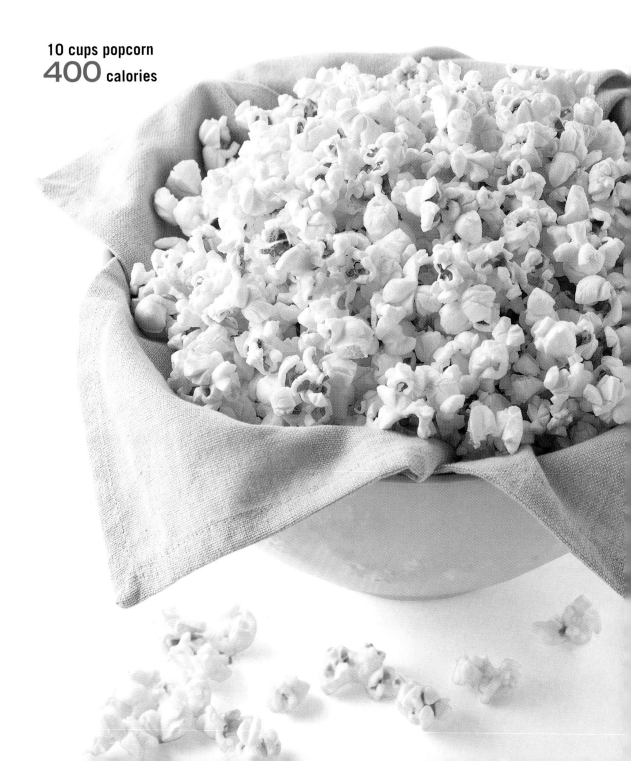

Steaked Out

High in saturated fat and cholesterol, this 8-ounce steak costs 600 calories. The plate of vegetarian Italian sausages with bell peppers totals the same number of calories—but look at how much you could eat! Those sausages could feed a family of five, plus its soy protein is a healthy choice.

1 steak (8 oz) 600 calories

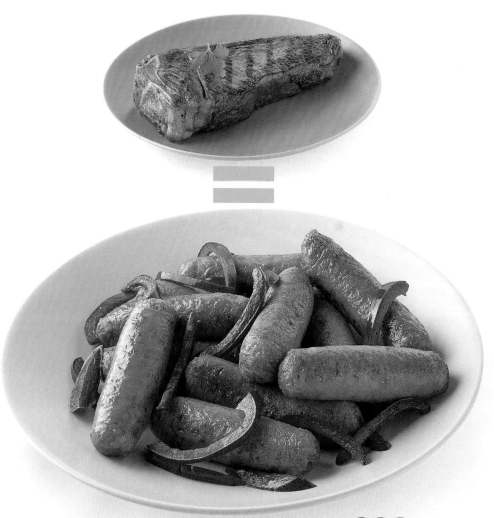

10 vegetarian Italian sausages with bell peppers 600 calories

Summer Treat

There's nothing like an iced coffee on a hot summer's day. The two drinks shown below may appear to be the same, but check out their calorie counts. A large latte—even with skim milk and no sugar—costs 180 calories. On the other hand, an iced hazelnut coffee with a small amount of milk and low-calorie sweetener has a mere 30 calories.

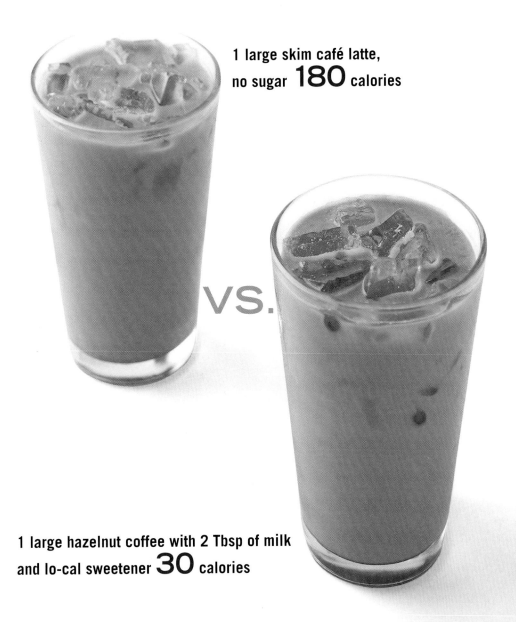

1 large skim café latte, no sugar 180 calories

VS.

1 large hazelnut coffee with 2 Tbsp of milk and lo-cal sweetener 30 calories

Sandwich Sweepstakes

The calorie count of a sandwich can be small or large, depending entirely on the ingredients. The turkey and mayo on rye weighs in at 740 calories. Compare that to the turkey/lettuce/tomato with mustard on rye, and you'll see that you'll get fewer than half the calories.

But there's another option, as you can see—the veggie salami on light rye with lots of trimmings. That one will cost a mere 190 calories.

Turkey and mayo on rye
8 oz turkey **400** calories
2 Tbsp mayonnaise **200** calories
2 slices rye bread **140** calories

TOTAL **740** calories

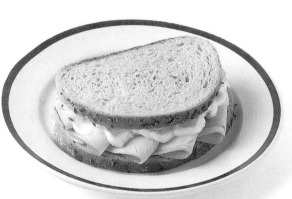

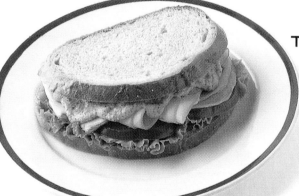

Turkey/lettuce/tomato with mustard on rye
3 oz turkey **150** calories
lettuce and tomato **10** calories
mustard **10** calories
2 slices rye bread **140** calories

TOTAL **310** calories

Veggie salami on light rye
3 oz veggie salami **70** calories
lettuce and tomato **10** calories
mustard **10** calories
2 slices light rye bread **100** calories

TOTAL **190** calories

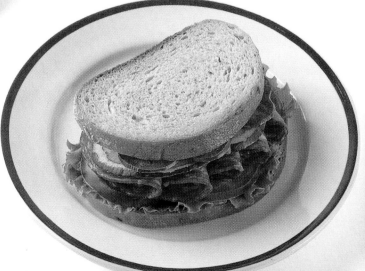

Bowled Over

Two bowls, two cereals, equal portions. Most weight-conscious adults probably assume the Grape-Nuts are a better choice for nutrition, while the Cheerios are what kids eat. If that's the case, kids are getting more nutrition with far fewer calories.

The next time you have a choice between cereals, you might want to recall the mini-lesson below. Sure, these bowls *look* like they hold the same amount of cereal. But in terms of calories, the Grape-Nuts are about four times as calorie-laden. A bowl of Grape-Nuts, one of the densest cereals around, costs 600 calories, compared to the Cheerios' 165!

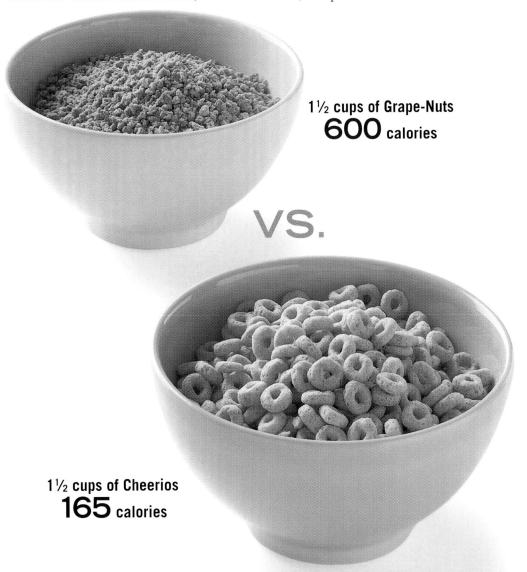

1½ cups of Grape-Nuts
600 calories

VS.

1½ cups of Cheerios
165 calories

Seven Cups

The variety in salad bars can be confusing as well as fun. All of these salads are widely available, but look at the differences in their calorie counts.

Next time you find yourself at your favorite salad bar, keep these pictures—and numbers—in mind.

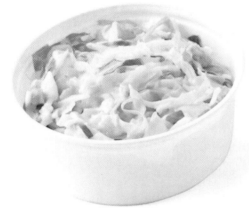

coleslaw (1 cup)
150 calories

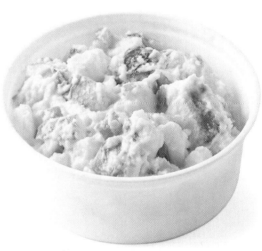

potato salad (1 cup)
300 calories

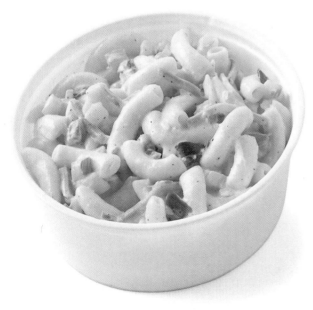

pasta salad (1 cup)
400 calories

Equal Portions, Different Calories

three-bean salad (1 cup)
180 calories

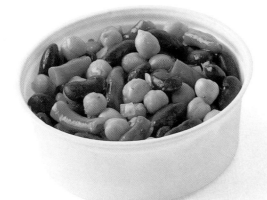

tuna salad (1 cup)
420 calories

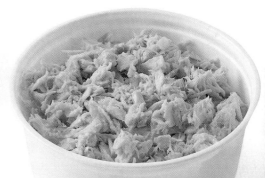

chicken salad (1 cup)
520 calories

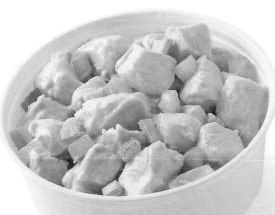

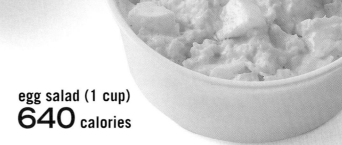

egg salad (1 cup)
640 calories

Skewed Skewers

A traditional skewer of lamb kabobs weighs in at 560 calories. But look at the photos below. Here's a tempting trade-off you're not likely to forget. For about one-fourth the calories, you can skewer the same amount of food in the form of scallops and mushrooms marinated in black bean sauce.

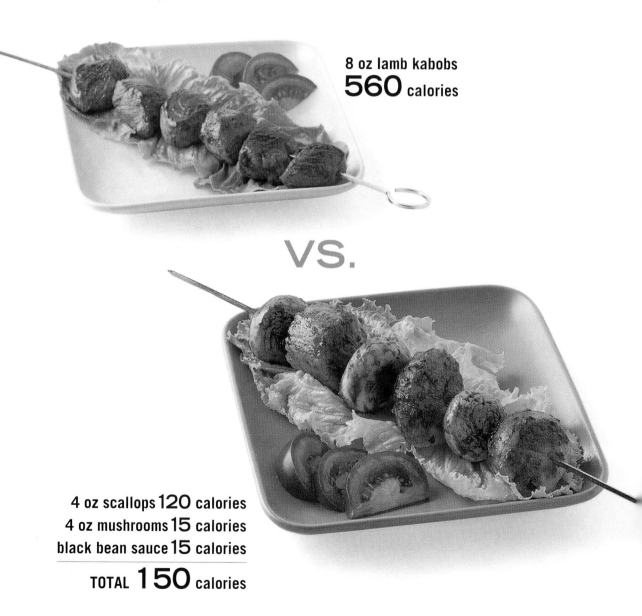

8 oz lamb kabobs
560 calories

VS.

4 oz scallops 120 calories
4 oz mushrooms 15 calories
black bean sauce 15 calories

TOTAL 150 calories

Buy by Weight

These three separate servings all weigh the same. So what's your best choice if you measure your selections in terms of calories?

The best caloric choice is the dried fruit, but not bananas (which are fried) and pineapple (which is sugar-coated). A dried fruit mix that includes pears, apricots, peaches, and prunes has the fewest calories for the weight. It also offers the most nutritional benefits. And its fiber-rich chewiness means it takes longer to eat, too.

6 oz pretzel nuggets
720 calories

6 oz banana chips and
dried sweetened pineapple
720 calories

6 oz assorted dried fruit
420 calories

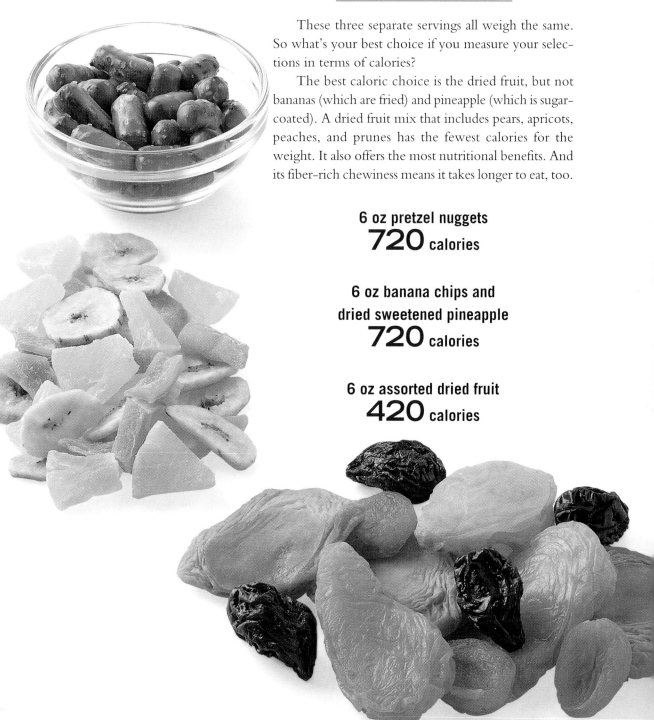

Fish Story

Sure, tuna is good for you. And it can be a real caloric bargain, too. But you may not realize that the benefits you get from tuna depend on how it's served.

The tuna melt on rye toast is calorically costly—a whopping 1,040 calories, in fact. If you have tuna on a sandwich roll, on the other hand, you'll be consuming about half that calorie count. You can lighten the sandwich even further by having light or nonfat mayo and light bread.

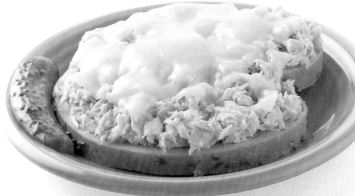

Tuna melt on rye toast
2 slices rye bread **140** calories
8 oz tuna **280** calories
3 Tbsp mayonnaise **300** calories
3 oz Swiss cheese **320** calories

TOTAL **1,040** calories

VS.

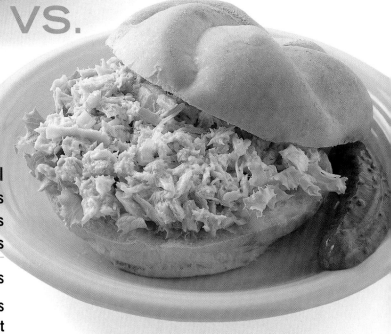

Tuna on a roll
roll **150** calories
6 oz tuna **210** calories
2 Tbsp mayonnaise **200** calories

TOTAL **560** calories

with light mayonnaise **460** calories
with nonfat mayonnaise on light
bread (not pictured) **310** calories

Deception in Glass Dishes

Can you guess which of these seemingly "nutritionally correct" sweet snacks is the best calorie buy? Before you actually go out and buy these snacks, don't forget the numbers you see here.

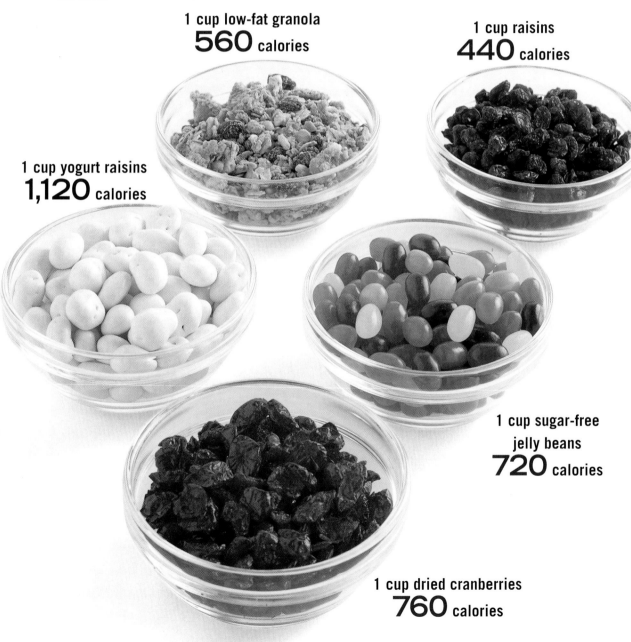

1 cup low-fat granola
560 calories

1 cup raisins
440 calories

1 cup yogurt raisins
1,120 calories

1 cup sugar-free jelly beans
720 calories

1 cup dried cranberries
760 calories

Playing the Pizza Wheel

No, pizza isn't roulette. But there are low-calorie bets as well as high-calorie ones on the pizza wheel pictured here. Traditional cheese pizza, not to mention cheese and pepperoni, hold no surprises: They're high in calories. Vegetable pizza, on the other hand, is a calorie bargain, as is a slice with tomato sauce and 12 pieces of vegetable pepperoni. Add the nutritional power of these two pizza slices, and the bargain gets even better.

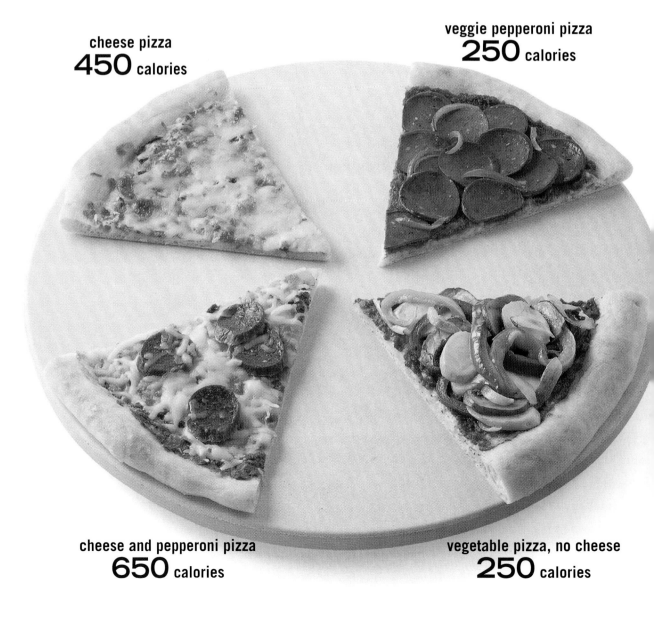

cheese pizza
450 calories

veggie pepperoni pizza
250 calories

cheese and pepperoni pizza
650 calories

vegetable pizza, no cheese
250 calories

Poppy Seed Poker

Poppy seed bagel: 400 calories. Poppy seed kaiser roll: 200 calories. The kaiser roll is twice as big but half as dense.

The moral? Next time you want bread, think about these tell-all images. You just might choose the kaiser roll—if you're thinking big.

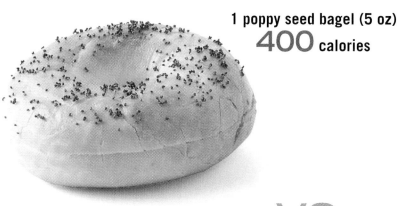

1 poppy seed bagel (5 oz)
400 calories

VS.

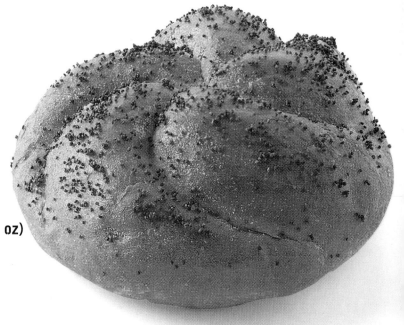

1 poppy seed roll (2½ oz)
200 calories

Parlay Pizza

A couple slices of pizza?

Well, maybe that's all you need.

But next time you order the second slice, you may want to conjure up the image of the many other foods you see here. Instead of two slices, you might prefer just one slice of pizza along with a bowl of minestrone soup and a big serving of salad. In short, you'll get fewer calories from a three-course meal with nearly a full day's supply of vitamins, minerals, and fiber.

More for less is always a good bargain, especially when you can get more food and more nourishment while getting one-third fewer calories.

2 slices cheese pizza 900 calories

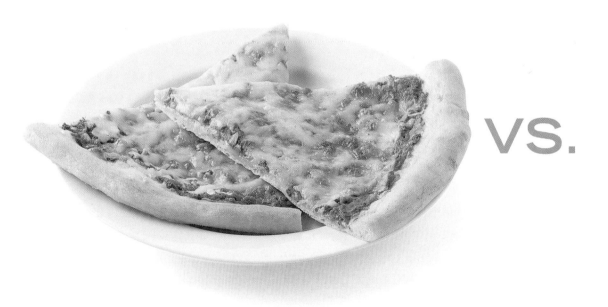

VS.

More for Less

1½ cups minestrone 110 calories
1 slice cheese pizza 450 calories
salad with artichoke hearts and tomatoes 40 calories

TOTAL 600 calories

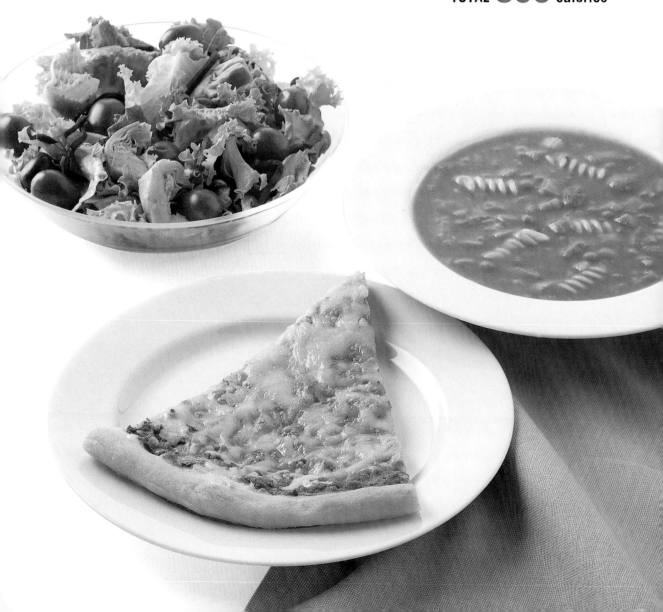

Salad Swap

Here are a couple of standard salad bar choices, but what a difference in size and calorie count! The small chicken Caesar salad has nearly twice the calories as the large gathering of vegetables, crabmeat salad, tofu, and a wheat roll. Next time you think about a Caesar salad, think about your alternatives, too.

Small chicken Caesar salad

romaine lettuce 10 calories
4 oz white-meat chicken 180 calories
3 Tbsp Caesar dressing 240 calories
1 oz croutons 130 calories

TOTAL 560 calories

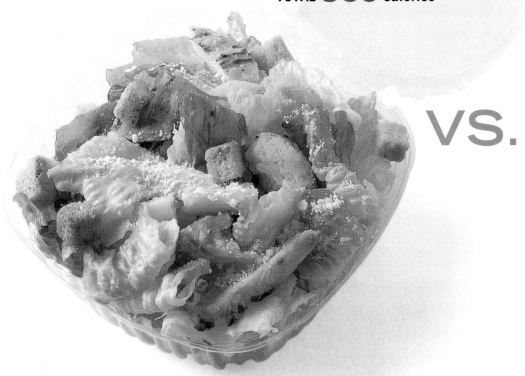

VS.

Large vegetable and crabmeat salad

1 quart mushrooms, red and yellow bell peppers, beets, artichokes, etc. 80 calories

½ cup crabmeat salad 120 calories

1 wedge stuffed tofu 30 calories

1 wheat roll (1 oz) 80 calories

TOTAL 310 calories

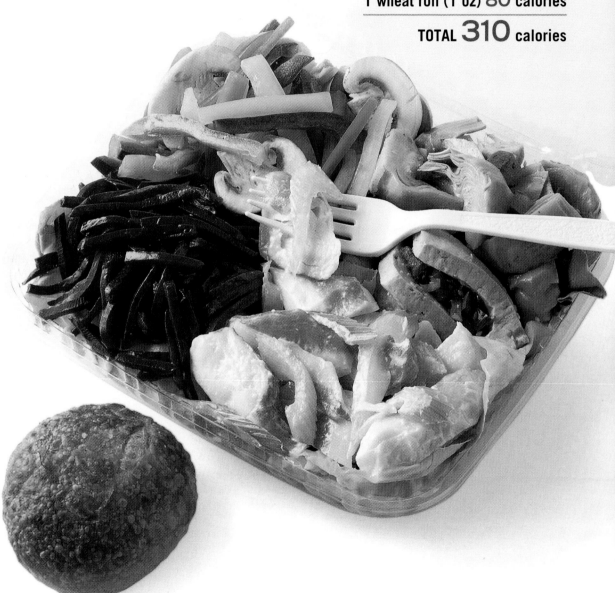

My Hero

Grab the hero sandwich on the left, and you're wolfing down 920 calories with those sausages and peppers. Consider the take-out items on the right: both overstuffed baked potatoes plus the two pints of soup. All together, they don't even come close to the calorie count of the sandwich.

Next time, before you choose your hero, think about the choices you see here.

Sausage and pepper hero
roll (4 oz) 320 calories
1 sausage (6 oz) 540 calories
sautéed bell peppers and onions 60 calories

TOTAL 920 calories

VS.

Potatoes and soups

1 pint tomato soup 120 calories
potato with broccoli and salsa 180 calories
1 pint vegetable soup 130 calories
potato with ½ cup vegetarian chili 240 calories

TOTAL 670 calories

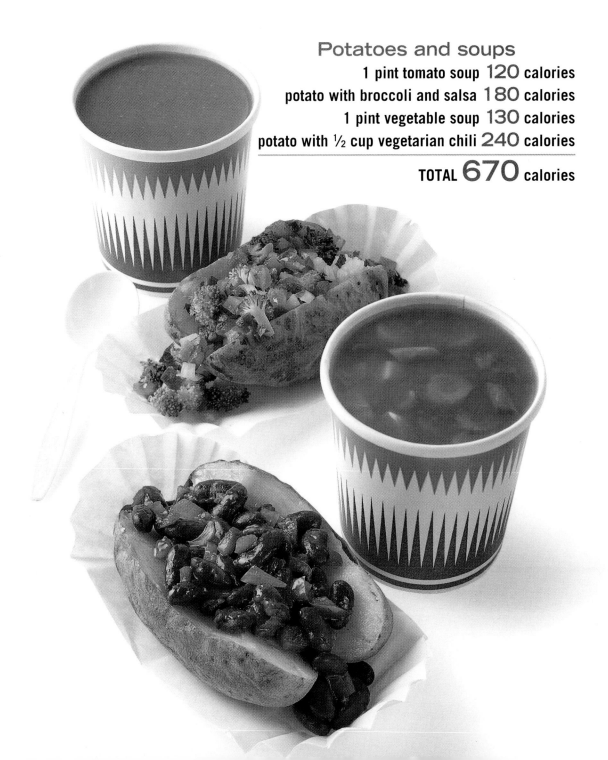

Not Enough Food on Your Plate

Who could feel deprived eating the platter on the right, with its range of well-seasoned vegetables and its plentiful helping of tomato sauce? True, the platter that's loaded with vegetables includes only 1 cup of pasta. But before you say, "I want more," consider all the other mouth-watering food that's shown in the meal at right—and then consider your choices.

3 cups pasta and tomato sauce 600 calories
zucchini 30 calories

TOTAL 630 calories

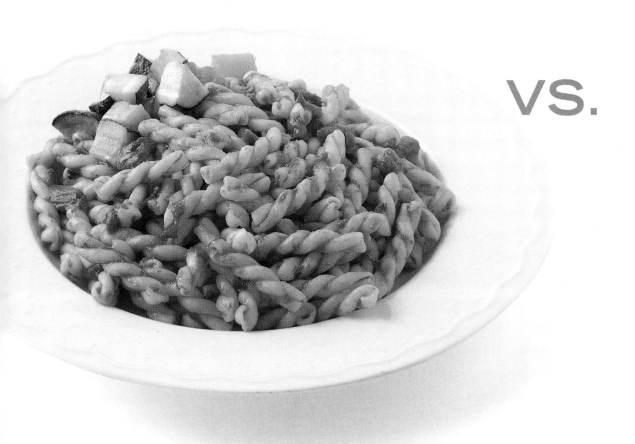

VS.

1 cup pasta and tomato sauce 200 calories
1½ cups zucchini and eggplant 60 calories
acorn squash and mixed bell peppers 60 calories
portobello mushroom 20 calories
additional tomato sauce for vegetables 30 calories

TOTAL 370 calories

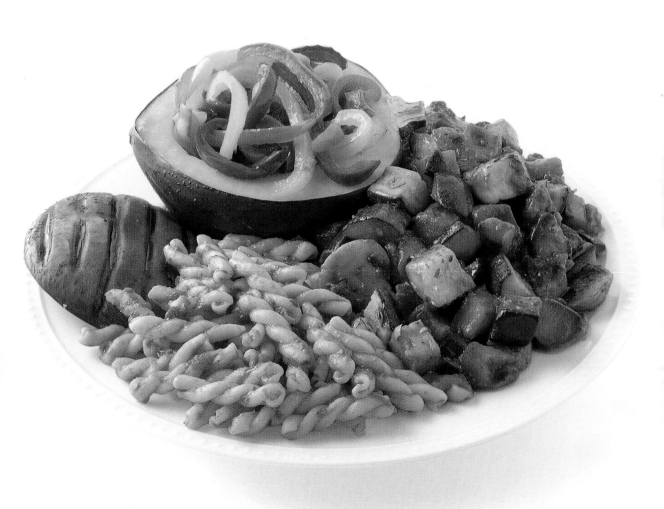

Cocktails or Dinner

Care for a drink before dinner? And perhaps a peanut or two while you're sipping? Picture this: The snack on the left contains far more calories than the full meal on the right. Have the soup, scallops, vegetables, salad, roll, and dessert, and you still won't match the drink and nuts. Add a glass of wine to your meal, and the calorie count is still 250 calories less.

Drink and nuts
2½ fl oz vodka **300** calories
½ cup mixed nuts **440** calories

TOTAL **740** calories

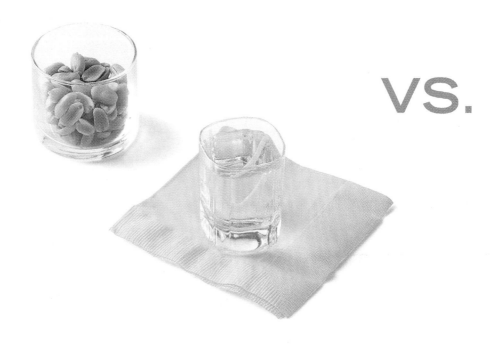

VS.

More for Less

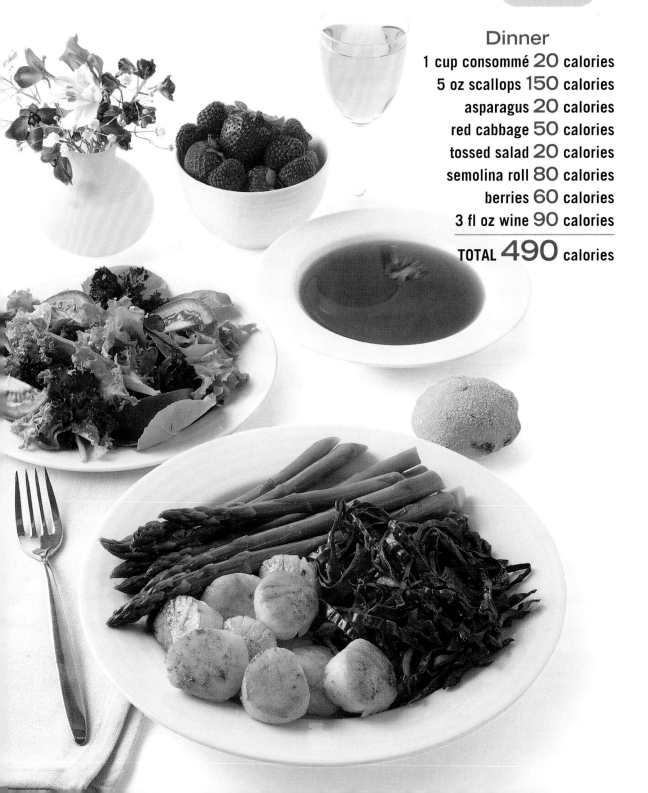

Dinner

1 cup consommé	20 calories
5 oz scallops	150 calories
asparagus	20 calories
red cabbage	50 calories
tossed salad	20 calories
semolina roll	80 calories
berries	60 calories
3 fl oz wine	90 calories
TOTAL	**490** calories

A Whole New Burger Ball Game?

What would happen if you tampered with the classic American burger? One result could be a dramatic savings in calorie count, not to mention a substantial uptick in health benefits. Here's how an all-vegetable Boca burger—with a whole lot of fixings—compares to the classic American hamburger. Check it out:

1 hamburger (6 oz) 480 calories
bun 110 calories
fixings 10 calories
TOTAL 600 calories

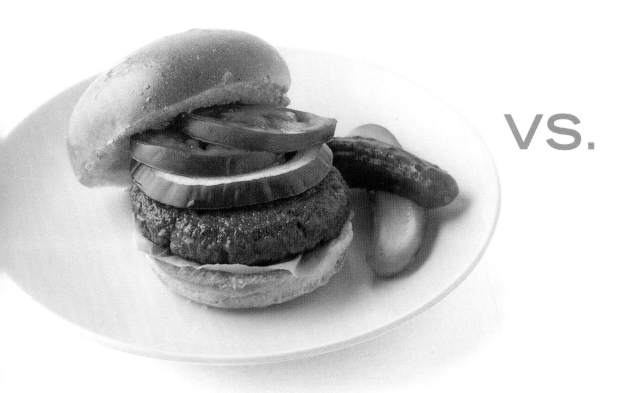

VS.

1 Boca burger (vegetarian) 85 calories
bun 110 calories
fixings 10 calories
2 portobello mushrooms 30 calories
2 slices eggplant 20 calories

TOTAL 255 calories

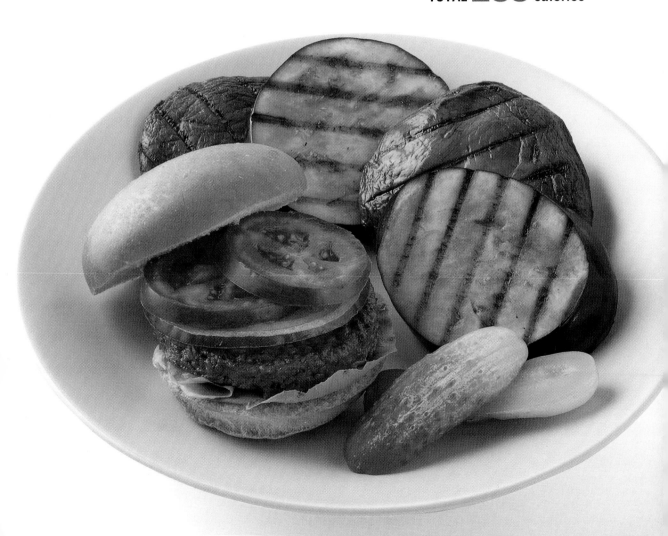

The Delicacy with a Diagnosis

Foie gras—literally, fatty liver—may be the only food that is actually a disease. Foie gras is produced by force-feeding ducks until their livers are abnormally enlarged about six times. That's why foie gras production has been outlawed for cruelty to animals in three countries and why legislation to that effect has been introduced in New York.

See for yourself: The health-destroying fat in a morsel of this "delicacy" is equivalent to seven packages of fast-food french fries and has the cholesterol equivalent of 20 tablespoons of pure lard.

So, even if it's a delicacy, cherished as far back as ancient Egypt and revered in haute cuisine circles, is this what you really want for an appetizer? Next time you reach for the foie gras, think of a very high number of calories in one tiny slice—450, to be exact.

1 slice foie gras (3½ oz)
240 milligrams of cholesterol
70 grams of fat

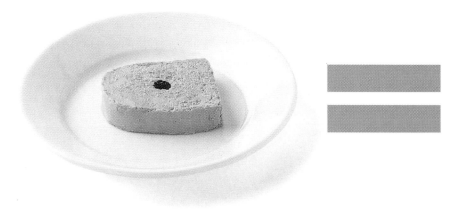

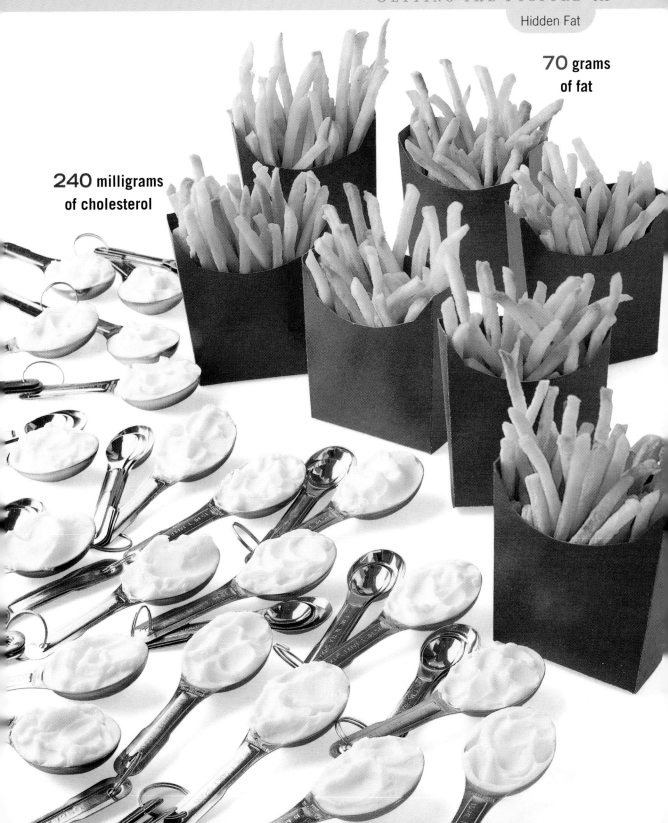

70 grams
of fat

240 milligrams
of cholesterol

Exploring the Hidden Fat

Of course, you always knew the foods in these pictures contained fat. But even with the most vivid imagination, could you really picture how much? Just contemplate the pats of butter next to each food item, and you'll find that these photos leave a lasting impression. Yes, those pats of butter represent the fat content in each food. A memorable sight?

Apple turnover (3 oz)

410 calories
24 grams of fat
216 calories from fat
5 pats of butter

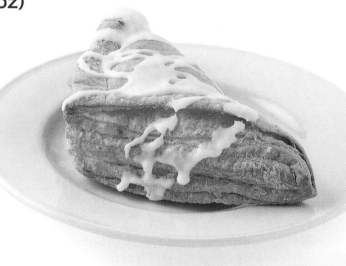

Semi-sweet chocolate (3 oz)

450 calories
27 grams of fat
243 calories from fat
5½ pats of butter

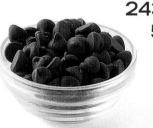
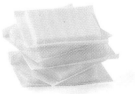

Cheddar cheese (3 oz)
340 calories
29 grams of fat
261 calories from fat
6 pats of butter

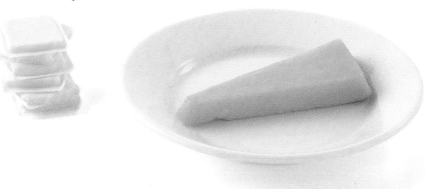

Super premium macadamia nut ice cream (1 cup)
720 calories
52 grams of fat
468 calories from fat
10 pats of butter

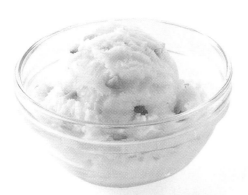
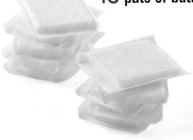

Little Caesar, Big Alternative

This small, compact serving of chicken Caesar salad looks like a dieter's delight, doesn't it? But put it up against all the food pictured on the right, and it falls short—by a lot of calories. So next time someone offers you a Caesar salad, think about your choices before you make a snap decision about that "diet special."

romaine lettuce 10 calories
4 oz white-meat chicken 180 calories
3 Tbsp Caesar dressing 240 calories
1 oz croutons 130 calories

TOTAL 560 calories

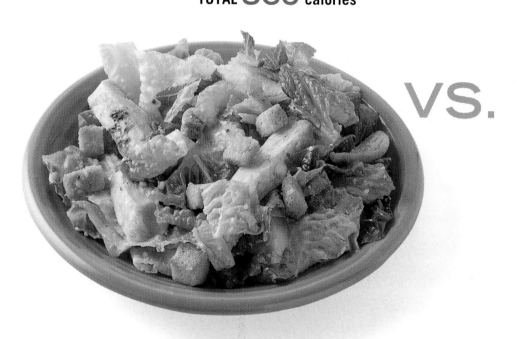

VS.

Looks like a Diet Meal

1⅓ cups black bean soup 120 calories
5-grain roll 100 calories
mixed salad 20 calories
1½ cups melon cubes 80 calories
5 fl oz sorbet 90 calories

TOTAL 410 calories

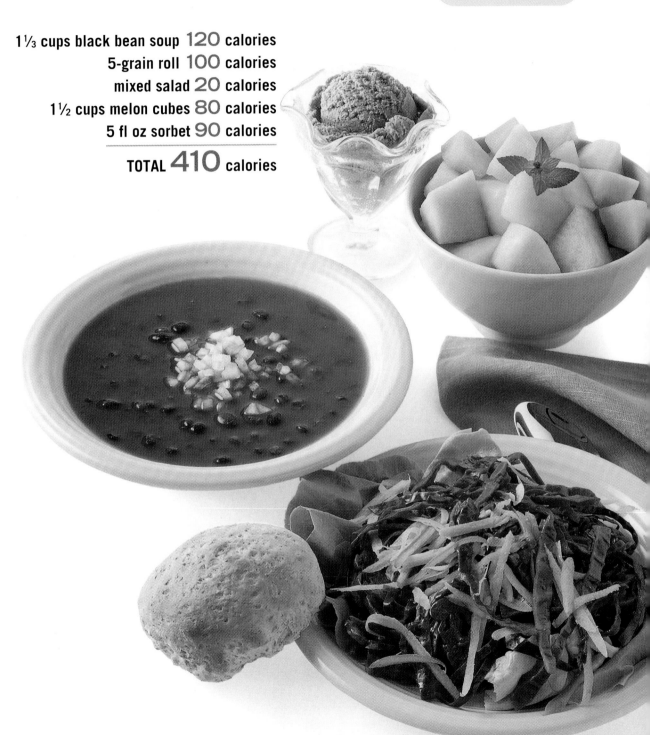

How Sweet It Is

One look at the butterscotch candies, and you may think you'll need to resist them with all the willpower at your command. These are forbidden foods, aren't they? Often, we think of candy as treats for children, not something for grown-ups interested in weight loss.

As for choosing between butterscotch candies and something as nutritious-looking as trail mix, you'd think, "No contest!" Isn't trail mix natural? Isn't it nutritious? Hence, it must be good for you. After all, trail mix is the power-up food that mountaineers and hikers consume to get them to the next peak.

For a little taste of Food Awareness Training, take a harder look. The candies are the caloric bargain: 32 of them are equivalent in calorie count to 4 ounces of trail mix. And while it will probably take a few fistfuls of trail mix to get you up the mountain, you can go for miles on just a few candies, as you keep each one in your mouth, enjoying the flavor for a long time. That's one reason hard candies are such a good snack where weight control is an issue.

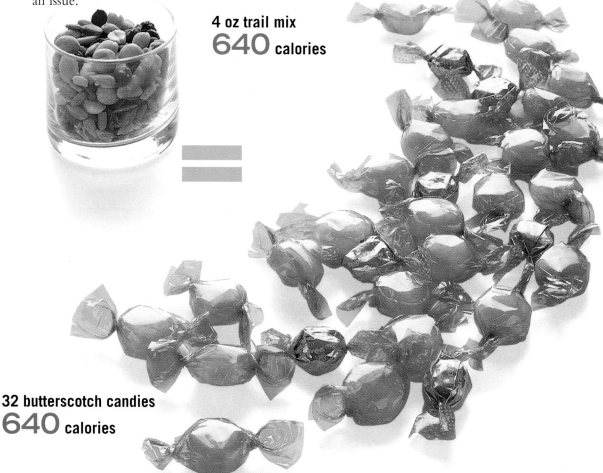

4 oz trail mix
640 calories

32 butterscotch candies
640 calories

Twisted Saboteurs

Think "yogurt" and you think "nutritionally correct," so a yogurt pretzel must be a better choice all-around than a plain old pretzel. You feel virtuous eating one. That reasoning, however, is as twisted as the yogurt pretzels. So look before you leap.

A yogurt pretzel has just as much fat and just as many calories as a chocolate-covered pretzel. From the minute portion you see here, you'll get 140 calories. Try two pretzel rods and a total of four plums—real foods, not saboteurs. In each serving of plums plus pretzel rods, you get the same number of calories as come from this small serving of yogurt pretzels.

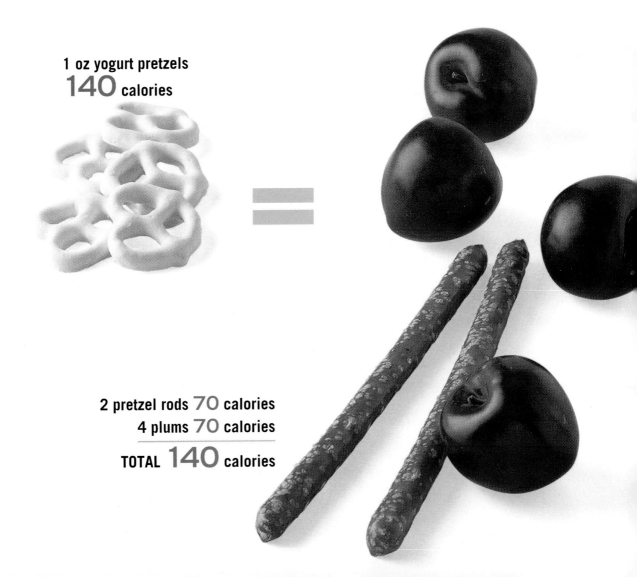

1 oz yogurt pretzels
140 calories

=

2 pretzel rods 70 calories
4 plums 70 calories
TOTAL 140 calories

Naturally Low-Calorie

If it says "natural" on the package, it must be a good choice for weight loss, right? Not necessarily. This cup of Quaker Natural cereal, for example, has as many calories as 16 low-cal frozen fudge bars. So before you automatically reach for the "natural" product with its high calories, you'll probably want to consider what's to the right of the equal sign.

1 cup Quaker Natural cereal 540 calories

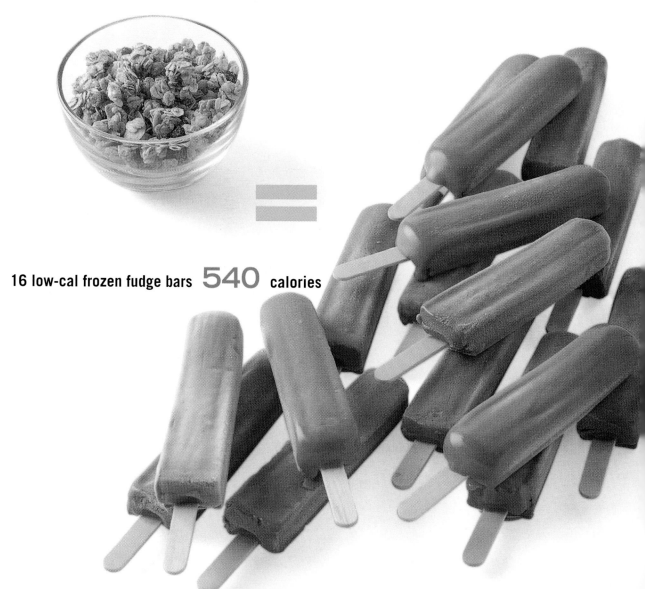

16 low-cal frozen fudge bars 540 calories

Devilishly Angelic

Angel food cake is fat-free and has a heavenly lightness that makes it seem virtually guilt-free as well. The result? We tend to eat a lot of it when it's around.

Now, looking at the photographs you see here, you might want to reconsider the wisdom of that choice. True, you could eat this small slice of angel food cake with just a bit of raspberry sauce. But for the same calorie count, perhaps you'd rather help yourself to a huge bowl of mixed berries with whipped topping!

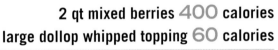

1 slice angel food cake (3 oz) 300 calories
⅓ cup raspberry sauce 160 calories

TOTAL 460 calories

=

2 qt mixed berries 400 calories
large dollop whipped topping 60 calories

TOTAL 460 calories

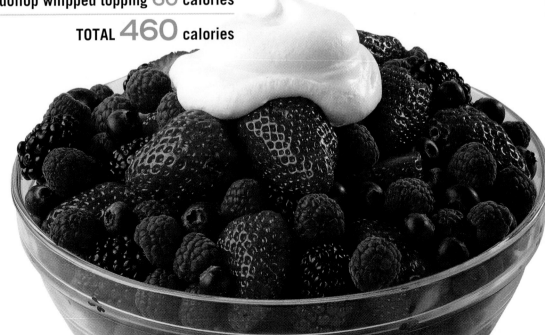

Wrong-Way and Right-Way Chocolate Binge

There's a wrong way and a right way to binge on chocolate.

For the wrong way, look at the meager portions of low-fat and low-sugar chocolate-ish snacks on this page. Each of them seems like a diet food. In fact, just taste any of them and you'll be *sure* you're dieting.

When it absolutely has to be chocolate, help yourself to a hefty portion of frozen yogurt, a chocolate shake made from a low-calorie mix, frozen fudge bars, a mug of hot cocoa, or classic Tootsie Pops or chocolate kisses. The chocolate feast on the opposite page is no calorie bargain, for sure—but still enough to satisfy the most committed chocoholic.

When it's chocolate you crave, eat chocolate—and enjoy it! Just keep in mind the picture lesson you see here: Those "diet" chocolates are really no bargain at all.

1 pack sugar-free chocolate caramels 360 calories
1 pack fructose-sweetened chocolate-covered raisins 540 calories
3 reduced-fat chocolate wafers 240 calories

TOTAL 1,140 calories

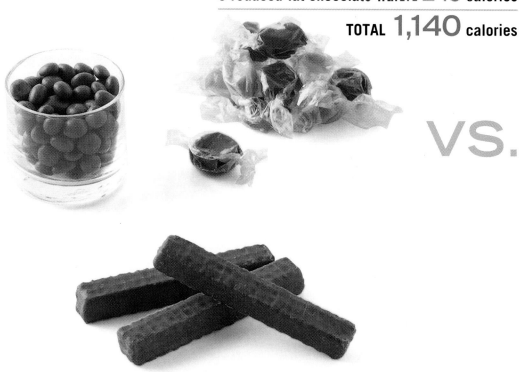

VS.

Saboteurs

12 oz chocolate frozen yogurt 240 calories
low-cal chocolate shake 70 calories
3 frozen fudge bars 90 calories
mug of low-cal hot cocoa 20 calories
2 chocolate Tootsie Pops 100 calories
3 Hershey's chocolate kisses 75 calories

TOTAL 595 calories

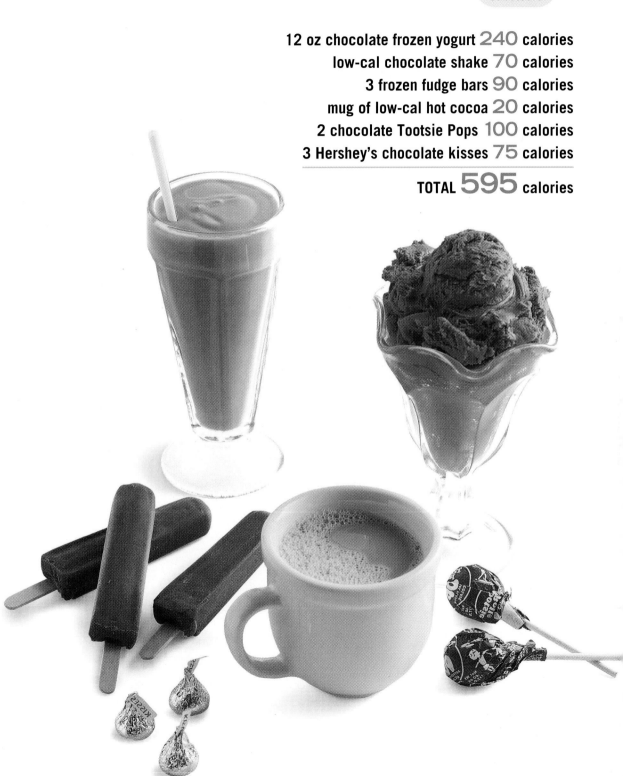

Looks Are Deceptive

Almost automatically, we see the 3 cups of bow-ties with cream sauce as being full of starch and fat. Don't you think it would be much better to have the pasta salad?

Maybe this page will change your impression.

The pasta salad shown here, for instance, has 3 cups of spinach-and-tomato pasta (vegetables are so good for us!). It's tossed with a quarter-cup of vinaigrette dressing. It looks cool, light, and healthy.

In fact, there's no calorie difference between the two dishes because the oil in the vinaigrette dressing brings the calorie count up to the level of the cream sauce. Each contains 920 calories. And, except for the lettuce leaf under the pasta salad, neither dish is a particular nutrition bargain. If pasta's what you want, have whatever pasta you like.

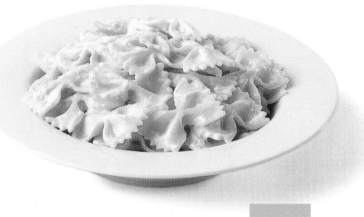

**3 cups pasta with
¼ cup creamy sauce
920 calories**

**3 cups spinach-and-
tomato pasta with
¼ cup vinaigrette dressing
920 calories**

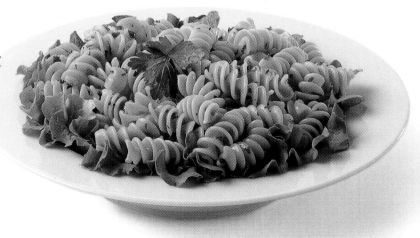

Eating on the Run

On the move? There are lots of food wagons that sell shish kebab, and you might be eager to have one. But before you settle on that choice, picture your alternatives—shown here. You can eat half a shish kebab—or, for the same calorie count, head for the baked-potato wagon and pile on the salsa and broccoli. And when you're done with that, you can have a container of cut-up melon as well.

½ shish kebab (3½ oz lamb) 280 calories

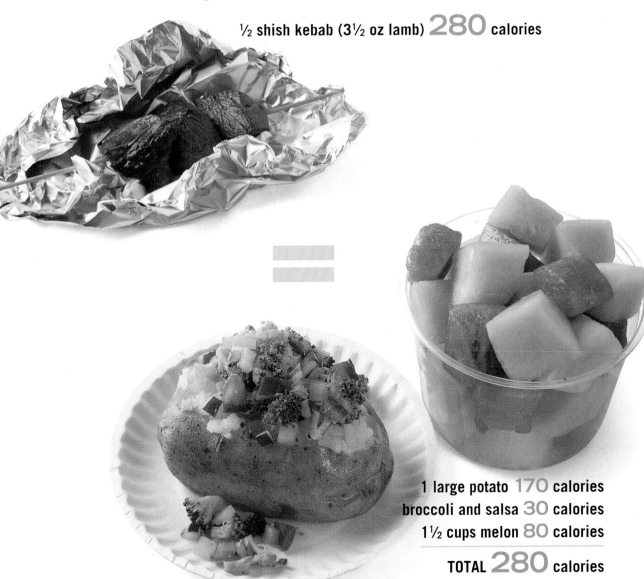

1 large potato 170 calories
broccoli and salsa 30 calories
1½ cups melon 80 calories

TOTAL 280 calories

New Yorker's Lunch

Uptown, downtown, New Yorkers are on the move—and eating as they go. Their city, however, offers them numerous choices in both taste and calorie count. You can have a hot dog on a bun with almost any style sauce. You might go for the classic potato knish for lunch. Or perhaps you want the increasingly popular soup-store offering. Whichever route you choose to go, you'll want to consider the calorie counts shown here.

hot dog on bun
280 calories

1 pint vegetable soup 120 calories
potato knish 160 calories

TOTAL 280 calories

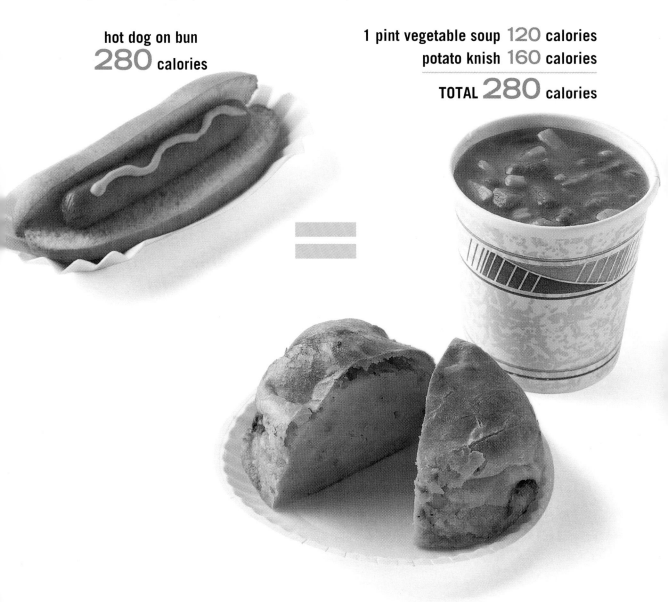

Phil-afel

Philly cheese steak or falafel? For the sake of both health and calorie count, if you're weight-conscious, you might want to pass the cheese steak and head for the falafel stand on the next corner. The falafel sandwich is less costly calorically—and many times more healthful as a protein source.

½ Philly cheese steak
1½ oz meat 120 calories
¾ oz cheese 80 calories
roll and sautéed onions 170 calories

TOTAL 370 calories

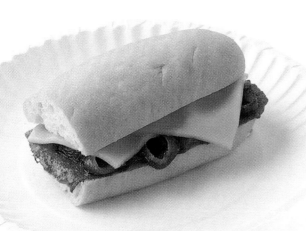

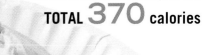

Falafel sandwich
pita bread stuffed with lettuce, onion, and yogurt dressing 140 calories
3 falafel balls 230 calories

TOTAL 370 calories

The Pretzel Paradox

Yes, this soft pretzel is low in fat, but at 470 calories, it's no great weight-loss bargain. In fact, for about the same calorie count, you could have 11 pretzel rods—if there's anybody who could manage that number. You could even have potato knishes—the classic New York "street food" that's usually considered highly fattening. In fact, you could have *three* knishes for nearly the calorie price of one soft pretzel.

Some other alternatives? For the same calorie count as the soft pretzel and with a much more powerful nutritional punch, try two 1-ounce packs of honey-roasted peanuts—full of fiber, protein, and essential fatty acids. Along with the peanuts, you can have two containers of mixed fruit—bursting with vitamins, minerals, fiber, and a variety of delicious tastes.

So take a good long look at this page—and remember, the next time you reach for a soft pretzel, there are other choices!

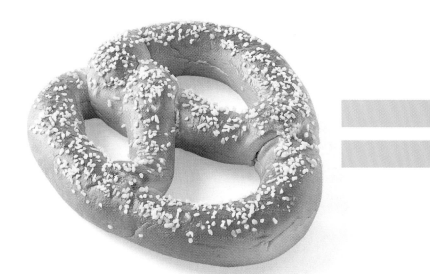

1 soft pretzel (6 oz) 470 **calories**

11 pretzel rods
40 calories each

OR

OR

3 knishes
160 calories each

2 containers fruit,
1½ cups each 120 calories
2 packs of peanuts, 1 oz each 350 calories
TOTAL 470 calories

"Coffee and . . ." at Starbucks

Wherever you turn in any large city and many small hamlets, you're sure to run into a Starbucks these days. Just to remind you of your pastry choices in a typical Starbucks, look at the photo-message below. And keep in mind that the lemon pastry, which looks innocuous, isn't the lowest-calorie choice you can make.

lemon pastry
420 calories

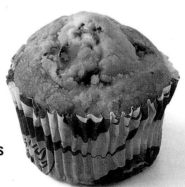

low-fat muffin
230 calories

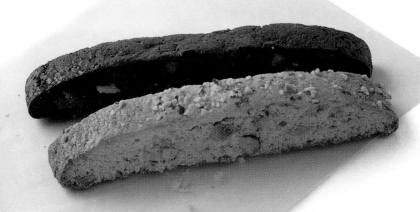

2 biscotti
180 calories

Fast Start

Breakfasting at McDonald's gets you off to a fast start, and it can be a lower-calorie start as well. Have a look at your choices.

The sausage-and-egg biscuit is easy to eat—and so is the cinnamon roll. Maybe too easy. You'll get 510 calories if you eat the sausage-and-egg biscuit, and 400 calories if you go for the cinnamon roll.

Maybe you'd prefer to dwell on another alternative. If you eat pancakes and syrup, you can get away with 360 calories. Just be sure to avoid the butter.

Better yet, what about the low-fat apple-bran muffin? It's just as easy to eat as any cinnamon roll, and just as convenient as a sausage-and-egg biscuit. But as you can see, the bran muffin gives you only about 300 calories, which easily beats out the competition at Mickey D's.

cinnamon roll
400 calories

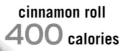

sausage-and-egg biscuit
510 calories

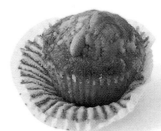

low-fat apple-bran muffin
300 calories

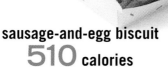

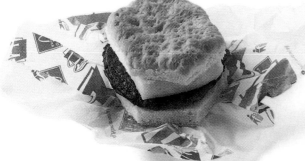

pancakes **310** calories
1 Tbsp syrup **50** calories

TOTAL 360 calories

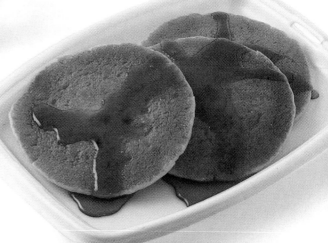

The Trick in the Treat

At 360 calories for this tiny portion, candy corn isn't much of a treat for the weight-conscious. But picture another choice.

Six Tootsie Pops total the same number of calories. And consider this: Each one takes so long to eat, you'll probably say "enough" after one or two. So, next Halloween, remember what else there is before you automatically reach for the candy corn. You might get all the candy you can eat, at just a fraction of the calories. Now that's a treat!

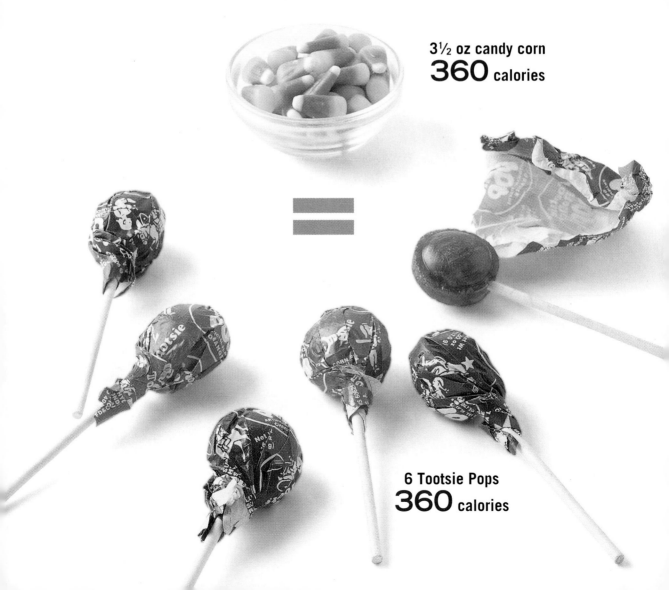

3½ oz candy corn
360 calories

6 Tootsie Pops
360 calories

Be My Valentine

Almost criminally delicious, chocolate truffles are also pretty much off the charts, calorie-wise. So . . . what about picturing something else for Valentine's day? Consider offering just a taste or two of truffles and satisfying your beloved's chocolate craving with chocolate-dipped strawberries instead. And don't forget the rose—no calories at all!

8 truffles (½ oz each) 560 calories

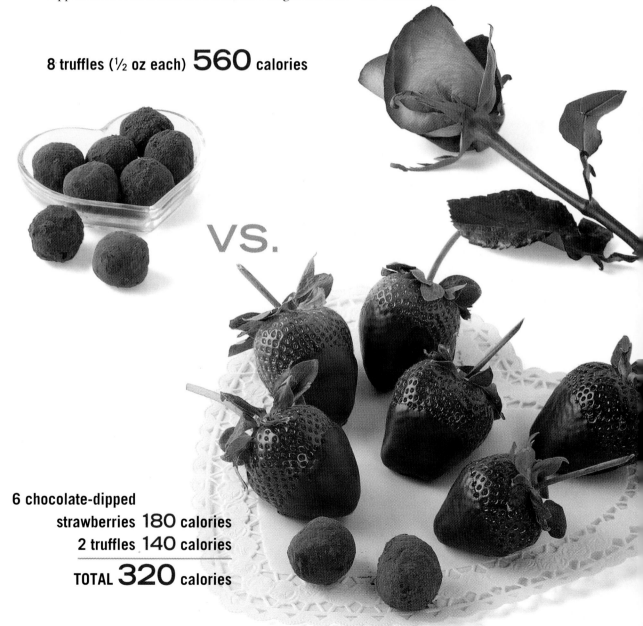

VS.

6 chocolate-dipped
strawberries 180 calories
2 truffles 140 calories
TOTAL 320 calories

Yankee Doodle Dandy

On the "Glorious Fourth," it's practically your patriotic duty to eat, but how can you eat a lot and still eat low-calorie?

Here are some choices to keep in mind before the fireworks go off. For the three items on the plate to the left of the equal sign—hot dog, sausage, and macaroni salad—substitute all the food on the three plates to the right. That's right—you can have the platter of shrimp, mushrooms, and vegetables, the corn on the cob, and all that watermelon. The calorie count is equivalent.

Small barbecue plate
2 oz hot dog **180** calories
2 oz sausage **200** calories
⅓ cup macaroni salad **150** calories

TOTAL **530** calories

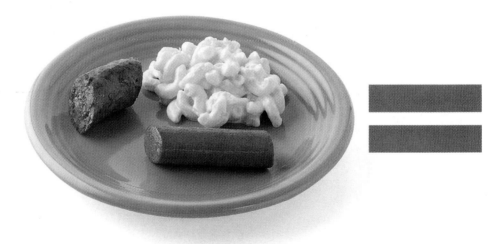

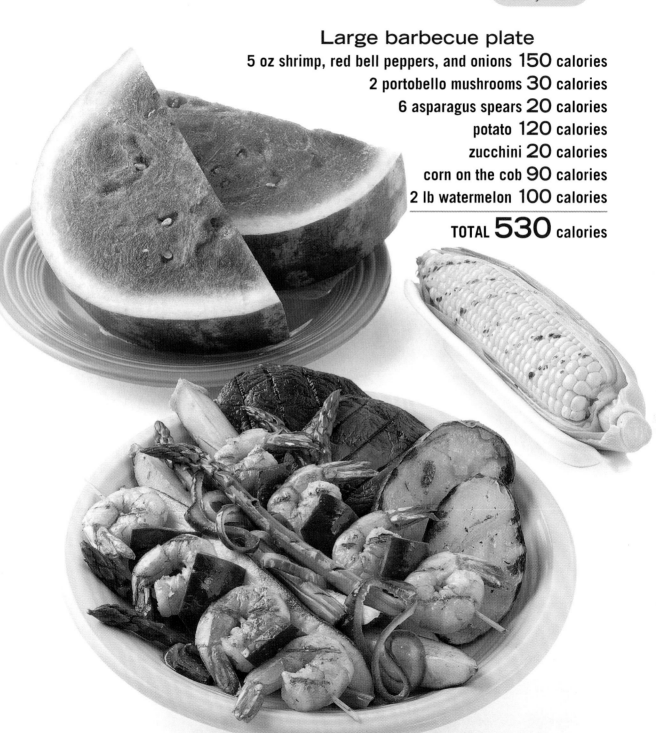

Large barbecue plate
5 oz shrimp, red bell peppers, and onions 150 calories
2 portobello mushrooms 30 calories
6 asparagus spears 20 calories
potato 120 calories
zucchini 20 calories
corn on the cob 90 calories
2 lb watermelon 100 calories

TOTAL 530 calories

A Gift for the Holidays

It's the holidays! And getting into the holiday spirit requires eating, doesn't it? But it helps to have a clear view of your choices as the season approaches.

Holiday meal 1 on the right is about as close to typical as you can get. You might have cocktails with peanuts, a couple of pastry hors d'oeuvres, and a tiny bit of cheese and pâté to start. If you're exercising restraint, you might have a few slices of turkey with trimmings along with one glass of wine and, of course, a wedge of pie. All in all, that's not a huge repast. But it certainly is a huge expense in terms of calories—a total of 3,710.

Can you do otherwise and still make merry? Turn the page, and check out the festive feast on page 189. From the champagne punch to the shiitake mushrooms, from the crudités and onion/chive dip to the several slices of turkey, from the scallops and tomatoes to the glass of wine and the pumpkin custard, holiday meal 2 is as tasty and filling as the one shown here. But meal 2 has 2,780 calories *less* than meal 1!

Holiday meal 1

2 glasses (2½ fl oz each) Scotch **400** calories
½ cup mixed nuts **440** calories
3 oz pastry hors d'oeuvres **380** calories
2 oz cheese **220** calories
2 oz pâté **240** calories
5 crackers **80** calories
6 oz turkey (light and dark meat with skin) **360** calories
4 Tbsp gravy **120** calories
1 cup sausage stuffing **400** calories
2 small candied yams **200** calories
½ cup buttered green beans **60** calories
6 fl oz wine **130** calories
wedge pecan pie **680** calories

TOTAL **3,710** calories

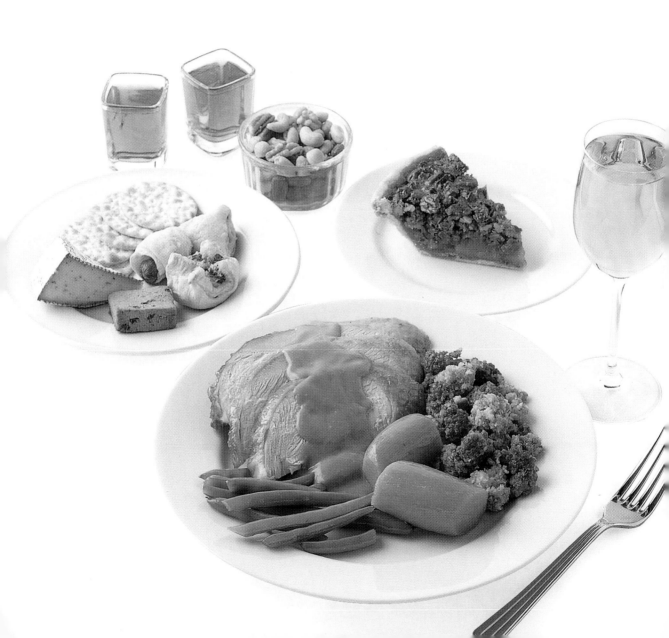

Holiday meal 2

2 cups champagne punch (made with champagne and low-cal punch) 40 calories

7 grilled shiitake mushrooms 30 calories

2 Tbsp soy dipping sauce 10 calories

2½ oz scallops 80 calories

5 cherry tomatoes 10 calories

2 cups assorted vegetables 30 calories

3 Tbsp onion/chive dip (low-fat) 30 calories

4 oz white-meat turkey (or vegetarian substitute) 200 calories

6 oz baked yam 150 calories

1 cup green beans with herbs 40 calories

¾ cup ginger-fruit stuffing (low-fat) 80 calories

2 Tbsp cranberry relish 20 calories

3 fl oz wine 60 calories

1 cup pumpkin custard 150 calories

TOTAL 930 calories

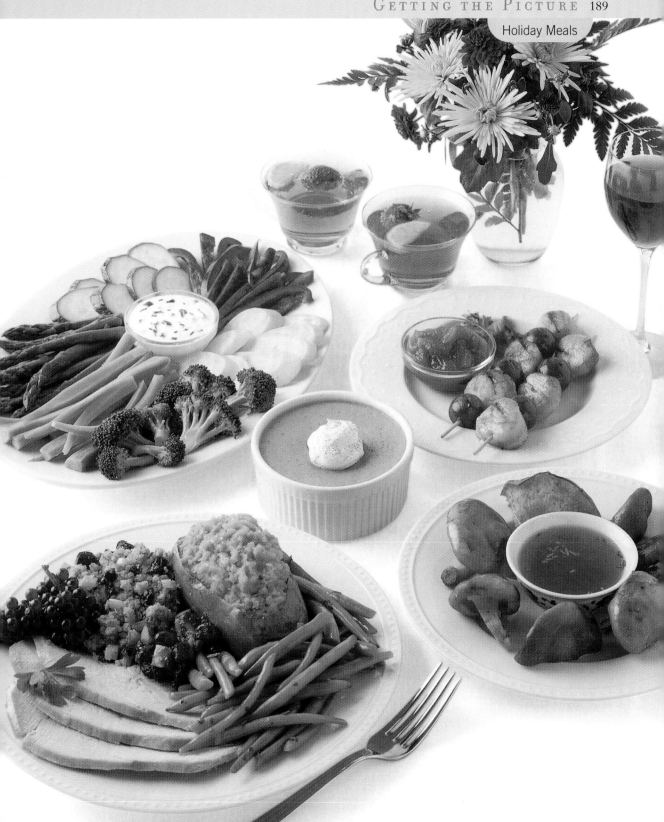

Dionysian Feast

Greek cuisine offers a range of exciting tastes. You can experience one of them—moussaka—for 520 calories. But is that really what you want to do?

Before you decide, picture what you can eat for the same 520 calories. The whole meal's worth of Greek food, shown at right, just might be a preferable choice.

6 oz moussaka 520 calories

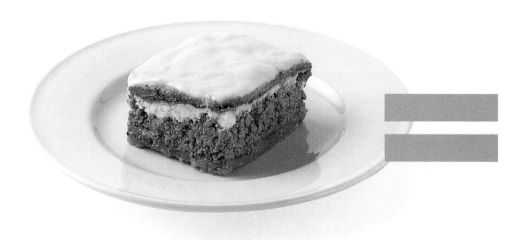

3 dolmathes (grape leaves stuffed with rice, pine nuts, and currants) 120 calories

4 oz shrimp Santorini 170 calories

1 cup tzatziki (cucumber and yogurt) 30 calories

½ cup melitzano (eggplant) salad 40 calories

3 fl oz retsina wine 60 calories

fig compote (3 figs) 100 calories

TOTAL 520 calories

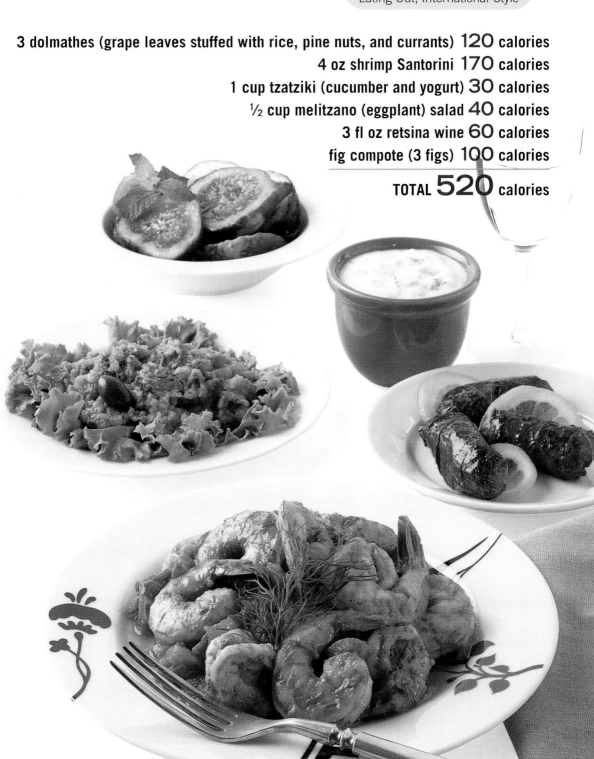

Burrito Bargain

These two offerings from the California Burrito chain look the same, but inside, they boast different personalities and substantially different calorie counts. On the blue plate is the Chula Vista burrito stuffed with meat, cheese, sour cream—and 1,050 calories. But now look at an alternative on the yellow plate. It's a burrito with lots of vegetables, accompanied by pico de gallo—and that yellow plate holds about half the calories as the blue one.

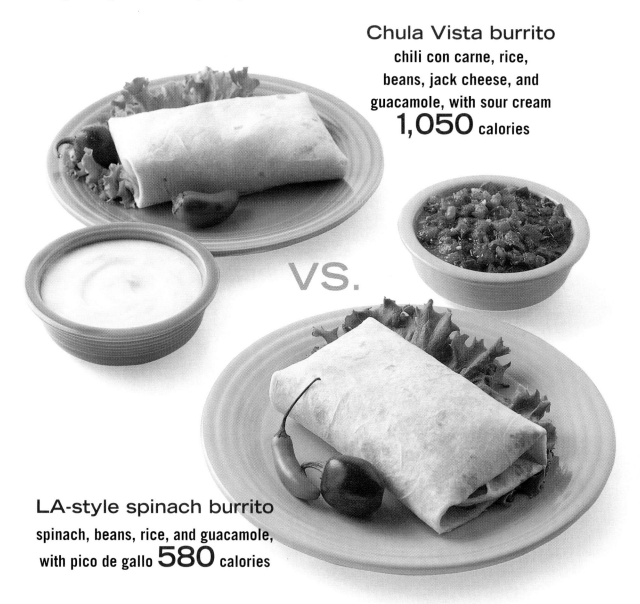

Chula Vista burrito
chili con carne, rice,
beans, jack cheese, and
guacamole, with sour cream
1,050 calories

VS.

LA-style spinach burrito
spinach, beans, rice, and guacamole,
with pico de gallo **580** calories

Portion Parsing

Because Japanese cuisine offers many low-calorie choices, it gives weight-conscious eaters an opportunity to enjoy large portion sizes. Here's a case in point that you might want to keep on hand for reference. One pork dumpling? Or one huge portion of miso soup with scallions and tofu? Either way, it's 70 calories—for a bite or a bowl.

1 pork dumpling (boiled)
70 calories

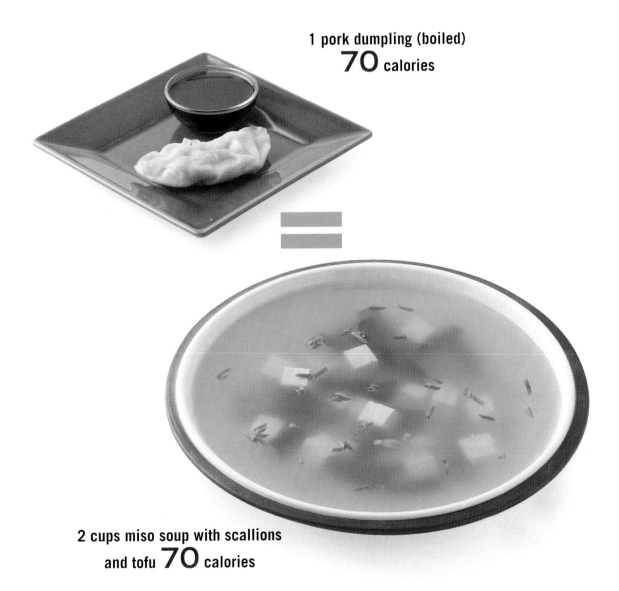

2 cups miso soup with scallions
and tofu 70 calories

Last among Equals

Here are three equally classic Japanese dishes in equal portions—tempura, teriyaki, and sushi and sashimi. But when you see equal portions, you can't assume equal calories. The portions of teriyaki and sushi/sashimi that you see here are equal in calories, but the tempura is another story. Choose the tempura, and you've selected a food with a stratospheric calorie count. For the weight-conscious who have a clear picture of the cost, tempura is probably the last choice.

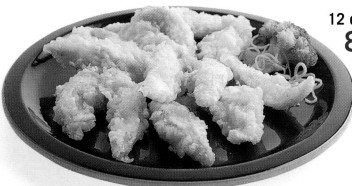

12 oz chicken tempura
860 calories

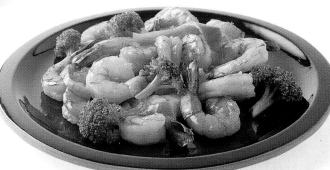

12 oz shrimp teriyaki
360 calories

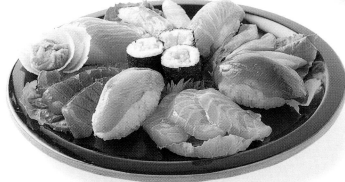

12 oz sushi and sashimi
360 calories

Middle Eastern Protein

Rice-and-meat balls—kufteh berenji—are a typical Middle Eastern treat, but even a meager portion tends to be high in calories. Now picture this instead: A filleted fish—mahi-ye tu por ba anar—offers a larger portion for far fewer calories. And you'll still get the calorie savings, even if you add a delicious Middle Eastern pomegranate sauce to that fish fillet.

6 rice-and-meat balls (1 oz each)
480 calories

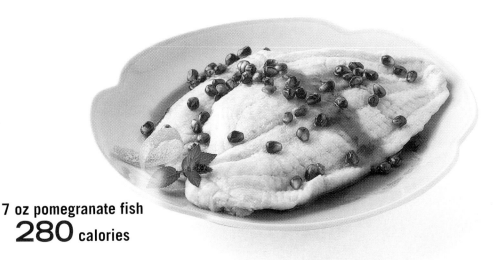

VS.

7 oz pomegranate fish
280 calories

A Mideast Feast

A small quantity of baklava—just 2½ ounces—may seem like a morsel. But accept that morsel, and you're getting 440 calories.

Picture this, instead—a full Middle Eastern meal consisting of eggplant-and-yogurt dip, two small wedges of pita bread, a butternut squash stew (khoresh), saffron rice, and a bountiful fruit plate that includes melon and figs.

One meager baklava with a load of hidden calories . . . or a Greek meal that's sure to satisfy your appetite? The choice is yours.

2½ oz baklava 440 calories

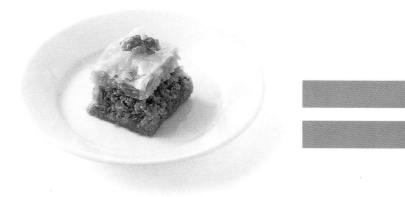

½ cup eggplant-and-yogurt dip 30 calories
2 small wedges pita bread 40 calories
1½ cups butternut squash stew 120 calories
½ cup saffron rice 100 calories
large fruit plate of melon and figs 150 calories

TOTAL 440 calories

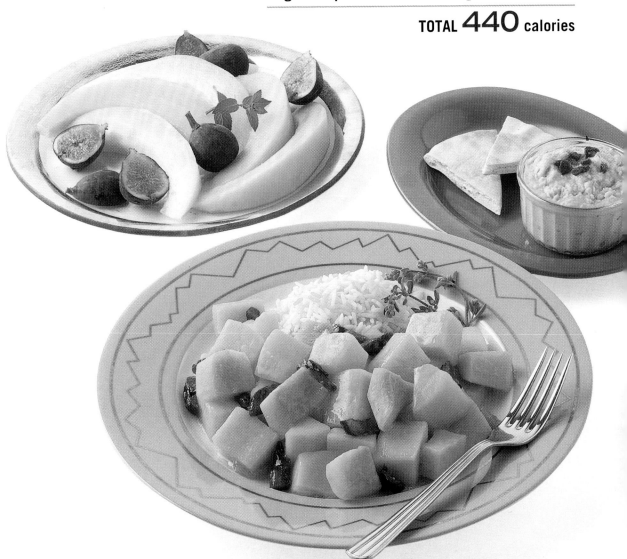

Appetizer Appreciation 101

Wolf down this small amount of prosciutto and melon or even the slightly healthier bruschetta—bread drizzled with olive oil and tomato bits—and you barely slake your appetite. Yet with either appetizer, you've already taken in 360 calories before even digging in to your meal.

But here's another picture to keep in mind. Contrast those small appetizers with this hefty bowl of mussels marinara. The calories are equivalent—360. But look at the portion size! Plus, you're getting a lot more nutrition with the mussels, which are a great low-fat source of protein and minerals.

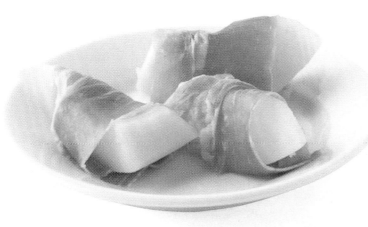

4 oz prosciutto and melon
360 calories

OR

3 oz bruschetta
360 calories

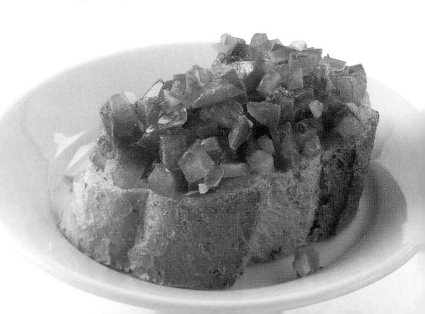

1 lb mussels marinara **360** calories

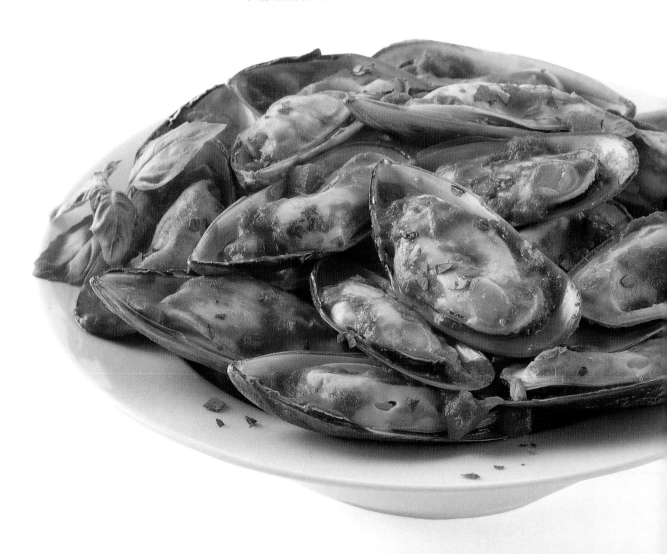

Italian Addition

Italian cuisine embraces such a wide variety of ingredients and tastes that it's easy to make low-calorie choices. For a quick reminder of one very easy choice, look at the comparison between a high-calorie pasta in cream sauce and some much-lower-calorie alternatives.

Here is a generous portion of *zuppa di pesce*, fish soup, and an equally generous serving of *pasta e fagioli*, pasta and beans. Together, these classic Italian foods add up to the calorie count of this small helping of tortellini in cream sauce.

Tortellini alla panna
15 small meat dumplings 500 calories
½ cup cream sauce 200 calories

TOTAL 700 calories

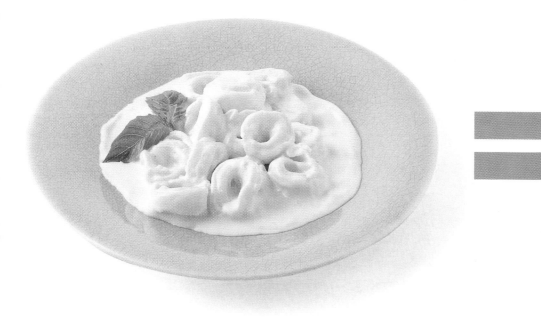

pasta e fagioli (made with 2 oz ditalini
pasta and ½ cup cannellini beans) 350 calories
zuppa di pesce (made with 8 oz fish) 350 calories

TOTAL 700 calories

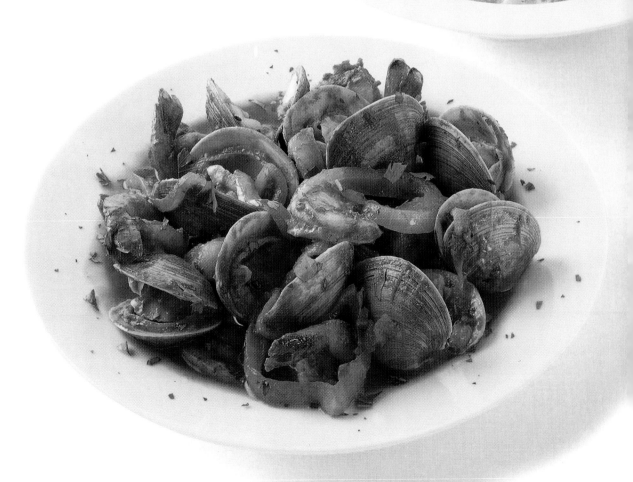

Fried Bread or Four Courses?

Here's another travel picture to help you with your choices when you're having Indian food.

Spiced, meat-filled Indian fried bread—keema paratha—has so many calories that it's really the equivalent of a full meal. It's fried in ghee, which is clarified butter. The photographs below show the contrast. A single serving of keema paratha has the same number of calories as the four-course meal pictured at right—a meal that includes mulligatawney spicy lentil soup, chana sag (chickpeas and spinach in spicy sauce), cool cucumber and yogurt raita, and a savory mango chutney with a chapati. The whole meal has 330 calories—the same as the single serving of keema paratha—plus it offers significant protein from lentils and chickpeas.

1 serving keema paratha
fried in ghee 330 calories

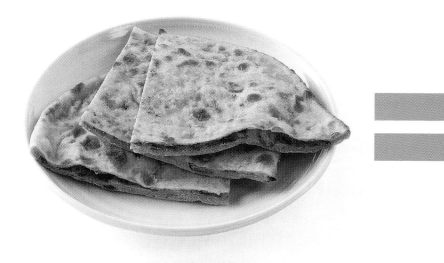

1 cup mulligatawney soup 80 calories
1½ cups chana sag 120 calories
raita and chutney 50 calories
1 chapati 80 calories

TOTAL 330 calories

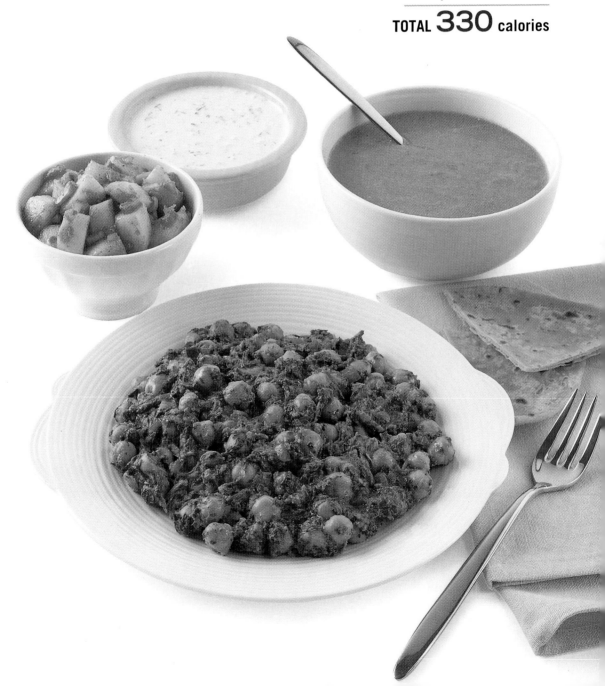

Eating Out, International-Style

The 450 Club

Each of these dishes holds 450 calories worth of food. You can have the bowl of lobster bisque *or* the single portion of quiche Lorraine as an appetizer: Either one of these, alone, has 450 calories. On the other hand, maybe you'd prefer a full meal for the same number of calories. You can have the platter of turbot, prepared with lemon, wine, herbs, and tomato concassé, string beans, and new potatoes with parsley. The next time you have a fish feast, keep these pictures in mind. Which club will you join?

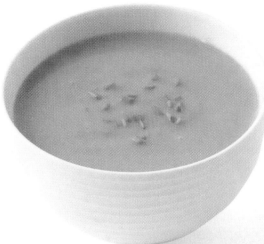

1½ cups lobster bisque
450 calories

OR

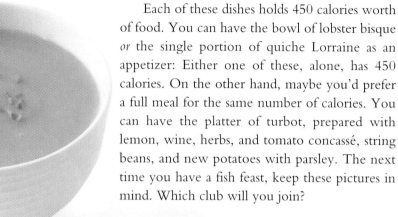

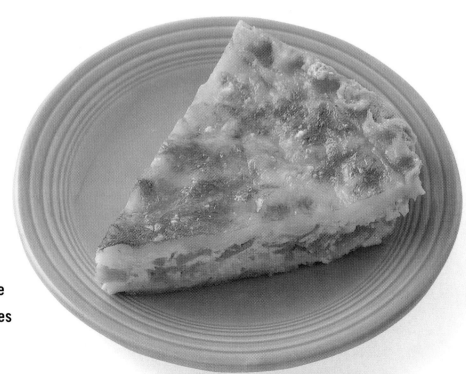

quiche Lorraine
450 calories

Eating Out, International-Style

7 oz poached turbot with lemon, wine, and herbs 230 calories
¾ cup tomato concassé 30 calories
1 cup string beans 40 calories
10 parsleyed new potatoes 150 calories

TOTAL 450 calories

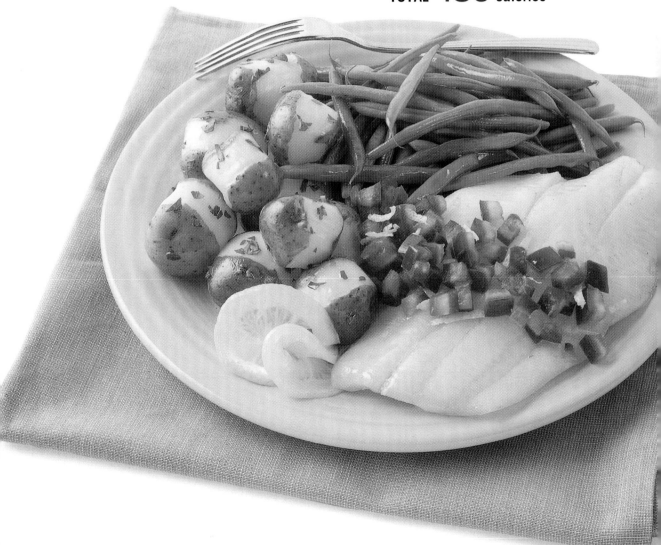

Vive la France!

French food is certainly superb when it's high-calorie. But low-calorie French food can be equally splendid—which means the weight-conscious can enjoy haute cuisine. Each of the desserts pictured on the left contains 460 calories: the apple tart, the small chunk of Roquefort cheese with a glass of cordial, and the small plate of assorted cookies. But now take a look at the four-course meal shown at right. It also contains 460 calories, and it includes marinated hearts of palm with artichoke hearts, a mixed salad, an entrée of salmon, potatoes, and asparagus, and a poached pear in red wine.

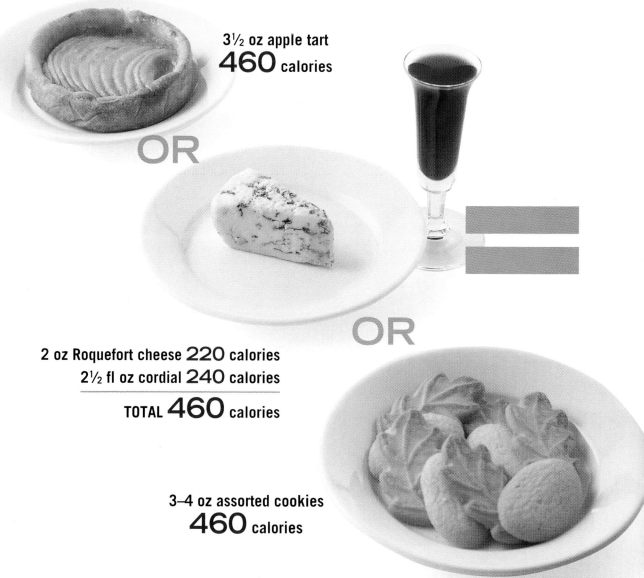

3½ oz apple tart
460 calories

OR

2 oz Roquefort cheese 220 calories
2½ fl oz cordial 240 calories

TOTAL 460 calories

OR

3–4 oz assorted cookies
460 calories

mixed salad with 1 Tbsp dressing 80 calories
marinated hearts of palm and artichoke hearts 30 calories
3 oz salmon 130 calories
asparagus 30 calories
oven-browned potatoes 90 calories
poached pear in red wine 100 calories

TOTAL 460 calories

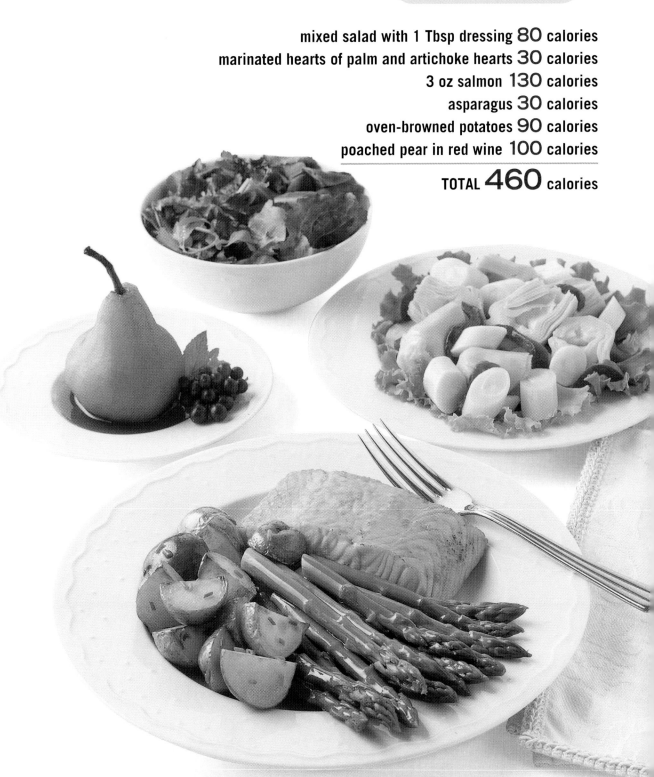

Characteristically Chinese

Chinese cuisine offers a range of tastes almost as vast as the country itself. For the weight-conscious, Chinese food offers a wide array of lower-calorie choices that are both delicious and distinctive. But you have to know what your choices are.

Before you contemplate your next Chinese meal, consider what you see in the food demonstration below. On your right—a whole meal consisting of soup, shrimp and broccoli in hoisin sauce, brown rice, and even a fortune cookie. It's certainly a good choice if you want to leave the table feeling satisfied.

That whole meal has the same number of calories as any *one* of the typical appetizers on the left—the single egg roll, the small portion of spareribs, or the crispy noodles. So you might want to turn to this page to remind yourself of your calorie alternatives before you order takeout or head for the nearest Chinese restaurant.

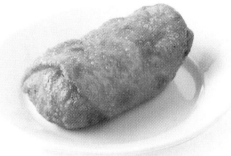

egg roll
400 calories

OR

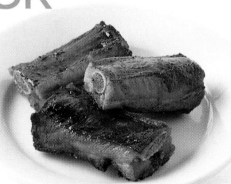

small serving of spareribs
400 calories

OR

dish of crispy noodles
400 calories

bowl of Chinese vegetable soup 40 calories
4 oz shrimp 120 calories
1 ½ cups of broccoli 60 calories
2 Tbsp hoisin sauce 20 calories
⅔ cup brown rice 130 calories
fortune cookie 30 calories

TOTAL 400 calories

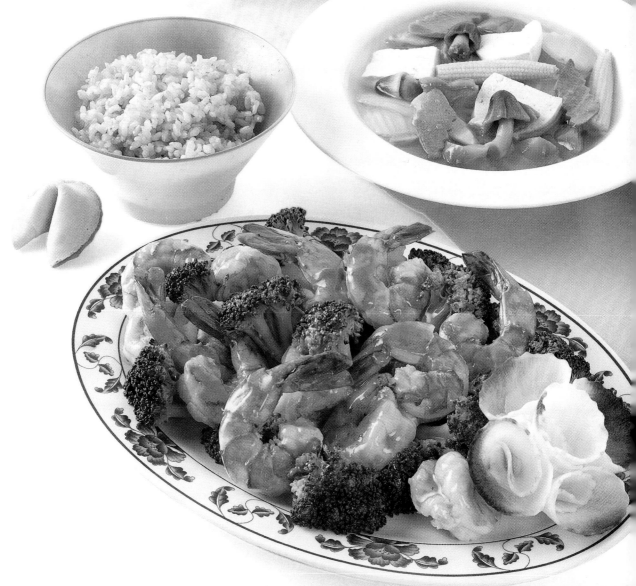

Descending Appetizers

Among the distinctive Chinese dishes below, the bigger the portion pictured, the more healthful the dish and the fewer the calories. Check the numbers. And keep these numbers in mind the next time you "order Chinese."

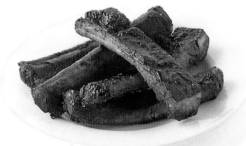

5 spareribs
1,000 calories

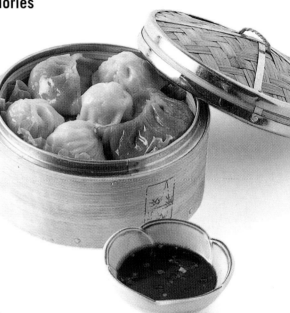

6 steamed vegetable dumplings
300 calories

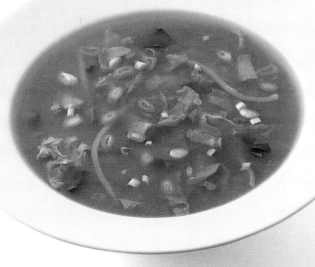

1 large bowl hot-and-sour soup
120 calories

Enlisted in Nutrition

Here's another comparison to keep in mind for your next Chinese dining experience. Look at the General Tso's chicken dish. The portion is certainly small, but General T's chicken packs a lot of calories. If, instead, you choose scallops and vegetables in black bean sauce, you'll be able to eat half-again as much food for about half the calories. And there are other benefits as well—including protein from the seafood and lots of fiber, vitamins, and minerals from the vegetables.

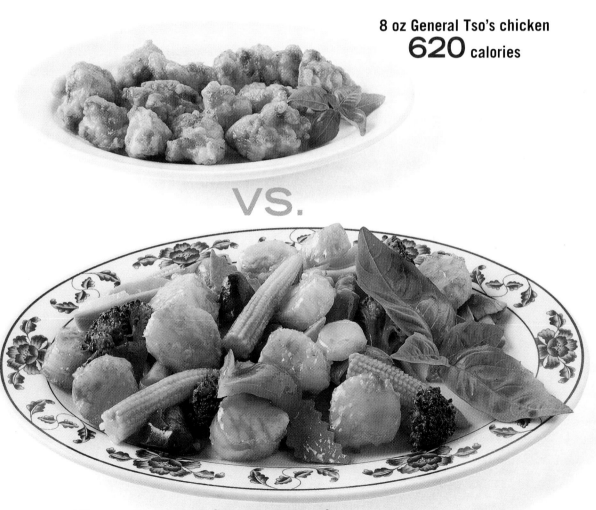

8 oz General Tso's chicken
620 calories

VS.

12 oz scallops and Chinese vegetables in
black bean sauce 320 calories

Tofu Trumps Chicken

They look almost the same—but for the sake of food awareness, you might want to look again. The dish of tofu and mushrooms in brown sauce at the bottom of the page costs less than half the number of calories of the chicken and mushrooms in brown sauce shown at top. And, of course, the tofu is a far better nutrition bet than the chicken.

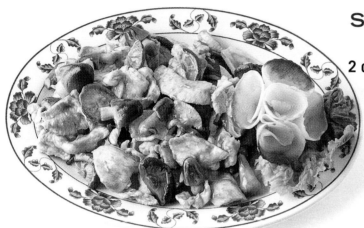

Stir-fried chicken
4 oz chicken 200 calories
2 cups mushrooms 80 calories
1 Tbsp oil 120 calories
brown sauce 30 calories

TOTAL 430 calories

VS.

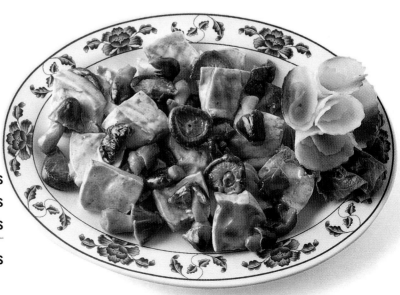

Steamed tofu
4 oz tofu 90 calories
2 cups mushrooms 80 calories
brown sauce 30 calories

TOTAL 200 calories

Indian Contrasts

Indian cuisine offers a range of contrasts in taste and calorie count. The next time you eat in an Indian restaurant, think about what these pictures are telling you.

Here are equal portions of lamb biryani and tandoori shrimp, but each of these portions has vastly different fat and calorie contents. The lamb biryani—cooked with raisins, coconut, and ghee—is high in saturated fats and costs 870 calories. Tandoori shrimp, flavored with vegetables and a savory marinade, is low in fat and high in good protein from seafood, and it weighs in at less than half the calories of the lamb.

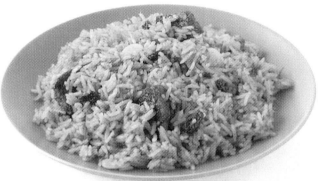

Lamb biryani

6 oz lamb 420 calories

1½ cups basmati rice 300 calories

raisins, coconut, and ghee 150 calories

TOTAL 870 calories

VS.

Tandoori shrimp

6 oz shrimp 180 calories

tomato 20 calories

marinade 20 calories

1 cup basmati rice 200 calories

TOTAL 420 calories

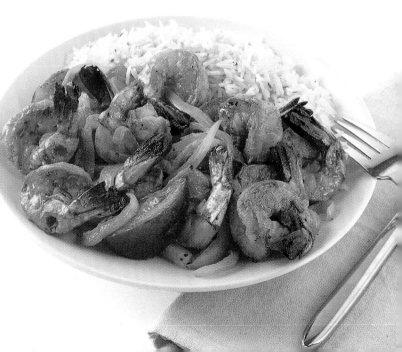

Chapter 7

SHOPPING LOW-CALORIE

*W*hen you begin to change your relationship with food, you'll find yourself making more low-calorie choices almost automatically.

But there's more to it than that.

You'll also change your relationship with food *shopping*. Whether you're a gourmet chef or someone who barely knows how to turn on an oven, you'll want to consider having a new set of ingredients in the pantry. And that will probably require some fresh thinking on the subject of cooking.

By stocking your pantry with the staples of a low-calorie life, you take responsibility for the weight-control choice before you ever sit down to a meal. Whenever you reach into the pantry or pull something out of the freezer, you have already assured yourself of getting the low-calorie option. *Shopping* low-calorie gives you a leg up on *eating* low-calorie.

If you are both mindful and creative in the way you prepare low-calorie food, you're demonstrating another level of commitment to weight control. It's another "right choice" for your health and your waistline.

Time to Go A-Marketing

Nearly all of us have access to supermarkets. Quality and size vary. But every super-

market—from one of the huge national chains to a smaller, regional establishment—offers some variety of choice. If you live in a large metropolitan area where you can also find specialty shops and health food stores, so much the better.

Let's have a quick look at some of your selections.

First, you'll need to shop for the low-calorie staples to go in your pantry and freezer. These are the foods that fit both your weight-control goals and your lifestyle. They provide all the basic ingredients for tasty, healthful, low-calorie meals in every season for any occasion.

Once your cabinets and freezer are stuffed with the basics, going shopping becomes pretty much a matter of buying the fresh foods—the vegetables and fruits or perhaps the fresh fish in season—that complete or are the focus of a meal.

The nucleus of your supermarket tours, any day of the week, any season of the year, will be what I call the Anytime List that you'll find on page 222. On the Anytime List are vegetables, fruit, and the lowest-calorie frozen desserts and candies available. This list has foods to keep on hand to eat anytime, in any amount, for any reason, either as a snack or as part of a meal. Make them the core of your eating, and you stand a superb chance of being thin for life.

Since I am a doctor and tend to think in medical terms, you can even think of the foods on the Anytime List as a daily remedy for weight control. My prescription? Take as needed.

So—What's Wrong with Packaged Foods?

As you scan the Anytime List, you'll notice that I don't have anything against canned, packaged, or frozen foods.

True, you may prefer the *taste* of fresh foods. But you don't have to avoid packaged foods out of fear of sodium, chemical preservatives, and other additives used in processing.

I meet many people who, in their yearning for all things natural, have come to distrust anything chemical. But it's worth reminding ourselves that some of the chemicals that are used in food may prevent food spoilage and improve flavor and texture.

As for fear of sodium—yes, for some people, there are medical reasons to limit sodium intake. (If you think a low-sodium diet might be a necessity for you, speak to your physician.) Unless you have such a medical condition, however, there's no reason to avoid sodium. It's simply a nonissue as far as fat loss is concerned.

What's Cooking in the American Diet

Are we eating more healthfully these days than we were a quarter-century ago?

Yes and no. What's certain is that we're definitely eating *differently* from the way we used to.

In 1970, for example, the average American consumed about 309 eggs, about 132 pounds of red meat, and some 26 gallons of milk every year. In 1995, those numbers had gone down to 237 eggs, 110 pounds of red meat, and just 9 gallons of milk per person per year. So it looks like we're cutting back significantly on high-fat, high-cholesterol foods.

During the same period, there was a trend toward lower-fat products. We started eating more fish, our consumption of poultry nearly doubled, and our consumption of nonfat milk tripled. We began eating more vegetables, fruits, grains, and seafood.

These statistics show a general shift away from high-fat meats toward foods with more phytonutrients—a slight improvement. Unfortunately, those 25 years also reveal a sharp increase in our consumption of sugars and fats. Between 1970 and 1995, our consumption of soft drinks doubled, and our consumption of cheese nearly tripled.

In short, we've come a long way. But we still have a long way to go in our shopping habits before we're really eating healthfully.

Scarce Nutrients?

Another misconception is the often-repeated mantra that canning, packaging, and freezing remove essential nutrients from food. Where canning and packaging are concerned, a very small amount of nutrients is lost in the process—not enough to keep you from using processed foods.

As for the freezing process, keep in mind that frozen food is usually of the highest quality. When you buy frozen fruits, vegetables, or fish, you're getting food that has been frozen at the peak of freshness. You lose nothing, nutrition-wise, when you eat frozen foods, and you gain all the advantages of variety, taste, and convenience.

Let's consider a couple of examples. A can of beans offers a wonderful source of protein along with such nutrients as folate, fiber, magnesium, iron, copper, and potassium. When you open a can of beans, you get all those advantages without having to go to the bother of soaking and cooking raw beans to make them edible.

Or consider your favorite brand and flavor of vegetable soup. (Remember, you probably do not have to select the low-salt kind.) Eating that vegetable soup can be a great way to take in vegetables. It's a meal unto itself, satisfying and filling as well as good-tasting and good for you.

In fact, the technologies for preserving food have brought enormous benefits. For the first time in history, wherever we live, we can enjoy fruits and vegetables all year round—tomatoes in December, berries in February. We can buy a supply of groceries that will last

for days—and some will stay good for weeks or months. We can cook up a whole meal just by boiling water or popping a frozen dinner in the oven.

For anyone making low-calorie choices over a lifetime, the variety and convenience of preserved foods can make a big difference in preventing boredom. And when you prevent boredom, you ensure that you don't end up with that deprived feeling.

Don't avoid such foods—embrace them! (Well, you don't have to actually hug them, but do eat and enjoy them without guilt and without worry.)

Organic—
A Separate Choice

As for organically grown foods, you can count on them being free of synthetic pesticide residues. You can also be certain that organic farming is gentler on the environment than farming that requires widespread use of synthetic pesticides. But just because these foods are pesticide-free does not mean they are any more nutritious than other foods.

Just like the first rule of practicing medicine, organic farming seeks to "do no harm." It returns as much to the soil as it takes out and does not contaminate the aquifers.

In other words, there are plenty of good reasons to "eat organic." But the promise of getting more nutrition from your food is not the compelling reason to go that route in your food-buying.

The Goods on Your Eating

Food labels are a great information source. They're the "study guide" to a lot of the foods that you're eating, and you'll find them on most food packages these days. If you've never really looked at one closely—or you want a quick refresher course—see "Getting the Hang of Your Label Lingo" on page 220.

But what can you do with the label information?

On the one hand, as New Yorkers like to say, having this data and a dollar-fifty will get you on the subway. In other words, knowing what it says on the Nutrition Facts label isn't much good by itself.

That's especially the case for people on my program, because Food Awareness Training does not entail calorie-counting, portion-weighing, or nutrient-measuring. There's no magic number of calories you should or should not eat every day, and no special serving size that will enable you to lose weight. I won't even tell you to eat a certain combination of nutrients that will produce the desired results.

On the other hand, this is information worth knowing. For example, by reading the Nutrition Facts label carefully, you can quickly learn how much of certain good-guy nutrients like vitamins A and C, calcium, iron, and fiber the food contains. At a glance, you can compare those figures with the percentage Daily Value for such "bad guys" as saturated fat and cholesterol. If the label reveals that you're getting just 2 to 3 percent of the good guys while you're getting 20 to 30 percent of the bad guys, you know immediately you're on the wrong side of the tracks.

Knowledge beats ignorance every time. Knowing the data on the Nutrition Facts label makes you a more mindful food shopper and a more mindful eater. That's reason enough to browse the Nutrition Facts labels when you're making your selections at the supermarket.

Read before You Buy

Caveat emptor! Let the buyer beware!

Not everything written on a package means what it says—or says what it means. Various advertising slogans and package descriptions are aimed at selling the product. Few rules apply.

Usually, the ads and slogans are in much

Label Lingo Lesson #1: "Enriched" vs. "Fortified"

If a food label says "enriched," it means some nutrients lost during the packaging or refining process have been replaced. In the process of refining flour for baking bread, for instance, some nutrients are removed. A number of these nutrients are later replaced to create "enriched" bread.

A fortified food, on the other hand, has its existing nutrient content topped off with additional dietary muscle. Vitamins, minerals, even fatty acids may be added to foods that never contained such nutrients. One common example is calcium-fortified orange juice.

Label Lingo Lesson #2:
"Low," "Reduced," "Light," and "Free"

Food-label terms have some strict definitions, but you won't find those definitions on most labels. The term *low* on a food package means that the food does not exceed dietary guidelines for fat, saturated fat, cholesterol, sodium, or calories. Before a food packager or supplier can put "low-something" on the label, the food must meet the following guidelines.

- A low-fat food has 3 grams or less of fat.
- A food that has low saturated fat contains 1 gram or less of saturated fat.
- A low-sodium food has 140 milligrams or less of sodium.
- If food is labeled "very low sodium," it has 35 milligrams or less of sodium per serving.
- Low-cholesterol foods have 20 milligrams or less of cholesterol and also have 2 grams or less of saturated fat.
- A low-calorie food has 40 calories or less per serving.
- To be described as lean, meat or poultry must contain less than 10 grams of fat, 4.5 grams or less of saturated fat, and less than 95 milligrams of cholesterol per serving.

- An extra-lean serving has less than 5 grams of fat, less than 2 grams of saturated fat, and less than 95 milligrams of cholesterol.

The word *reduced* on a package means something quite different from *low*. A nutritionally altered product with reduced fat, for example, contains at least 25 percent less fat than the "regular" food.

The word *less* has the same meaning as *reduced*, but a food with "less fat" or "less cholesterol" might not have been altered. A steak with all the fat trimmed off might be advertised as having "less fat."

Light or *lite* means that a nutritionally altered product contains a third fewer calories or half the fat of the original food. It can also apply to sodium, as in "lite salt," meaning that a low-calorie, low-fat food has its sodium content reduced by 50 percent.

The term *free* means that a product has virtually no fat, saturated fat, cholesterol, sodium, sugars, or calories. "Virtually" none means only a trace amount. "Fat-free," for example, means less than 0.5 grams per serving. "Calorie-free" means fewer than five calories per serving.

---

larger type and more prominently displayed than the food label. So you might be inclined to believe what's printed in the biggest, boldest type.

But that's not the only way you can be led astray. Even the claims listed on food packages

about the ingredients the items contain may or may not be covered by government standards or regulations.

Consider the kind of slogans that are most likely to lure you to the shelves.

No cholesterol! proclaims the brightly col-

Label Lingo Lesson #3: What's "Healthy"?

Thanks to federal guidelines, the word *healthy* on a food package now has a mandated meaning. A "healthy" food must be low in total fat and saturated fat, cholesterol, and sodium. And, in most cases, a healthy food must provide at least 10 percent of the recommended amounts of vitamins A or C, iron, calcium, protein, or fiber.

---

ored package of potato chips. Of course, no potato chip *would* have cholesterol, since cholesterol isn't in any food that comes from a vegetable. But those chips are likely to have hydrogenated fats and lots of calories from fat.

What about *sugar-free*? It's true that sugar-free candies probably have no sugar, but what about other sweeteners? The candy might contain honey, corn syrup, fructose, sorbitol, or mannitol. To find out, you'll need to check the small print on the ingredients list. But the other thing to remember is that *sugar-free candies have the same number of calories as "real" candy*. So why go for the sugar-free? From the all-important vantage of taste and avoiding feelings of deprivation, you're much better off eating the real thing.

Mind-Boggling Claims

Some advertising tactics can be misleading without even trying very hard. Consider this doozy, which you can probably find in any local market: A jar of Smucker's Simply Fruit—Strawberry proclaims that it contains "spreadable fruit." On closer inspection, the fine print admits that it contains "100 percent fruit sweetened with concentrated fruit juices." An admission in even-smaller print—

not for those with myopia—concedes that the product has more "clarified white grape juice concentrate" than it does strawberries.

Another one of my favorites is the snack pack of chocolate-covered raisins advertising "70 percent less fat." Look more closely, and you'll see that the snack pack contains 480 calories. At that rate, you're better off eating a solid chocolate bar. From that, you get about 200 calories.

Some Original Sins

If Eve had offered apple chips to Adam, their garden would have needed a weight-control program. You might think these chips are simply the shriveled-up version of the fruit on the tree—an impression that's often reinforced by offering the apple chips right in the produce department. After all, the claim on the bag is "30 percent less fat than potato chips."

But apple chips are a far cry from the fresh apples in the bin next to them. The chips have added sugar and hydrogenated fat, and they deliver up to 140 calories per serving. Of course, all those chips in a bag are quite easy to eat. And since the bag holds three servings, you could end up munching about 420 calories at a sitting.

Getting the Hang of Your Label Lingo

Food labels are your friends. But to get the most from a food label, you have to read it correctly.

Start at the top with serving size. It's the basis for all the other facts and figures on the label.

Sometimes overlooked, often neglected, serving size is the most important item to check before you go on. Once you read the serving size, take a moment to think about what you *really* eat, and compare that to the serving size described on the label. On a jar of olives, the label might indicate that three olives is the serving size, but if you usually eat six, you need to double the calories and all other nutritional figures to find out what you're actually getting when you eat those half-dozen olives.

On the other hand, a box of shredded-wheat cereal might say "two biscuits" is the serving size. If you like just one shredded-wheat biscuit for breakfast, you'll be getting half the calories but also half the fiber. All other nutritional values on the label also need to be cut in half.

Government regulations require certain other information—such as total calories, calories from fat, total fat, saturated fat, cholesterol, sodium, total carbohydrate, di-

Nutrition Facts		
Serving size: 1 container		
Amount Per Serving		
Calories 120	Calories from Fat 0	
		% DV*
Total Fat 0g		**0**%
Saturated Fat 0g		**0**%
Cholesterol 5mg		**2**%
Sodium 140mg		**6**%
Potassium 380mg		**11**%
Total Carbohydrate 22g		**7**%
Dietary Fiber 0g		**0**%
Sugars 16g		
Protein 8g		
Vitamin A 0%	●	Vitamin C 8%
Calcium 35%	●	Iron 0%
* Percent Daily Values (DV) are based on a 2,000 calorie diet.		

etary fiber, sugars, protein, vitamin A, vitamin C, calcium, and iron. Though not required, the label may also include information on calories from saturated fat; polyunsaturated fat; monounsaturated fat; potassium; soluble and insoluble fiber; sugar, alcohol, and other carbohydrates; and other vitamins and minerals.

The label shown at left is for a brand-name strawberry-banana yogurt. While the calories are shown as plain numbers, all the nutrients are expressed as plain numbers as well as percentages of the Daily Values (DV). Those Daily Values are based on a reference intake of 2,000 calories per day. If you eat one serving of a food that has 20 percent of the DV of total carbohydrate in each serving, then you're fulfilling one-fifth of your daily requirement for total carbohydrate *if* you get about 2,000 calories of food every day.

As you assess these DV numbers, keep in mind that you're going to be eating a variety of foods in the course of a day. You don't need to grab a huge amount of the Daily Value of any one nutrient right away. A food that has even 20 percent of the DV can probably be considered high in that nutrient.

Fishing for Customers, the Hue Is the Lure

There's a reason the lettering on that package is yellow. Yellow is a proven attention-getter. It's the color the brain processes fastest.

So say the researchers who have done extensive studies of colors on mood, attitude . . . and buying habits.

And there's another thing about yellow. It's happy.

So if you see a food that's packaged in a bright yellow box—or it's wearing a bright yellow banner—you know why. Cheerful shoppers are more likely to happily buy it.

This is all part of the subtle art of marketing, of course. Experts in consumer research have studied our responses to colors in detail, and they package accordingly. Here's what the findings tell them about our responses.

- Red is a color that increases blood pressure and stimulates appetite.
- Green suggests food products that are environmentally sound and probably healthful.
- Orange is easy to find. And people find it easier to pay for orange-colored packaging, experts say.
- White means pure, and it also means low in calories.
- Brown is simply a rich background color. (It's unlikely you'll find it at the forefront of any supermarket sale.)
- Blue means fun.

Check out these colors the next time you're in the supermarket. It will help you be aware of what foods, in which packages, are luring you toward them. And why.

The fact is, the apple chips don't hold a candle to the fresh apples, which are not only easy to eat but also free of added sugar and fat. Munch an apple, and you're getting a healthful, nutritious treat in an extremely efficient delivery package.

I think my favorite marketing claim, though, is the use of the word *natural*. For most foods, natural means absolutely nothing. (The exceptions are meat and poultry: "Natural" on a meat or poultry package means there are no artificial colors, preservatives, or synthetic ingredients of any kind. But even

without artificial colors, preservatives, or synthetic ingredients, meat and poultry have a negative impact on health.)

True, many natural foods are healthful and nutritious. A fresh apple, for instance, has bountiful nutrients. But what's *labeled* as natural is not necessarily good for us. After all, sugar is natural. Cholesterol is natural. Saturated fats are natural. So are tobacco and alcohol.

Also, there's no reason to think that a food made from "natural ingredients" is the best choice for weight control. When I see "nat-

(continued on page 224)

Dr. Shapiro's Anytime List

The following foods are the best bets for any time of year. If you have these foods at the ready, they'll be the first that you reach for when you're hungry. So here's my prescription for the foods that you should keep on hand.

Vegetables

- All kinds of vegetables—raw, cooked, fresh, frozen, canned, or in soups

Condiments and Seasonings

All the flavorful ingredients listed below are low-calorie. Use them creatively to spice up your vegetable courses, treats, and snacks.

- Oil-free or low-calorie salad dressings
- Nonfat or lite mayonnaise, nonfat sour cream, nonfat yogurt (plain or with Nutrasweet)
- Mustards: Dijon, Pommery, and other kinds
- Tomato puree, tomato paste, tomato sauce
- Clam juice, lemon or lime juice, tomato juice, V–8 juice
- Butter Buds, Molly McButter
- Nonstick sprays in butter or olive-oil flavors, such as Pam
- Vinegars: balsamic, cider, tarragon, wine, or other flavors
- Horseradish: either red or white
- Sauces: A-1, barbecue, chutney, cocktail, duck sauce, ketchup, relish, salsa, soy, tamari, and Worcestershire
- Onion: fresh, juice, flakes, or powder
- Garlic: fresh, juice, flakes, or powder
- Herbs: all kinds, including basil, bay leaves, chives, dill, marjoram, oregano, rosemary, sage, tarragon, and thyme
- Spices: all kinds, including allspice, cinnamon, cloves, coriander, cumin, curry, ginger, nutmeg, and paprika
- Extracts: including almond, coconut, maple, peppermint, and vanilla
- Cocoa powder
- Dried soups as seasonings

Beverages

Help yourself to any low-calorie beverage. Be sure to avoid all beverages that are labeled "naturally sweetened" or "fruit-juice sweetened." Beverages to keep in stock include:

- Coffees and teas
- Crystal Light, Diet Mystic, Diet Nestea, Diet Snapple, and other brands of iced tea
- Diet sodas—any preference of flavors
- Seltzer: plain or flavored (If the product is labeled "naturally sweetened," be sure to check the calorie count.)
- Hot cocoa mixes (Look for mixes that have 20 to 50 calories per serving, such as Carnation Diet and Swiss Miss. Avoid cocoa mixes that have 60 calories or more.)
- Milk shake mixes (You want the kinds that have 70 or fewer calories per serving, including brands such as Alba Fit and Frosty and Weight Watchers.)

Fruit

All fruits—raw or cooked, fresh, frozen, or canned (But avoid any packaged fruit with added sugar.)

Frozen Desserts

Any nonfat yogurt or sorbet is good to have in your freezer. When selecting brands, be sure to keep an eye on the calories. Here are some that I like.

- In soft-serve, up to 25 calories per ounce, as in Columbo Lite, Skimpy Treat, TCBY nonfat, and Tofutti
- In hard-pack, up to 450 calories per pint, as in Dannon Lite, some Sharon's Sorbet, Sweet Nothings, Tofutti Lite, and all brands of Italian ices
- In Creamsicles, frozen fudge bars, and popsicles, up to 45 calories per bar, as in Tofutti Chocolate Fudge Treats, Weight Watchers Berries 'n Cream and Orange-Vanilla Treats, and Welch's Fruit Juice Bars, and chocolate mousse by Dolly Madison, Weight Watchers, or Yoplait
- In individually packaged frozen bars, up to 100 calories each, as in FrozFruit, Häagen-Dazs bars, and Starbucks low-fat bars

Candy

- Any chewing gum
- Any hard candy, including candy canes, gumballs, lollipops, and sourballs, as in Blow Pops, Hershey's Tastetations, Jolly Rancher, Tootsie Pops, and Werther's Butterscotch

ural" applied to food, I assume it's nothing more than a marketing tool. I'm afraid it can mean just about anything the advertising department wants it to mean. A "naturally sweetened" beverage or cookie, to take just one example, has the same number of calories as a drink or cookie made with refined sugar.

The Meaning of More

While we're on the subject of labels and advertising, I might as well bring up one more supermarket inducement that can easily lead you to overbuying—and get in the way of your weight-control objectives. All the in-store inducements to buy *more* can be very seductive, but such offers are not for you.

If an item is marked "Two for $4.70"—and one of that item costs $2.40—why not just pick up two? You'll save a dime, and that seems like a sensible bargain as long as you're in the store.

Like bargain offers, suggested quantities can be persuasive, too. "Buy two packages of muffins and freeze one today" sounds good—but maybe you don't need a second package of muffins gathering freezer burn, just waiting for you to eat them.

Putting limits on quantity is another lure. "Just four to a customer" has almost magical powers to sell at least eight to a customer. After all, shoppers want good value for their money. But you're not getting any bargain at all if you're filling a cupboard with unwanted goods.

Remove Temptation

There's no dark conspiracy in this advertising. Food manufacturers hope you will eat more because they want you to buy more. Simple.

But you have to be aware of what many studies have shown: You *will* eat more when there's more to eat. If you buy the family-size package of potato chips, you'll eat more chips than you would have if you'd just bought the snack size. One recent study showed that people eat as much as 50 percent more of "hedonistic foods"—popcorn, chips, candy—when they come in bigger packages. (The same principle, by the way, applies outside the supermarket. If you buy a big bucket of popcorn in the movie theater, there's a good chance you'll finish it down to the last kernel whether you're hungry or not.)

The lesson from all this? Read the package and know what you're reading. And be aware of the inducements being used to influence your buying.

If you're an informed food shopper, you're more likely to be a mindful eater. And a mindful eater has a better chance of taking responsibility for a lifetime of weight-control choices.

A Tour of the Premises

Just about everyone who comes into our office will be taken on a shopping tour with one of our on-staff nutritionists.

Makes sense, doesn't it? If you went to see a personal trainer in the gym, you'd be taken on a tour before you touched the equipment. While you're not "going into training," and you may feel as if you know your supermarket pretty well, perhaps new discoveries await you in the next aisle or two.

A tour of the supermarket is really a how-to lesson. On our program, each person gets to have a personalized, customized tour with a dietitian.

While I can't quite match that level of individualization in this book, you already have two tools you can use when you begin surveying your supermarket. First, you have your own objectives. Second, you have your food diary. With those to guide you, I can come close to giving you a personal tour.

Stock Up

Let's start with those foods you can stash away for weeks or months—the ones on my Anytime List. The staples that belong in your cupboard or freezer include:

- Canned foods, including vegetables, beans, and fruit
- Low-calorie beverages
- Low-calorie frozen desserts
- Hard candy
- Condiments

With a good supply of these foods on hand, you can be ready to put together a meal at any time. Then just add to it with what's fresh that day or what's in season that week. Finally, consider the condiments to add creativity to your cooking and variety and excitement to your eating.

Begin your tour by wheeling your shopping cart down the aisles of canned or packaged soups and vegetables. These items are a must. Remember: Your eating program from now on is about choice. Give yourself plenty of it by stocking up on a range of options. Be limited only by the extent of products available on the supermarket shelf. While a bowl of soup can be a meal unto itself, you'll find that soups, like canned vegetables, have numerous uses in a broad range of other recipes. Stock up.

Be sure to get canned fish, too. I recommend tuna, salmon, or sardines packed in water or in tomato or mustard sauce. Besides

The Supermarket Psych-Out Layout

There is method to the apparent madness of supermarket layouts.

First, by dispersing staples all over the place, supermarket management forces you to walk past all sorts of attractively packaged and magnificently displayed food products. You have to pass by them before you get to the food you came for.

Food that's displayed at the end of an aisle is not necessarily on sale, even though that end-of-the-aisle rack may look like a special offer. Supermarket managers know that people notice those displays more than products on the rest of the shelves. So products with the highest markup are carefully positioned to catch your eye.

Shelf level counts, too. The first things you see are products at your eye level. If you have kids along, eye level is lower for them.

Notice where the children's candy and snacks are located—just about your waist level, where the kids will be transfixed by the sight of them.

being low-calorie, most seafood is rich in omega-3 fatty acids that are beneficial to heart health. In fact, any way it comes—fresh, canned, frozen, even smoked—fish is a winner for health and weight control.

Chill

Now the frozen food aisle. If you're the type of person who needs a quick meal occasionally, you may wish to toss a bunch of frozen low-calorie complete meals into your shopping cart, along with a generous supply of frozen vegetables and fruits.

The options are numerous—frozen light pancakes or waffles, light lunches, low-calorie and low-fat multiple-course dinners, and of course, low-calorie, low-fat desserts. Above all, don't forget frozen seafood.

In the Amber Fields

It's a good idea to have some packaged grains in the pantry. Choose whole grain, high-fiber products. These are becoming easier to find. Commercially packaged whole grains are available in many different varieties. Bulgur wheat, millet, and quinoa used to be found primarily in health food stores. Now you'll see them in many supermarkets.

Of course, whole grain breads, pasta, cereals, and crackers all have excellent nutritional benefits. They are good carriers of iron, fiber, and the B-complex vitamins. From the point of view of weight control, they're also very satisfying and filling—good "comfort foods."

But they also tend to be high in carbohydrate calories. My recommendation is to look at the starches as a lower-priority food—far below vegetables, fruits, legumes, and seafood in the hierarchy of best choices.

In fact, I recommend that you look for the light breads now offered by nearly every major bakery in every form—rye, wheat, sourdough, oatmeal, and Italian. Such breads are offered by the major brands like Pepperidge Farm, Arnolds, D'Italiano, and Wonder. All have 40

Multigrain? Look Again

In the lexicon of "natural foods," many descriptives are used to suggest that you're getting an overwhelming abundance of whole grains in bread or other food products. Some packages advertise "seven grain." Others laud the contents as "Made with natural brans," or "stoneground." "Unbleached flour" is often mentioned—as if every other kind of flour was mere chaff by comparison.

What it all comes down to, unfortunately, is absolutely nothing. If you want to find out whether a bread is whole grain—meaning that it's also high in fiber and other nutrients—look for the words "100 percent whole wheat (or other grain)," or be sure the whole grain flour is the first and only grain product in the bread. While whole grain products contain more nutrients than refined products, refined grain products—light bread, English muffins, and the like—are still good choices for the weight-conscious.

What's in a Lite Suds?

What's light in "lite" beers is the calorie count. To be considered light, a beer must have at least 25 percent fewer calories than regular beer. Most brands of light beer have about 100 calories in 12 ounces, versus regular beer with anywhere from 140 to 200 calories per 12 ounces.

But while calories are substantially reduced, alcohol content is only slightly reduced. That's something to keep in mind before you get behind the wheel of a car. Light beer may spare your waistline, but it can still make your head spin.

to 45 calories per slice. What's more, the slices are regular-size, not those wafer-thin slivers that turn to mush at the first touch of tuna salad.

As for cereals, try to find one that's a good fiber buy for the calories. Fiber One, at 60 calories with 13 grams of fiber per ounce, and All Bran/Extra Fiber, at 50 calories with 14 grams of fiber per ounce, are excellent choices for the calories.

You may also want some refined grain products such as rice, pasta, couscous, grits, polenta, and the like—but enjoy them in moderation. Have a small bowl of linguine, for instance, or a light helping of rice. Of course, you can add as many vegetables as you like.

Something to Drink

Check the Anytime List and stock up on a good range of beverages that suit your tastes. In addition to having diet iced teas, coffees, and low-calorie cocoas in the cupboard, you'll probably want unsweetened or artificially sweetened diet drinks, plus water, both flavored and plain.

Be sure to check the labels to make sure that no sugars have been added. As I've men-

tioned, you should avoid beverages labeled "naturally sweetened" or "fruit-juice sweetened," since they tend to be full of calories.

There is a profusion of low-calorie cocoa and coffee mixes available—from plain to exotically flavored. Most range from 20 to 50 calories per packet—a good thing, since it's probably best to avoid hot beverages that carry more than that.

Milk shake mixes are usually at the higher end of the calorie range. Look for those that don't exceed 70 calories.

For Your Sweet Tooth

In the frozen-food aisle, you'll find many nonfat frozen yogurts and sorbets that are on the Anytime List. Remember to look for the kinds that contain approximately 25 calories or fewer per ounce. Creamsicles, frozen fudge bars, popsicles, and individually packaged frozen fruit bars—at 20 to 80 calories per bar—are fine. Look for frozen fruit marked "no sugar added."

At the candy shelf, you may be attracted by the offerings of dietetic or sugar-free candies. The labeling is enticing, but while these candies may help avoid tooth decay, they usually have the same number of calories as

Sugar Surprises

You know there's sugar in such foods as chocolate bars, Coke, and Pepsi. But did you ever suspect that orange juice, applesauce, and most flavored yogurts also have sugar? Lots of it, in fact.

In addition to the sugar that occurs naturally in these foods, much more may be added.

Each half-cup of Mott's applesauce, for instance, has an additional 5 teaspoons of added sugar, which means one serving of that applesauce is more "sugarful" than a bar of Hershey's milk chocolate.

An 8-ounce glass of Tropicana Pure Premium orange juice naturally contains 22 grams of sugar—10 more than occur naturally in a 5-ounce orange. A cup of Dannon's French vanilla low-fat yogurt with raspberries has as much as 51 grams of sugar.

The whole story may not be apparent from the label. Since sugar comes in many forms, check the label for corn syrup, fructose, honey, molasses, sorghum, even fruit juice concentrate. It's perfectly true that there are many high-sugar, low-calorie foods that can be included in a weight-loss program—think of sorbets or hard candies—but beware foods that contain hidden sugar calories.

---

regular candy. Besides, eat too many of them, and they can cause bloating or have a laxative effect.

As you can see from my Anytime List, I recommend the real thing instead: chewing gum or any hard candy—lollipops, sourballs, gumballs, butterscotch, or candy canes. Like gum, these candies last a good while, so there's little chance you'll overdo the calories. The fact is that the longer something is in your mouth, the longer your brain thinks you're eating, so you can become mentally "full" by chewing a stick of gum or sucking on a Tootsie Pop.

Spice for Your Life

Load your shopping cart with low-fat condiments of every variety. If you've been hung up on plain yellow mustard—the kind that you squirt on hot dogs—now is the time to scan the mustard shelf and begin testing some of the incredible number of varieties that are now available. Or go for the ketchups, relishes, chutneys, barbecue sauces, steak sauces, fat-free and reduced-calorie dressings, fat-free or light mayonnaise, and flavored vinegars.

And don't miss the condiments in the Asian cuisine section. You have your choice of soy sauces as well as other sauces like hoisin, miso, black bean, oyster, and wasabe.

Like hot? You can get as fiery as you want with horseradish, cocktail sauce, and many kinds of salsa.

Anything that can add flavor and variety to food will be beneficial and important to your weight-control program. After all, enjoying your food is essential for both weight loss and a lifetime of weight control.

What's for Dinner?

Once your pantry is well-stocked with staples from the Anytime List, you can concentrate on fresh food when you stop by the supermarket or fruit-and-vegetable stand during the week. Just look for the food you're going to eat today or over the next few days.

In the produce section of the supermarket, you'll find the freshest in-season food. The more you eat of this food, the better. The more you can make fresh vegetables the basis of your diet, the thinner and healthier you will be. The reason is simple: Just about everything in the produce section offers the fewest number of calories—and the biggest fiber punch—relative to the quantity of food you eat.

If your idea of vegetables is limited to a salad with iceberg lettuce or the spinach your mother made you eat as a child, think again. Now within our global reach is food that's imported from all over the world. Each new season brings a new feast. And there are always new ways to deal with the old, familiar favorites.

How about Dijon coleslaw? Or curried pumpkin soup? Have you ever made a meal of a marinated, grilled portobello mushroom? All of them are culinary treats by any definition—and they're all made with fresh produce.

Branching Out

If you see the less-than-familiar in your produce aisle, why not take the opportunity for a new taste sensation? The global market offers many new opportunities. Try chayote from Latin America, a pear-shaped, mild-tasting vegetable you can steam, sauté, bake, or eat raw. From Japan comes the daikon radish—crisp and pepper-hot and looking somewhat like a white carrot. It's superb in salads, dressings, soups, and stir-fries.

Look for bok choy from China. Its stalks and leaves have a crisp texture and mild taste. Add it to stir-fries or soups.

Or what about these foods, now finding their way into the produce aisle? Jicama. Okra. Taro root. They're good news for any vegetable-eaters who savor new tastes.

Of course, it's fine to stick with the old standbys if you prefer. Have some beans, peas, brilliant-yellow peppers, deep-purple egg-

In Praise of Beans

Beans offer the person trying to lose weight a double dose of benefits. First, they are low in fat and packed with nutrients: fiber, phytochemicals, folate, protein, magnesium, potassium, zinc, copper, iron, and vitamins. Second, the potential they offer for culinary creativity is as staggering as their variety. From Cuban black beans and rice to Indian dal (lentils), from Israeli hummus (chickpeas) to Egyptian foole (fava beans)—not to mention all the old American standbys such as baked beans, chili, and navy bean soup—you can eat a different bean dish virtually every night of the week.

plant, bright-orange baby carrots, mushrooms, Brussels sprouts, turnips, broccoli, watercress, parsnips, cucumbers, and many kinds of squashes. The range of tastes is almost as staggering as the recipes possible.

Yes, They're Good for You

My recommendation for fruits and vegetables is simple: The more the merrier. Nothing is better for weight control or better for your health.

All vegetables and fruits are high in fiber and full of all the vitamins, minerals, and phytochemicals that not only keep us healthy but also help stave off disease.

The high fiber content is particularly helpful for weight control. High-fiber foods can take the edge off appetite. Fiber is not digested or absorbed. They take up space in the intestine, thus contributing to a sense of satiety. So eating a lot of vegetables and fruits keeps your calorie intake low and reduces your hunger.

Better This Than That

There are a couple of myths about vegetables that I'd like to dispel right now. One myth is that vegetables like corn and peas, which are high in starch, are fattening. It is true that these and other vegetables are higher in calories than, say, lettuce or spinach. But they are highly satisfying and are great sources of fiber.

The bottom line? It's better to get your starch from corn and potatoes than from bread and crackers.

The other myth is that cooking vegetables destroys the nutrients. Not necessarily. In some cases, in fact, some nutrients in vegetables are more easily absorbed by the body after the vegetable is cooked.

Certainly, raw vegetables are very, very good for you. They're also convenient snack food, especially if you buy prewashed and precut salad greens, baby carrots, and the like. But that doesn't mean the raw kind is the only nutritious kind. Any style of vegetables—raw, cooked, canned, or frozen—is full of what's good for you. For a lifetime of weight control, you can't go wrong if you stock up on whatever fruits and vegetables are available. Eat them whenever you're hungry.

A Quick Tour of Fruit

Like vegetables, fruit is high in fiber, rich with nutrients, and low in calories. And like vegetables, they've gone global. In fact, the names of the most nutritionally dense fruits may surprise you. They are, in order, kiwifruit,

Try This Substitution

Instead of one 6-ounce hamburger, try two 3-ounce veggie burgers. What you give up are fat and cholesterol—about 20 grams of the former and 150 milligrams of the latter. What you gain is fiber and most of the other nutrients contained in the vegetables that make up the veggie burgers.

papaya, mango, and orange. Other tropicals, such as guava and kumquat, are also high in fiber and rich in nutrients.

Kiwi, the leader of this high-nutrient pack, is loaded with vitamin C. In fact, this fruit contains about twice as much vitamin C as an orange. It also has hearty amounts of potassium, magnesium, and numerous phyto-chemicals.

Once considered exotic, most of these tropical fruits are now available at nearly every supermarket.

Another option is dried fruit. Chewy and sweet, dried fruit is so delicious that you might wonder whether it has any of the good qualities of fresh fruit. And what about calories?

Well, many kinds of dried fruit have the same calories as fresh. A plum has 25 calories, and so does a prune. A fresh apricot has 16 calories, and so does a dried apricot. Unsweetened figs, dates, and pears have no more calories when they're dried than they did when they were fresh-picked.

But you have to check the labels on some other kinds of dried fruit. Dried pineapple and papaya, unless labeled "no sugar added," usually contain a lot of sugar and more calories than the fresh fruit.

And stay away from banana chips. They're not simply dried—they're fried in fat, like potato chips. As a result, they have about the same number of calories as potato chips, in the neighborhood of 150 calories per ounce.

Banana chips, like fresh bananas, do have potassium, and that's certainly a plus. But you're far better off getting the potassium from a fresh banana instead of the fried, high-calorie chips.

Dairy Do's and Don'ts

In the dairy aisle, you may hear the echo of your mother's voice. Remember when you were a kid and she kept telling you, "Milk is good for you"? Well, it turns out this may not be the case.

Recent research has turned up evidence that milk and other dairy products may contribute to breast cancer, ovarian cancer, even diabetes—and substituting nonfat dairy products will not eliminate these risks. Two substances in milk seem to be linked to breast cancer—estrogen and an insulin-like substance called IGF-1. When estrogen and IGF-1 come together, each one increases the effect of the other. Unfortunately, this harmful combination occurs in low-fat and fat-free milk as well as whole milk.

In the case of ovarian cancer, the risk comes from galactose, a break-down product of lactose. New studies show that women who consume a lot of dairy products are more likely to suffer ovarian damage—resulting often in infertility, endometriosis, and sometimes ovarian cancer.

Finally, early exposure to cow's milk has been shown to increase the risk of insulin-dependent diabetes later in life.

In addition to posing these health risks, milk may also be less helpful in preventing bone loss than we once thought. Since milk and many other dairy products are high in calcium, doctors long assumed that dairy products could help prevent osteoporosis that frequently makes our bones more fragile as we age.

New evidence contradicts this assumption. In countries where people consume the most dairy products, doctors have reported the

Soy Subs

Keep soy products in mind as substitutes for milk products. Instead of enduring the taste of fat-free cheeses, for instance, you can enjoy a delicious soy replacement like scallion tofu cream cheese. Soy products are good replacements for many other kinds of dairy products as well, including milk, yogurt, and sour cream. Even if the soy replacement contains a small amount of fat, it's the good kind; soy oil is extremely healthy. With so many potential problems associated with milk, there are many compelling reasons to find substitutes for dairy in your diet.

highest incidence of osteoporosis-related hip fractures.

Now we're beginning to understand the reason: Animal protein (including dairy) actually stimulates the loss of calcium through the kidneys. And it's this loss of calcium that can help accelerate the pace of osteoporosis.

Fatter

Another issue with dairy products is their fat content. Unless they're fat-free (like skim milk), dairy products contain highly saturated fat. This is the very worst kind. Many dairy products, such as milk, yogurt, sour cream, cream cheese, and other cheeses, come in very low fat and nonfat versions. This can make a significant difference. Fat-free Cheddar cheese might have 35 calories per ounce, while regular Cheddar has more than three times that amount—about 110 calories per ounce. (Unfortunately, many fat-free dairy products leave something to be desired in the flavor and texture department. My own view is that fat-free mozzarella, for example, serves only one purpose: to plug the hole in the sole of your shoe.)

If you choose to eat dairy and think you can dodge the fat issue, be sure to read the labels carefully. Some low-fat cheese is really just lower-fat. The range can be confusing. A "light" cheese might offer as little as 40 calories and 2 grams of fat per ounce. Another, "reduced-fat" cheese might have 90 calories and 6 grams of fat per ounce—which puts it in the range of a really good Brie.

Go Fish!

Because fish carry a considerable amount of muscle on their spindly little skeletons, and since protein comes from muscle, they are an exceptionally good source of complete protein. They also supply a wealth of iron and other minerals.

In addition, fish are rich in vitamins. And they contain essential fatty acids—like omega-3's and omega-6's—that your body requires for turning food into energy (the process of metabolism). In fact, fish are the only animals that carry these good kinds of fat. And the richer the fish, the more good fat there is.

To top off all these benefits, fish are low in calories. So, for purposes of weight control, they're almost a perfect food. You can eat fish any way you like—filleted, skinned, or whole, fresh, smoked, frozen, or canned. Or help yourself to sushi.

Tuna and shrimp are the two most popular kinds of seafood in the country—and both are fine. But why not try monkfish, skate, tilefish, smoked whitefish, smoked trout—and on and on? They, like all fish, are very low in saturated fat.

Meet the Meats and Poultry

I am not going to lecture you on the benefits of a vegetarian diet. I *am* going to tell you that it's certainly a very healthy way to eat, and I am going to try to acquaint you with tasty meat and poultry substitutes.

An increasingly wide range of soy products is available today to replace meat and poultry foods like hot dogs, hamburgers, Italian sausage, meatballs, even turkey salad. Tried any recently? They're surprisingly tasty. Even the leanest meat or poultry cannot compete with these products for low calories and health benefits.

If and when you do eat meat, look for particularly lean cuts. I recommend round, top, or loin cuts for ground meat. Look for labels that say the meat is 95 percent lean or higher. If you want cold cuts, look for fat-free versions. The maximum should be 2 grams of fat per serving.

Skinless poultry is somewhat better for you than red meat because it's lower in fat. But I have trouble giving wholehearted endorsement to chicken because it has a higher concentration of certain cancer-causing substances than red meat. Again, soy replacements make more sense.

In general, there are better sources of protein and iron than you'll find in red meat and poultry. So when you eat a meat or poultry dish, eat sparingly.

Why Soy So Often?

As you can probably tell, I'm a great fan of soy products for everyone—but especially for anyone trying to lose weight. There are a number of reasons for my enthusiasm.

Soybeans, despite the name, are members of the pea family and were first discovered more than 5,000 years ago in Asia. Their in-

Concealed Calories in "Reduced-Fat"

When you see the label "reduced-fat," you may think you've found something that can help you lose weight. But before you take the product to the check-out counter, check the calorie count. Manufacturers tend to compensate for the lower fat in many of these products by loading them with sugar and other carbohydrates.

The result? Often, the calorie reduction is minimal. For example, 2 tablespoons of reduced-fat Skippy Super Chunk peanut butter has 12 grams of fat and 190 calories. The regular version has 17 grams of fat—but the same number of calories.

A Bone to Pick with Chicken

A number of research reports have warned that cooked red meat may contain cancer-causing agents called heterocyclic amines. Many people assumed that these substances were found only in red meat.

Now there's evidence that chicken may carry the same risk—perhaps even higher. The National Cancer Institute has reported that chicken has even more of these carcinogens than red meat. Whether you broil, fry, or barbecue the chicken, the level of these amines climbs steadily upward the longer it's cooked.

troduction revolutionized the region's diet, and soybeans came to be regarded as a sacred crop. During the past 5 millennia of experimentation and invention, Asian chefs have perfected the art of working with soybeans, steadily expanding the range of foods made with this excellent culinary product. Although soybeans have only been cultivated in the United States since 1765, their health benefits and culinary potential are finally beginning to catch on with the public at large.

Today, we can get soy milk, tofu, tempeh, miso, and, of course, soy sauce. But there's far more as well. More than 2,000 new soy products can be found on the shelves of supermarkets. If you're in search of soy, you can find a food fit for almost any taste and any occasion.

More Bean Benefits

In a study that included people from 59 different countries, researchers showed that the incidence of fatal prostate cancer was inversely related to the intake of soy products. In other words, the more soy that people ate, the lower the rate of fatal prostate cancer.

Soy was four times more likely to prevent prostate cancer than any other ingredient in the diet.

In Asian countries where soy has long been a culinary staple, the incidence of breast and prostate cancer is far below that of Western countries. Recent studies in the United States, Japan, and China confirm that even one serving of soy per day can halve the risk of colon, rectal, lung, and breast cancer.

The key weapon appears to be genistein, an important estrogen-like substance that seems to suppress the growth of certain cancer cells. In addition to prostate cancers, the genistein in soy may lower your risk of breast cancer, colon cancer, and lung cancer.

Genistein may also be the secret weapon protecting calcium in the bone and thereby helping to prevent osteoporosis. Compare this to dairy products, in which the animal protein is now thought to promote osteoporosis by inducing calcium loss through the kidneys. Soy protein, on the other hand, has just the opposite effect: It helps protect the calcium in your bones.

Say "Soy"

These days, you'll find more healthful, low-calorie soy products than ever before. Check your local market for hot dogs, sausage, and Canadian bacon—all made with soy. You can also find lunchmeat, jerky, and a number of different kinds of burgers, including the Boca burger.

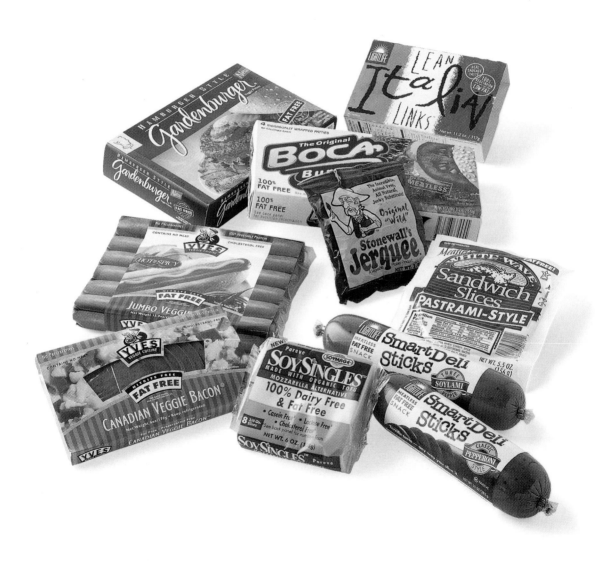

This legume is also cost-effective. A single acre sown with soybeans can produce sufficient protein to sustain a person for 7 years. (For the sake of comparison, consider that an acre of grazing range for cattle produces only about 58 pounds of meat—just enough protein to keep someone well-fed for about 2½ months.)

In addition to its other virtues, soy packs a sensational nutritional wallop. As a protein source, it is comparable to meat and eggs. It also contains iron, B vitamins, calcium, and zinc.

With soy, you'll get a power-packed supply of good health. And nearly all soy foods that are considered "substitutes"—like soy burgers—have fewer calories than the foods or ingredients they're replacing.

The Gourmet in Your Soul

This is not a cookbook, and I am not a chef. I am far more at home in the medical office than in the kitchen. But there are some tips on food preparation that make sense even to me.

First of all, it seems to me that the shopping tour we've just been on offers plenty of room for culinary creativity. Even I could probably put together a tasty meal out of a package of soup, a can of beans, and salad fixings. And I can imagine how a real cook, someone with an understanding of herbs and spices and an appreciation for the use of condiments, could turn a plain old bowl of soup and a bean salad into the gourmet's equivalent of a smash hit.

So my first cooking tip is this: Be willing to explore the possibilities.

Second, as we said back in chapter 3, grill, steam, bake, poach, or sauté your food; don't fry it. Frying by definition is a fat-adding, high-calorie cooking process. It's bad for your health and bad for your waistline. (Notice how frequently the two go together!)

My third cooking tip has to do with taste—all-important for achieving weight control over a lifetime—and it focuses on all those condiments in the Anytime List. The tip itself it simple: Open the bottle. Open up the Worcestershire sauce or hoisin or salsa or the jar of Pommery mustard or the can of tomato puree and use the contents liberally.

Brush your own version of a sauce or marinade over vegetables before putting them on the grill. Spice up a tomato paste with tamari sauce and lemon juice instead of using just plain old ketchup on your soy burger. Doctor your bottle of low-calorie creamy ranch dressing with grated Parmesan cheese, mustard, or salsa. Perhaps add some curry or maybe a touch of ginger to season your salad.

If you constantly try out these condiments, you'll soon find out what tastes good—even without the help of a cookbook. You'll discover that you can use that low-calorie ranch dressing as a marinade for a fillet of fish, then sprinkle on garlic powder and onion flakes and other herbs and spices. Try mixing a can of black beans with a can of corn kernels, add some chopped-up red pepper and onions, cover with mustard and balsamic vinegar—then eat as a salad or a salsa. Poach a salmon fillet and eat it chilled with low-fat sour cream and dill or with an Indian raita made of low-

Some Medium-Rare Problems with Meat

We've long known that undercooked meat can pose a threat to your health. Some meat contains the dangerous E. coli bacteria. A new and particularly aggressive strain of salmonella bacteria is also a potential danger. Found in raw or undercooked poultry, eggs, or meat, this form of salmonella is proving resistant to antibiotics.

On top of that, now comes news that cooked meat can also cause problems. Certain carcinogens in cooked meat can lead to colon cancer and breast cancer. The culprits are the heterocyclic amines, which are generated by the process of heating meat, whether it's being broiled in the oven, pan-fried, or barbecued on the grill. Studies in both Finland and the United States confirm that it's the carcinogens in well-cooked meat rather than the fat content that create a higher risk of breast cancer.

In fact, meat consumption in general is now thought to increase the risk of cancer in both men and women. A long-running study of 22,000 health professionals showed that men who made meat their main dish five or six times a week were 2.5 times more likely to get prostate cancer than men who ate little or no meat. Another study showed that the risk of colorectal cancer was greater in people who ate a substantial amount of meat.

In general, the health care costs for people who eat meat are far higher than the medical costs for vegetarians or even semi-vegetarians. It's something to chew on.

fat yogurt, cucumber, cumin, lemon, and garlic.

In short, be creative. You may discover a superb new dish, a hidden talent for creating chutneys, or a special liking for Brussels sprouts. The point is to not feel deprived, to not be bored. With a pantry and freezer stocked with all the vast array of choices on the Anytime List and in the market, you'll be able to prepare food that's tasty as well as low-calorie and healthful.

Eating is a pleasure as well as a necessity. Being mindful of calories may be a necessity—but that shouldn't take anything from the pleasure.

Chapter 8

THE EXERCISE COMPONENT

*E*very health professional in the country advises patients that exercise is important. Every new piece of research confirms it. Every reader of newspapers is aware of it.

Exercise helps prevent disease by strengthening your immune system. It makes you feel better, sleep better, work better. It improves your appearance. It raises your energy level. It even lifts your mood. And, proven beyond all doubt, exercise helps you lose and control weight.

The connection between exercise and weight control is as simple as it is obvious: Exercise burns calories. Specifically, exercise builds and strengthens muscles, and muscle cells burn calories more efficiently than fat cells do. And since weight loss is a matter of using up more calories than you take in, exercise is an important part of the weight-loss battle.

But there are other factors as well—some hidden but proven virtues that also play a big role. Exercise can actually decrease appetite. And, just as important, exercise can reduce the stress that so often *influences* appetite.

In fact, the ultimate equation for weight loss in this book can be summed up pretty simply: lower-calorie food choices + walking and/or light home exercise (and/or structured exercise) = weight loss and weight control for life.

Research increasingly confirms that even short bouts of exercise, spaced intermittently throughout the day, enhance your overall fitness and contribute to weight control. A brisk walk up and down stairs, 10 minutes of lifting homemade weights, a quarter of an hour on the stationary bike all provide boosts to your system. And, say researchers, what counts is the total accumulation of exercise in a 24-hour period. In other words, whenever you exercise, it's beneficial.

Starting on the Right Foot

If you're starting the weight-loss program in this book and you're not now involved in regular exercise, it's time to start an exercise program as well. Together, exercise and healthful, low-calorie food choices can help you control your weight for the rest of your life—and can also help keep you fit, trim, vigorous, and the picture of health.

Of course, say the word *exercise* and the picture that inevitably comes to mind is that of the professional athlete. That's not what I expect. It's both unrealistic and unnecessary for you to become Jackie Joyner-Kersee lofting into the air for the long jump, or Lance Armstrong looking like he barely feels the strain as he heads his bike uphill in the French Alps. Both of these athletes are certainly

238

worthy standards to aim for, but that level of training and fitness isn't what you need to help you with weight loss.

In fact, for the kind of exercise I'm suggesting, you don't need to join a gym or buy fancy equipment. You don't even need to take up a sport. All of those are fine ideas, but if you don't particularly like sports, or you don't like the expense and ambience of a health club, or you're not into exercise equipment, you still have lots of opportunities for exercise. There's only one slight challenge: getting enough of it.

I want you to approach physical activity with the same awareness with which you're now learning to approach your food choices. The information and the photographs in this book help you understand your low-calorie options among foods. In the same way, with some awareness of your exercise options, you can get in the habit of choosing the energetic, more physically demanding option among available activities.

Choose to Move

The fact is that we live in a sedentary age.

Once upon a time, our forebears had to hustle just to live. Eating meant going out on hunting and gathering expeditions every day. To get enough food, our ancestors had to do a significant amount of walking, running, and climbing. The necessity for warmth and light meant gathering fuel. This entailed more walking, more gathering, plus the furious activity of rubbing together two sticks—humankind's first non-regulation exercise equipment.

Of course, driving to the supermarket doesn't involve the same caloric burn as hunting wild bison. And we're paying a price for our indolence. We've also come a long way from the era of our grandparents. They at

Exercise and Triglycerides

Some recent studies are shedding light on the effects of exercise on triglycerides, a type of fat that contributes to cardiovascular disease. It has long been suspected that the influx of these fats into the bloodstream after eating—especially after heavy eating—actually damages blood vessels. The more rapidly the triglycerides can be cleared out of the blood, therefore, the lower the risk of heart disease.

Exercise, it has now been shown, increases the body's enzyme that breaks down triglycerides and thus gets them out of the bloodstream fast.

In one study conducted in England, researchers measured the triglyceride levels among two groups of women both before and after they walked. The first group was asked to walk at a moderate pace for 1 hour while the second group walked for 2 hours. The next day, all the women were fed a high-fat meal. Those who had walked for 1 hour showed a 12-percent lower trigylceride level, while the 2-hour walkers reduced their postmeal triglyceride levels by 23 percent.

The equation is simple: More walking equals faster breakdown of triglycerides, which equals lower coronary risk.

Flexing through the Next Traffic Jam

Cut the stress of your road trip and burn calories at the same time. While waiting at a light or while you're stuck in a traffic jam, try these exercises.

- Press your lower back into the seat and tighten your abdominal muscles for a few seconds. Work your "glutes"— that is, squeeze your buttocks together.
- Stretch your neck down toward your left shoulder, then toward your right.
- Squeeze the steering wheel. Release. Squeeze again.

- Set your hands at nine o'clock and three o'clock on the steering wheel. Press your elbows together.
- Lift both shoulders. Hold. Then release.
- Leaning forward in your seat, press your shoulders back, trying to make your shoulder blades touch.
- Move your head forward and from side to side.
- Tighten every muscle in your body. Relax.

These are also great exercises if you're in an airplane!

least had to get up out of their chairs to change the channel on their TVs. Pretty soon, according to researcher James Levine at the famed Mayo Clinic in Rochester, Minnesota, "we won't even need to expend the energy to push a button. We'll just say 'bring me the food' and computers will operate on voice recognition. We'll become immobile blobs."

Organized, regular physical activity can help avoid the "immobile blob" fate. But the real antidote is not strenuous effort. Rather, it's getting more physical activity into our lifestyles. In other words: Move, and make movement a part of just about everything you do.

I call this lifestyle physical activity. As with food, it is all about awareness and choice. It means parking as far as possible from the supermarket and walking the rest of the way. It means taking the stairs whenever

possible. It means mowing or raking the lawn yourself instead of hiring the kid down the block to do it.

I'll also recommend some exercises you can do easily, right in your own home, to extend and expand the benefits of physical activity for weight loss. As with changing your relationship with food, the change in your relationship with physical activity is not aimed at overturning your lifestyle. The idea instead is to make exercise an integral part of what you do every day. Some form of exercise can become as much a habit as low-calorie food decisions.

When you are automatically mindful of both your food choices and your activity choices—when your routine consists of walking the three blocks to get a low-calorie lunch and then walking back—you'll be set to control your weight for life.

Exercise Basics

The experts divide exercise into three components—aerobics, strength training, and flexibility.

Aerobic exercise—walking, jogging, dancing, cycling, even climbing the stairs—uses your large muscle groups and works your heart, lungs, and circulatory system. By definition, aerobic exercise releases energy through the use of oxygen; it requires endurance more than power.

Strength training or weight-bearing exercise builds muscle tissue, and bigger muscles burn more calories. What's more, since we lose muscle mass as we age—about 30 percent of our total number of muscle cells between ages 20 and 70—anything that counteracts that loss also counteracts the effects of aging. And despite the name, strength training isn't just about lifting weights. Any activity in which your muscles work against resistance counts. That includes everything from playing soccer to learning the tango.

Finally, flexibility exercising—stretching—not only helps "lubricate" the body for effective exercise and for injury prevention, but it also improves balance and coordination while enhancing your physical performance. A regular program of stretching can also help retard some of the most immobilizing effects of aging.

Think of your muscles as springs. If they're short and tight, they have little room for range

Strength Training for Weight Loss

Human metabolism slows as we age. In fact, it's estimated that with each passing decade, the body needs 100 fewer calories per day. This would be an argument for eating fewer calories the older we get.

But there's an additional way to compensate for the reduced calorie needs that accompany aging. Since exercise speeds metabolism, we'll burn more calories if we get more intense physical activity.

As we get older, however, we probably have to strategize if we want to increase exercise and calorie burn. After all, we're inclined to "slow down" rather than "speed up" as we get older—aren't we?

So what's the solution? How can we get more of that "burn" going?

One solution is strength training. By counteracting muscle loss, strength training helps increase metabolism—by as much as 10 to 15 percent by some estimates. Just two or three strength-training sessions a week can help.

And strength training is *not* weight lifting. You're not going for a a bodybuilder's physique. It just means lifting weights in a very slow, controlled way to build muscle tone and burn calories.

Along with its other benefits, strength training can help you feel more youthful. While nothing can actually halt the aging process and its effects on weight, strength training seems to retard the process and mitigate the effects.

Table Tennis, Anyone?

The only racquet and ball game you can play in the house, table tennis is a highly effective calorie-burner, blitzing about 300 calories an hour. That's equivalent to a brisk walk, but table tennis also exercises the playing arm in addition to the heart and legs.

of motion when they're contracted. But if you stretch your muscles—slowly, easily, deliberately—they'll respond with power. Muscles that are more flexible and powerful also allow you wider range of motion. That can make quite a difference as you get older.

In addition, a slow, focused stretching routine is a great relaxation technique. It reduces anxiety along with muscle tension and lowers blood pressure along with your breathing rate.

Not surprisingly, the best exercise program includes all three types of movement—aerobics, strength training, and flexibility exercises. The perfect workout starts with a simple warmup. Then stretch. After that, do some aerobic and strength-training exercise. Finally, cool down and finish with another stretch at the end. You can do just about all of this in one perfect exercise that I call POW—Plain Old Walking.

Off and Walking

The perfect exercise is as close as your feet. The more we learn about the benefits of walking, the better it gets.

Walking is superb for heart health and for maintaining muscle mass. It is low-impact; it strengthens bones, it doesn't hurt them. It helps improve your coordination, speed, and agility.

Where weight is concerned, you can almost literally "walk it off," not to mention the fact that walking can give you lean, shapely thighs and buttocks. And, of course, walking will put roses in your cheeks, clear the cobwebs out of your mind, and give you deep sleep and, more likely than not, pleasant dreams.

But there's more. We also know that walking can help prevent cancers of the colon and prostate. It runs interference against gall bladder problems. It aids metabolism. It helps prevent osteoporosis.

Walking has been proven to be an important preventive against adult-onset diabetes—type 2 diabetes. A recent study by the National Institutes of Health showed that brisk walking helped keep diabetes at bay and/or blunted its effects. The study covered 1,500 people, and the results held true whether the study subjects had the disease, were predisposed to it, or were free of it. All it took was a brisk, half-hour walk several days a week.

We're also learning that walking for exercise need not mean a lengthy "power walk" or an all-day mountain hike. Even brief, intermittent walks—say three 10-minute walks interspersed throughout the day—can make an enormous difference to your overall health and to your weight-control efforts.

For a while, it was popular to carry hand

weights or strap on ankle weights to enhance calorie burn and strength building. But I don't advise it. Carrying weights when you walk for exercise adds little in the way of aerobic intensity and may actually alter your gait, put pressure on your neck and shoulders, and even make you injury-prone. For more aerobic intensity, walk uphill, quicken your pace, or walk a greater distance.

Taking It in Stride

How can you get started? Just lace up a pair of comfortable, sturdy shoes, open the door, step outside, and go. You don't need special equipment for walking; you can do it anywhere; you can do it alone or with company, and the neighbors won't think you're loopy when they see you treading briskly past their front windows. After all, you're just out for a walk. Best of all, this is an exercise you already know how to do.

As with any exercise, start slowly at first. Move at a comfortable, easy pace for at least the first 10 minutes—or until you feel ready to pick up the pace.

If it's cold outside, dress in layers—long underwear (if it's really cold), then street clothes or workout clothes, topped with a sweater or windbreaker. You'll warm up as you go, and you can shed the outer layers—tying the sweater or jacket around your waist.

Count on getting thirsty. Pack a water bottle in a pocket or waist pack.

And the rest . . . well, just enjoy it. Swing your arms. Stretch your legs. Loosen your shoulders. Look at the scenery; it changes with the seasons. Hum. Whistle. Sing. When you get back home, stretch your body. Feel how loose and strong you are.

That's all it takes—just going for a walk two or three times a week. If you find yourself getting bored with the walk in your neighborhood, drive to another neighborhood or into the countryside. Try some other kinds of changes. Alter your pace. Speed up for 2 minutes, then slow down and stroll. Go into long strides, then drop back to a short, quick pace. Change the distance you walk.

Or try some hills. Pump your arms on the uphill, keep your knees soft on the downhill.

If it's raining or snowing, or the weather is unpleasantly hot and humid, you can drive to the nearest mall and join the early-morning walkers. Just before the shops open is a perfect time to stride through the mall—and you always have perfect conditions.

A Risk-Reducer for Men

A recent study involving 51,000 male health-care professionals has demonstrated that physical activity can lower the risk of benign prostatic hyperplasia, BPH, an enlargement of the prostate gland that causes frequent urination and is particularly common in older men. Walking 2 to 3 hours per week lowered the risk by 25 percent—not to mention its benefits to weight loss and overall fitness.

Of course, there's nothing wrong with walking in the rain. It's only water, after all. Just buy some good protective clothing so you don't get chilled.

The Work/Walk Options

Many people drive or take public transportation to work from door to door, but there are ways to introduce some extra steps in your travels.

If you take public transportation, you can get off one stop early or a few blocks from work—then walk the rest of the way.

If you drive to work, you may find yourself jockeying for the parking space that's nearest to the front door. What about reversing that trend? Park as far away as possible and walk to the office. It will clear your mind for the day ahead as well as help with fitness and weight loss.

Once you're there, can you walk upstairs for that meeting? Or at least walk at a fast clip from office to office?

What do you do on your breaks? If you get an hour for lunch, why not spend 30 minutes on a light meal and the rest on a brisk walk?

Exercises at Home

In addition to walking, there are many exercises you can do at home for minimal cost or none at all. In the same National Institutes of Health study where doctors looked at the effect of walking, they also discovered benefits from simple household chores and activities. Such light "exercises" as gardening and cleaning the bathroom carry many of the same benefits as walking.

Apart from routine activities, you can get special benefits from simple weight-lifting exercises. Not only do these exercises build strength, but they can also help sculpt your arm and leg muscles at the same time.

All you need are 3- or 5-pound weights. These are available at most sporting goods stores. Alternatively, take a couple of old socks and fill them with dried beans or even with pennies. Or fill a pair of empty 1-liter plastic bottles with sand or water.

Another alternative for strength training is the elastic exercise band. You can get these bands for about $3 a band in sports stores.

Be Happy—Exercise!

Research studies confirm what people who exercise regularly have long suspected: Physical activity can actually make you happier. Some long-term studies suggest that physical fitness and the ability to be active may make people less likely to become depressed. They also even suggest that exercise might be used to treat depression.

People who exercise exhibit a more positive outlook on life, studies have shown. And if you walk regularly, you're more likely to have a greater sense of well-being on a day-to-day basis. It stands to reason: With exercise providing the benefits of weight control, high energy, and feeling good, who wouldn't be happier?

Different Strokes

Swimming—or any water workout—is the perfect high-aerobic, low-impact exercise. It works the quadriceps, hamstrings, biceps, triceps, abdominals, and gluteus muscles while building stamina.

Swimming is often a good alternative for people who have chronic pain. When you're swimming, there's no jarring or shock to the body. With the water keeping you buoyant and supporting your body weight, there is no pressure on your joints or tendons. What's more, you don't have to know how to swim like an expert—even a workout in the shallow water can be beneficial.

They're sold under such brand names as Thera-Band, Dyna-Band, and Can Do. The bands have different ranges of resistance. In a package of three bands, the resistance ranges from easy to medium to high. The package typically includes an illustrated booklet on how to use the bands.

A workout of half a dozen exercises with these bands strengthens and tones virtually every muscle in the body. Further, the bands can travel with you. Just toss them in your briefcase or suitcase when you travel.

Hops, Skips, and Jumps

Did you ever jump rope as a kid? This may be a good time to try it again. It is superb for building cardiovascular endurance, working the upper-body muscles as well as the legs, and burning lots and lots of calories. It's also an activity you can do in the dead of winter.

Jumping rope is not the knee-cracking bone-crusher some people think it is. When you do it right, you're only jumping a little way off the ground, making jumping rope a fairly low-impact exercise. Plus, all you need is a rope.

Video Guides

If you haven't checked out the health/exercise collection at your local video store, be sure to have a look. The number and variety of aerobics program tapes are staggering. Aerobics isn't just jumping in place while moving your arms anymore, either. You can find exercise sessions modeled on everything from African dance to martial arts, from disco nights to belly dancing, from military boot camp to grade school recess.

If you think the same tape will eventually become boring (and it might), just turn on the television. Cable networks are chock full of exercise shows.

Stretching and/or yoga videos are also easy to come by. You might also want to check your local library or bookstore for books and tapes.

One caution, however. Remember to warm up before stretching and to warm up and stretch before exercising, then cool down and stretch afterward. Often the warmups and stretches are part of the video, but even if they're not, you need them to prevent in-

Monitoring the Monitor

If you're accustomed to watching yourself burn calories—literally—on the monitor on your exercise machine, be aware that the reading you get on the monitor is not really accurate. Even if you've entered your age and weight, there are many other variables that affect how many calories you actually burn. The monitor can't give you a precise calorie count.

What the machine monitor can provide, however, is a relative assessment of calorie-burning. In other words, if you continue to use the same machine, you'll be able to compare today's results with the results you get a week or a month from now during the same period of exercise. That way, you can see your improvement over time.

jury and to get the most benefit out of your exercise.

Static stretching is the safest kind. Do the stretch through the muscle's range of motion until you feel resistance—in the form of tightening or even the first stirrings of discomfort. Hold the stretch at that point for at least 10 seconds, then relax. Never go past the point of pain or discomfort.

Your Stairs Are Your Friends

If you live in a two-story house, you have a built-in health club. Walk up those stairs. Then walk down; then up again. Increase the number of times you go up and down.

Over time, you may want to speed your pace as well. If you live in an apartment building, walk up as many flights as you can; you'll find that the number increases as you become more fit.

Even if you live in a one-story house, you can get the same benefit from "step exercising." Buy a step from your local sports store. It may seem like a simple exercise to

step up and down from a single step—but if you pace yourself, you'll get all the benefits of stairclimbing.

Exercise Unlimited

If you want to go beyond these home exercises, you can, of course, choose from among a greater range of activities, including many that are more rigorous. Joining a gym is great—if you go regularly. Learning to play a sport is wonderful—if you can find teammates and if you enjoy it. And bringing high-powered equipment into your home, such as treadmills, stationary bikes, and the like, can be a big help—if you use the equipment.

Above all, don't be limited by the obvious, traditional exercise activities. There's a world of alternatives out there: interesting activities that are fun, that stretch the mind and soul along with the body, that feel less like working out than like undertaking an adventure.

Some examples? Pilates comes to mind. This is a program of precise, controlled movements that improve strength and flexibility without bulking up your body. Once the almost-secret province of dancers like George Balanchine and Martha Graham, Pilates has recently come into its own. Its non-jarring movements and stretches, often machine-assisted, are based on the theory that the abdomen is the body's power center and that its muscles can anchor strengthening exercises.

Then there's contact yoga. This variation on traditional yoga—itself superb exercise for balance, flexibility, and relaxation—is practiced with a partner. Nateshvar, the inventor of contact yoga, began as its sole practitioner—though others are being trained. Resistance comes from your partner's body, as you are lifted, pushed, and pulled through various stretching, strengthening, and relaxing positions. The fashion and Hollywood celebrities who have done contact yoga say it's like having had a deep-tissue massage. As I write this, Nateshvar is training yogis to carry the contact yoga word to studios and gyms across the country.

If you're more into forced discipline than New Age, you might want to try boot camp.

Yes, that's exactly what it is: an exercise regimen that imitates the basic training activities usually reserved for 18-year-old Army recruits. You'll run the obstacle course, hit the ground for pushups, jump rope, and run sprints before it's all over. It's great for the heart, and it's great for people who like a challenge and not just more of the same.

In other words, exercise, so essential for weight loss and weight control, isn't just dull old calisthenics or 20 minutes on a stationary bike anymore. And the new world of possibilities means there's really no excuse for not exercising.

The Spa Experience

Vacations, I think we can all agree, are a time when you should pamper yourself. You want to relax. You want to come back refreshed. You want a break from the everyday whatever-it-is-you-do.

But that doesn't mean a vacation has to be totally sedentary, does it? There are many pleasurable, amusing, and leisurely activities to

Going in Cycles

Did you know that cycling is one of the best forms of exercise available? It offers a great workout for the heart and circulatory system. With cycling you burn from 400 to 700 calories an hour. While you're pedaling away, you strengthen your quadriceps and even your abdominals.

Cycling puts little stress on your joints, except your knees. And if you keep the seat high, you can even reduce pressure on your knees.

As for bikes, you have your choice. Ranging from fat-tire mountain bikes to skinny racers, bikes come in a range of sizes and shapes. Just be sure to get "fitted" for the right bike at a good cycling shop—and also get a helmet that fits right. Once you're outfitted, cycling is a sport you can do just about anywhere, in just about any season.

enjoy on your vacation. Far from stressing you out, this is the kind of exercise that can give you a tremendous sense of relaxation and well-being. It's the kind of exercise that's of-fered at many destination spas throughout the United States and other countries.

You can visit a spa for just a few hours or for as long as several weeks or more. Among

The Martial Arts: Ancient Practices, Modern Variations

Most of the martial arts—developed thousands of years ago in the Orient—evoke images of high-speed punches and whiplash kicks. But that's only part of the picture.

Actually, to perform martial arts correctly, you need training to master the controlled movements. Even *judo*, the classic martial art, means "gentle way." Despite the grappling and throwing, what judo really teaches is the flexible use of balance, leverage, and movement. As an exercise discipline, judo develops body control, power, flexibility, and coordination while also enhancing self-confidence and concentration.

Karate, all the rage among suburban youngsters, offers a great cardiovascular workout while teaching self-defense techniques. It enhances coordination and strength. In karate training, students learn to develop a sense of fair play. After every contest, contestants bow to one another in a demonstration of mutual respect.

In *Tae Kwon Do*, students learn how to use their feet for kick-fighting rather than relying on their hands for defense. The discipline provides an intense strength-building workout that is good for cardiovascular fitness and for flexibility.

Like all the martial arts, Tae Kwon Do also helps relieve tension while improving balance and coordination.

Tai chi originated centuries ago in China as a self-defense technique—as well as a religious ritual—but has become the perfect gentle exercise for people of all ages. Part graceful dancelike movements, part slow-motion karate, tai chi is often called moving meditation. As that phrase implies, it's a great mind-calmer, but it also works the lower body and, of course, the cardiovascular system.

A sequence of tai chi forms takes your joints through their full range of motion. This martial art also improves coordination and balance, tones muscles, aligns your posture, lowers blood pressure, and helps you relax.

In addition to these and other classic martial arts, there are contemporary variations on the theme. Some exercise programs combine techniques from a range of martial arts disciplines. Others combine martial arts with other aerobic exercises such as dance, running, and boxing. Taebo, cardio kickboxing, and stepboxkickjump are just some of the names these programs use. Check your local health club or look in the Yellow Pages under "martial arts."

the 1,600 spas in the United States are day spas, resort spas, and destination spas. A day spa offers beauty, wellness, and relaxation programs on an hourly or daily basis. A resort spa has an "à la carte" program that's offered by the resort. A destination spa—the crème de la crème of spa experiences—is devoted exclusively to nutrition, fitness, stress-reduction, and wellness. Most destination spas offer an all-inclusive package for several days or weeks.

But why should a spa—any spa—attract you?

First, spending time at a spa is a great way to "get going" on an exercise program or to take a refresher course if you've allowed yourself to slack off. Second, the spa experience provides a wonderful vacation. It includes as much activity as you choose, along with training from experts in case you'd also like that.

Dining policy? Spas specialize in healthful, nutritious meals that taste delicious. If you happen to like cooking, take some classes while you're there, or bring home a backlog of favorite spa recipes to make in your own kitchen.

The other plus, of course, is what spas are famous for providing—all the pampering you want. Help yourself to a deep-tissue massage. Have a facial. Or what about a head-to-toe steam cleansing of every pore while you bask in the fragrances offered by aromatherapy?

Spending time at a spa is also a good way to accustom yourself to incorporating exercise into your lifestyle. Even though the spa experience is truly a vacation—time off from "real life"—you can still get into the habit of making physical activity an integral part of your existence.

In fact, integrating healthful habits into your everyday life is the whole idea behind the spa experience—the one thing all 1,600 of them have in common. What differentiates one spa from another is the way the experience is approached and presented, the spa's special style or primary emphasis.

Given the number of spas today, the variety of their styles, and their geographic range, it's virtually impossible not to find the one that's just right for your own needs. For the weight-conscious, I recommend choosing a spa that emphasizes not just the gym workout but outdoor activities as well. That's the best way to begin to make exercise an integral part of your everyday lifestyle.

Spa Shopping

Which spa should you choose?

You can find "the perfect spa" in every corner of the continent—from southern Florida to northern California, from the hills of New England to the beaches of Mexico. There are day spas, resorts with spa offerings, and all-out spas. There are spartan "boot camps" and super-indulgent luxury resorts—and everything in between.

The recommendations of friends probably come first. But there are other ways to track down a spa that has what you're looking for. And whether it's the super-expensive Golden Door in Escondido, California, or a single day at the Spa at Atlanta's Peachtree Center Athletic Club, or the Canyon Ranch Health Resorts, the idea, as one spa enthusiast has put it, is "to change your lifestyle." Following are some representative choices.

The Classic

At Canyon Ranch Health Resorts, you'll find what I think is the essence of the spa experience. These resorts are located in the desert foothills of Tucson, Arizona, and the pastoral Berkshire Mountains of Lenox, Massachusetts.

Canyon Ranch focuses on the commitment to a healthier lifestyle. But there's nothing spartan about this lifestyle. You get every amenity that a paying guest could desire.

There are facilities for a seemingly limitless array of workout activities. You can try aqua aerobics, weight lifting, boxing, cross-training, or even squash, depending on your preferences.

Headed outdoors? At Canyon Ranch, you can start the day paddling in a canoe or taking a hike. You can get in a bike ride before lunch. In fact, it is quite possible to stay physically active every moment of the day.

Apart from the rope challenges, there are many other things you might never have tried before. Maybe you've never even heard of them. You can have *chi gong* therapy. Take a seminar where you learn about Chinese herbs. See a specialist in acupuncture and find out whether the therapy helps some of your aches and pains.

Luxuries abound. That's the nature of spas. You can get a sage-scented body wrap. Experience a scalp massage. Or sink into a lawn chair and just absorb your beautiful surroundings.

The total package, in short, is an integration of physical activity and personal pampering. You get sound health advice for your life in general—and if you want advice on a

specific question like weight loss, you can get that, too. In short, this is just what the spa experience is supposed to be.

Patients' Picks

Clearly, I like what both of the Canyon Ranch spas have to offer. But many of my patients have traveled farther afield, and here are some of the favorite spas that they recommend.

- Cal-a-Vie, in Vista, California, is in the hills just north of San Diego. You start the day with some vigorous all-American activities—an early-morning hike, maybe water sports, then some strength-training classes—and spend the afternoon undergoing European-style treatments. Seaweed wrap, anyone?

- The Greenhouse, in Arlington, Texas, near Dallas, offers as many as 20 different classes in physical exercise. It also provides intense pampering and candlelit dining on healthful haute cuisine.

- In Catalina, Arizona, outside Tucson, is the Miraval, where you can ride horseback or pedal a mountain bike through the desert hills. Rock climbing and landscape photography are other activities that take advantage of the special topography. Or try some hot-stone massage, in which lava stones are kneaded into your muscles. People who have experienced Miraval tell me it's sensational.

In addition to these full-time "destination spas," as they're known in the travel business, many resorts have added spa facilities as an accompaniment to their mainstream facilities. My patients love the spa at the Doral in Miami, Florida—with 25 fitness classes and European body treatments, plus a separate dining room so you don't even have to look at the double-vodka-Martini-linguine-in-cream-sauce crowd.

Business travelers in particular should take note: Many of the luxury Four Seasons hotels worldwide now offer spa facilities.

Get Wet and Chill Out

The word *spa* comes from the town of Spa in the Ardennes Forest of Belgium, where crowned heads of state and VIP celebrities have been "taking the waters" since ancient Roman times.

But the custom of soaking in "healing waters" is also a tradition in the United States. Near many of America's natural springs, you'll find hotels—some very famous—that have spa facilities. These are great places to find stress relief and utter relaxation, in addition to receiving all the physical exercise and body pampering you seek at any spa. Here are some choices.

- The Greenbrier Spa and Mineral Baths in White Sulphur Springs, West Virginia, specializes in the private mineral-springs soak.

After your soak, you're welcome to take a steam bath or sauna, then a shower or spray.

- The Homestead Spa in Hot Springs, Virginia, features the century-old Dr. Goode's Spout Bath. But other activities are abundant. Among the outdoor activities are golf, tennis, and shooting.

Come on! "Relaxez-Vous!"

Okay, a French spa isn't for everyone. But this one is certainly nice to dream about.

A variation on the natural springs type of treatment is thalassotherapy—a range of treatments that make use of the therapeutic qualities of seawater to relieve stress and help you relax. If you find yourself near Paris one day and would like to try this therapy, head for Quiberon and the spa known as Thalassa Quiberon.

Spend some time in their jet bath, or undergoing hydromassage, or doing dynamic swimming exercises in the saltwater pool. If you just feel like stretching out, you can languidly breathe seawater mist charged with negative ions. Whatever your choice, you'll emerge with an exquisite sense of well-being.

Dance It Off

Want to work your heart, lungs, and circulatory system while also learning graceful movement, maintaining low impact, and having fun? Try dancing.

Here are just some of the dance exercise programs available at today's health clubs:

African dance, Afro-Caribbean dance, Jazz dance, Latin dance, Middle Eastern folk or belly dancing, and Reggae. All burn calories along with shoe leather, and all are great mood-lifters. Plus, you'll get inside another culture when you dance to their tune.

For the Calorie Counter

Want to know how many calories you're burning when you rake leaves? How about when you play a set of tennis? While calorie-burning results vary from individual to individual—and depend on a number of factors—the following chart gives at least a relative idea of how effectively you burn calories when you're doing different activities.

Activity	Calories per Hour	Activity	Calories per Hour
Cycling	400–700	Weight training	420
Running at 6 miles per hour	700	Gardening	350
Cross-country skiing	490	Low-impact aerobics	350
Tennis	490	Walking at 4 miles per hour	315
Pushing a lawn mower	420	Raking leaves	280
Swimming	420	Tai chi	280
		Yoga	280

After your Quiberon experience? Well, just return to Paris, head for the nearest superb restaurant, and feed your sense of well-being with healthful, low-calorie food choices!

The "Do It" Factor

Whatever exercise you choose, whether it's a walk in the neighborhood or a daily session with a personal trainer, the impor-tant thing, as a certain commercial says, is to just do it. It needn't take a lot of time, and it needn't leave you dripping with sweat and panting for breath. Quite the contrary. Research increasingly demon-strates that brief periods of even low to moderately intense physical activity have benefits. Where your weight loss is con-cerned, exercise is a necessity.

Chapter 9

THE PSYCHOLOGY FACTOR

Why do we eat?

Everyone knows the answer to that question: We eat to stay alive, to nourish our bodies, to gain energy, and to preserve our health.

We also eat for a range of different reasons. There's the social reason—lunch with a friend, perhaps, or a dinner party. There are cultural reasons—the Fourth of July picnic, Thanksgiving dinner, midnight supper on New Year's Eve.

Meals can be the focus of a religious observance—like the Passover Seder, to take one example, or the Easter dinner of lamb. We eat to celebrate—what's a birthday cake, after all?—and we even eat when we mourn, such as at a funeral lunch. And, of course, eating plays a role in romance—the dinner date and, to be sure, breakfast in bed.

But why do some of us overeat? Or eat when we know we're not hungry? Or eat ill-advisedly? Or eat when there's no obvious need or reason at all? The answer to those questions is not so simple. It has to do with emotions, with our own very individual, very personal psychology.

Emotional Eating

Of course, everyone eats for emotional reasons some of the time. You have an argu-

ment with your spouse, and you storm into the kitchen to fix a sandwich. Your boss reams you out for something, and you take yourself to a lavish lunch—you deserve it after that. You're waiting for your habitually late friend to join you for dinner at the local Mexican restaurant, and the minutes drag by like hours, and by the time he arrives, you've eaten a bowl of chips and downed two beers. Anger, humiliation, boredom—at the time, each seemed like a good reason for eating, as if food could "fix" the feeling.

For some of us, however, the psychology factor influences the totality of our relationships with food—the entire pattern or habit of our eating. That's why, in my practice in New York City, psychology often plays an important role in the weight-loss program. In fact, whenever a new patient comes through the door, we perform three "intakes" (a term used by health professionals). The primary intake is medical, looking at the problem of overweight as a total health issue. The second intake is by a staff nutritionist, who analyzes the patient's eating habits and relationship with food. The third intake is offered by a psychotherapist, who can help a patient identify the psychological factors that may have contributed to the weight problem, understand the influences on the person's eating

253

decisions, and manage the responsibility for making better decisions in the future.

Of course, no book can do that for you. A single chapter can't even identify, much less diagnose, the particular issues that are the psychological factors in your eating habits. But what is certain for everybody is that psychology is a factor. Knowing how it might be influencing your eating choices is an important component of the awareness that is at the heart of this book. To make mindful choices about food, it helps to look not just outward at the food options you have, but also inward at the influences that may be impelling you toward one option or another.

In my practice, patients have the option of working with a psychotherapist to help with the "looking inward" part. Ideally, everyone would have that option. I think psychotherapy sessions can help many people identify the possible root causes of their eating habits and deal with those causes once and for all, in a supportive, nonjudgmental setting. Certainly, that's a highly advisable thing to do. But even if you don't have that option, it can be extremely helpful to be aware of the psychological factors that may be influencing your eating habits.

Awareness for Action

Awareness is only the beginning. Once you're aware of an emotional issue affecting your eating habits, you can actually turn that awareness into action to control the issue. Every personal insight you glean thus becomes an opportunity for a mindful choice. And mindful choice is the key to losing weight and keeping it off.

For example, food obviously can't "fix" a fight with your spouse. Only honest and open communication can do that. What if you simply turned around in the kitchen doorway and went back upstairs to try to work things out? Or at least, what if you took a walk around the block to cool off? Those are two other choices—and for the weight-conscious, better choices.

Nor can food change the humiliation of being yelled at by your boss. Only doing better the next time can fix that problem—or finding a boss who doesn't use humiliation as a management tool. Until either happens, however, why not choose to spend your lunch hour getting rid of your frustrations at the gym?

And certainly, eating a bowl of chips and ordering yet another beer will not make your friend arrive any sooner or make the time move any faster. Wouldn't you be better off asking the waiter if there's a spare newspaper around, or using the time to jot down your to-do list for the week? And maybe next time, couldn't you choose to carry a paperback, or adjust the time you tell your friend you'd like to meet, or show up late yourself?

Mindful choice, in other words, isn't just about choosing among food options. It's also about being sufficiently in touch with your feelings that you know why you're making some of the choices you make—and can perhaps step back and choose not to choose. If you do decide to make the sandwich, go out to lunch, or order the third beer, your food choices will likely be more mindful as well.

Seeking Comfort, Finding More Stress

In the cases I've just talked about, the real reason for eating was to find comfort. The angry spouse, the humiliated employee, and the bored friend all felt frustrated, upset, and stressed out. They wanted to take their minds off what was really happening, and they sought a soothing substitute to do that. What they found was food—familiar, handy, easily available.

For the weight-conscious, however, finding comfort in eating is like rubbing salt in a wound. You're already angry or stressed or hurt. Eating mindlessly only brings you more of what you don't want: added weight and, as a consequence, extra guilt. For you, the soothing effect of food is so momentary as to be illusory. It's instant gratification, not lasting satisfaction. Mindless eating will not change the problem that stressed you out in the first place. That problem still exists, but now

Impractical?

Over the years, I've heard almost every conceivable explanation of people's reasons for eating. Unfortunately, some of these explanations are what I would call, simply, excuses. Here are some of the classic excuses for not eating right—and some responses.

Excuse #1: Health food—even fresh food—is simply too expensive. Eating "right" just costs too much.

Response: Actually, it costs less, according to experts at a number of research institutes. An experiment involving people with high blood cholesterol showed that eating heart-healthy food for 9 months cut more than a dollar a day off the food bill. For a family of four, that amounts to $1,600 a year in financial savings—as well as significant reductions in cholesterol level and weight, and significant gains in health.

Excuse #2: I don't have the time to eat right, and I certainly don't have the time

to cook right or to prepare elaborate meals.

Response: Well, how much time do you spend watching television? The average adult American watches 22 hours per week, and it's safe to say that not all of those hours are illuminating or even interesting. What's more, preparing healthy meals need not be inconvenient or time-consuming; see chapter 7 for some shopping suggestions. Further, eating right when you're dining out is increasingly easy; see chapter 12 for tips on dining in restaurants.

Excuse #3: In my work, I depend on fast food too much to eat right at lunch.

Response: Chances are your local fast-food place now offers low-calorie, reduced-fat sandwiches and salads. Or try combining a fast-food entrée with a more healthful side dish than an order of fries: maybe a salad from the nearby deli's salad bar, or even something brown-bagged from home.

you've added bad eating choices and the burden of guilt to the problem.

When you're tied up in knots, food won't unravel you. How can it? In fact, if weight loss is your aim, using food as a substitute for comfort often just ties the knots tighter.

Finding Another Way

There are ways to find comfort besides eating high-calorie foods—other activities, other strategies, and always, other foods.

Start by trying to substitute another activity. It should be something other than eating that will provide you with an equivalent gratification while you lower the temperature of your anger or hurt.

I've already mentioned the cooling-off walk around the block, the frustration-busting session at the gym, the paperback or notebook permanently stashed in the handbag or briefcase. Do this kind of comfort-seeking substitute activity often enough, and it will become just as familiar, handy, and available as those quick trips to the kitchen, the company cafeteria, or the fast-food counter at the mall.

As another alternative, you could work out a strategy for dealing with the cause of the stress—especially the kind of stress that you know from past experience is likely to send you looking for the bag of potato chips or the linguine with pesto sauce. Whatever the specifics, make the strategy one that works for your benefit, not against it. Then maybe next time, armed with the strategy, your awareness of the psychology factor at work will empower you to pass up the potato chips for the fruit cup—or even for a brisk walk in the park.

From a practical standpoint, having the right foods on hand is a big help. If you're well-stocked with the foods on my Anytime List on page 222, when you storm into the kitchen after an argument with your spouse, you'll find food that will give you comfort in a low-calorie way.

As for that friend of yours who's always late: Maybe it's time to stop meeting him in restaurants altogether, but if you do, at least it's time to insist that if he's late on this occasion, you're simply going home. Then be sure you stick to your resolve. Your time is too valuable to waste mindlessly scarfing up high-calorie snacks.

Strategic Thinking

Having time on our hands is the classic spur to mindless eating, overeating, and high-calorie food choices. As one patient put it, "When I have nothing to do, I eat to fill the time between meals."

The same thing goes for the lawyer who retires after 40 years of 12-hour days, only to find himself home, at loose ends, with nothing to do but make trips to the refrigerator . . . or for the young mother who at last has all three kids in school and finds that time moves at a glacial pace . . . or for the athlete with the broken leg who won't be able to work out again for 3 months.

Understanding the cause of the stress lets each of these people create a strategy for dealing with it—and keeps them away from the food pantry.

What is the cause of their stress? For all three, the thing that gave real meaning and purpose to their lives is gone, and they need to strategize a replacement, something other than eating that will add to their lives.

Maybe the ex-lawyer can volunteer his time and expertise to a local nonprofit organization that couldn't otherwise afford legal counsel. Perhaps the young mother can persuade herself to see her "empty days" as a blank slate on which she can write a new chapter of her life—maybe by going back to school, or volunteering at the hospital, or training for a career. As for the athlete who can't use his legs, he can still use his arms, and he can certainly still use his head. Maybe the local Little League could use another coach, or perhaps it's time to build up those arm, shoulder, and pectoral muscles with hand weights.

Finally, let awareness of how your own emotions work become part of your overall mindfulness about food. After all, it isn't wrong to eat a bag of potato chips or some penne à la vodka, a classically delicious dish, when you're in touch with your feelings about eating it. Simply knowing why you've made a particular choice may lead to another choice next time.

As always, I am not telling you not to eat nor asking you to deprive yourself of any food. Quite the contrary. I am asking you to be aware of a range of factors when you make your food choices. One of those factors is psychological.

Psychology Saboteurs

There's another way in which the psychology factor may play a role in your weight-loss program. Just as there are foods that can sabotage your efforts to lose weight and keep it off, there are emotional saboteurs as well. Sometimes the saboteurs are family

The Pressure to Eat:
Don't Take Orders from a Cookie

In just about all cultures, food has social meaning. It is the centerpiece of family festivities, even of national celebrations. As a result, there is pressure to eat the way everyone does.

Food can also have personal meaning. For some people, it is their best friend. When they feel alone, food is there to comfort them. As a result, many look forward to being alone with their food at night; it offers the comfort and assurance that they're not getting from other people.

In addition, billions of dollars' worth of advertising urges us to eat at any time of day—all day long. Television, billboards, and magazines are constantly pushing mouth-watering images of food for every occasion. Often, the "reason" for eating is no reason whatsoever. But advertisers would love for us to be constantly thinking about breakfast, snacks, movie popcorn, a hot dog at the ball park, fast foods, fresh foods, quick lunches, meals in a can, meals in a candy bar, meals in a tart, and lavish dinners. We can't get away from it.

and friends, but sometimes we do it to ourselves.

A classic example of self-sabotage is the I've-killed-the-day-so-I-might-as-well-really-blow-it syndrome. You're trying to lose weight, and one day at lunch, you can't resist temptation, so you eat a piece of chocolate cake. That kills the day. Since you're having a bad day anyway, you might as well throw caution to the wind and eat that piece of pecan pie you think you crave at supper. Since the whole day has then become a failure, you might as well forget the week. After a while, you stop trying to lose any weight at all.

That's a long way to travel from one chocolate dessert. What about just accepting the fact and moving on? You haven't "killed" anything. You've eaten a delicious dessert. There's nothing bad about it.

Think of trying to push a car up a hill. If it slips a bit, and you catch it and keep pushing, you haven't lost much. If it slips and you let it slide, you'll have to go back down the hill and start all over again. All that earlier effort will have been wasted.

It's the same in weight loss. If you eat the chocolate cake at lunch and keep pushing, you haven't lost much. If you let the chocolate cake kill the day for you, you're back at the bottom of the hill. You then have to "make up" the entire killed day before you're even at the point where you slipped just a bit. Why climb the same hill twice? Accept the tiny slip, and keep on pushing.

Besides, what's your hurry? This isn't a race. You have undertaken a lifelong commitment to a changed relationship with food. You can afford to lose weight slowly. If

things have become uncomfortable for you, wait for a while—even stop until you're comfortable again. Remember: Anxiety is natural, and weight loss is a change that can provoke anxiety.

When the Saboteur Is Someone You Love . . .

It happens more frequently than you think. The husband who has long nagged his wife to lose weight suddenly finds himself living with a glamorous butterfly. She's confronting the world in a whole new way now, and the dynamics of her relationships—with friends, partners, and spouse—have changed. You don't have to be a psychologist to know that a change like that can be scary—especially to the husband who lives with the butterfly.

Consciously or unconsciously, he begins acting in ways that actually undermine his wife's weight-loss efforts. He might start bringing home her favorite dessert or insisting on taking her out for lavish restaurant dinners. Maybe he just wants to "celebrate" her weight loss and doesn't realize that this particular kind of celebrating subverts her success.

Most likely, however, he simply doesn't understand the focus of her weight-loss effort. He doesn't understand that she's doing this for herself—for her sense of health and well-being, for her self-esteem, for her own very personal reasons.

She needs to tell him. She must open up those all-important lines of communication and explain exactly why she's doing what she's doing. She needs to assure him that she's not out to attract another man, that he's the one she loves, that she understands his discomfort but that he's reading more into the situation than is there.

Here's a perfect case where the individual can use psychology to overcome psychology, where the wife's awareness of what's going on can empower her to take action that actually helps bring about a new level of closeness in the marriage. When wife and husband communicate clearly, there's a good chance they can work together toward the joint goal of healthful, nutritious, low-calorie eating.

Awareness and Action

Have you ever noticed how many extremely accomplished individuals are overweight? I have. My patients include some of the most talented, cultivated, successful people you could ever want to meet. There's no question in my mind that every single one of them—along with every single person reading this book—is capable of losing weight and keeping it off. By understanding the choices available to you, you can be empowered to choose in different ways.

Adding mightily to that understanding is an awareness of the reasons for many of your choices, and an appreciation for how past choices may have led to current eating habits. Once you have that awareness and appreciation, you'll be even better equipped to eat amply, wisely, and well for life.

Food, after all, is not the culprit. On the contrary. Food can be—ought to be—a pleasure. The romantic, candlelit dinner . . . the festive Christmas meal . . . the blueberries you and your best pal picked together as kids . . . the haute cuisine banquet in an elegant restaurant. You want to enjoy to the fullest all the reasons for eating that this world has to offer. And you can. Knowing how your own psychology works gives you the power.

Chapter 10

Meeting Resistance— And Overcoming It

*S*talled?

Well, what happens when you know you're not losing weight anymore?

You were going along nicely, shedding pounds at a safe, steady pace. Then nothing. Not last week, or the week before last, or this week. Something has happened. Your forward movement has come to a halt. What can you do about it?

The first thing to do is to recognize that a slowdown in the pace of weight loss—even a complete stop—is normal, natural, and to be expected.

Part of the reason is physical. The fact is, your appetite actually increases after you've undergone weight loss. It's a natural reaction: Your body is simply fighting like mad against what it experiences as a "disruption" to its equilibrium.

Picture the fat cells in your body sending SOS messages to your brain—"Help! We're shrinking! Send fat!"—and you have the picture.

How does the brain respond? By increasing your urge to eat either larger portions or higher-calorie foods. Or both. You answer the urge—often without even being aware

that the urge is there—and that, in turn, can slow or stop your weight loss.

Part of the reason for the slowdown in weight loss is also simply that weight loss is a journey. Like any journey, it has gradual curves and steep climbs as well as speedy straightaways. It has slow lanes as well as fast tracks. This may just be your time to be stuck in traffic on a one-lane hill.

What Kind of Stall?

So there you are, creeping along. Or perhaps you've actually come to a dead stop. Is this a brief delay, or a total breakdown? A logjam you can break to get the flow going again—or a stone wall you can't get over, under, through, or around?

Maybe you're still doing everything you set out to do when you undertook your weight-loss program. It could be that you're making the same low-calorie choices and exercising just as regularly and vigorously as you did when you started. But suddenly, the things you did that let you lose weight before are not letting you lose weight. If that's the case, you may indeed have hit a wall.

Other things might be happening, though. Maybe you're making different choices. Maybe there's a subtle, almost imperceptible change in the kinds of foods you're deciding on, or in your eating patterns. Perhaps you're simply bored with the foods you ate with gusto when you started your weight-loss program. Or you're bored with making choices all the time.

Or perhaps for some "very good reason"—there's always a very good reason—you're exercising less than you used to. Maybe a project at work is keeping you in the office from morning till night, too early and too late to get to the gym. Is tennis the game that keeps you active? Well, maybe the problem is that winter is setting in, and you haven't been able to arrange for an indoor court—or figure out another kind of indoor sport that could replace tennis.

At any rate, something may have changed, and the change has slowed or put a halt to your weight loss. This kind of halt is probably a logjam. Find the snag, unblock it, and you can be on your way again.

When Good Enough Is Good Enough

If what worked before is no longer working, if you've been losing weight steadily and now can't do it, then here's something to consider. Maybe you've gone as far as a weight-loss program can take you.

And if your goal was a certain number on the weight scale—a number that now seems unattainable? What should you do?

Maybe you should remind yourself that this is the real world. Wherever you are right now might be the right weight for you. This may be it.

Does that come as good news? Well, not if you secretly long for a certain weight that you think is ideal.

Maybe that ideal weight is where you were 5 years ago. In fact, it might not even be a number. If you're a woman, the ideal is being able to fit into a particular dress that you want to buy—or were able to wear a few years ago. For a man, it might be a pair of trousers that you'd just like to be able to wear comfortably.

But if this is *it*, if you've lost all the weight you can reasonably lose—congratulations! You have succeeded in changing your life in enormously positive ways.

First of all, if your weight was substantial enough to have put you at risk for such diseases as heart failure, certain cancers, and diabetes, even a relatively moderate weight loss will have significantly reduced the risk. You will have dramatically improved your health and will have guaranteed yourself a better quality of life for the rest of your life.

You have also empowered yourself to make the choices that can continue to offer you a high quality of life. Never again will you have to fight the battle you fought before—and for much of your life.

You have done wonderful things for yourself. You have made an important investment in your future. Now keep it up—and enjoy the returns the investment yields: increased energy, enhanced self-esteem, and an improved appearance. The job of lowering your weight and maintaining good health by changing your relationship with food has been accomplished.

The Big If

There's another possibility. And only you can really evaluate what's going on.

If your weight loss has consistently slowed or stopped altogether because you started making *different* choices, you'll need to stand back and re-evaluate the dynamics affecting your weight-control program.

Is something else going on? Perhaps your relationship with food has changed. Or it's possible that you have made changes in your personal or professional life that are affecting the food you eat, the amount of exercise you're getting, and your motivation.

After all, you cannot solve a problem until you have analyzed it. If you think you've gone off track in your weight-control program, you need to figure out where that happened—and why.

Step back, take a breath, and prepare for a close look at your eating, your life, your work, and your motivation.

Re-Evaluating Your Relationship with Food

Is something changing your relationship with food? It may be an outside influence, or it may be something from within.

To find out what's happening in the case of a stall in weight loss, I've devised a special food diary. This is a kind of guerrilla tactic to help you find the resistance to your further weight loss. This tactic also helps you undermine the resistance once you've discovered it. I call it the Direct Action Food Diary.

As with your first food diary, you'll note the date and time that you ate and provide a description of what you ate, including the amount. Then you'll rank your degree of hunger or appetite on a scale of 0 to 4, where 4 is the hungriest. I also want you to write down what your mood or feelings were before you began eating the food, and the reason why you are eating this food now.

But there's a distinction between the first three columns as opposed to columns 4 and 5. In columns 1, 2, and 3, fill out the date and time, what you're eating, and your degree of hunger for *everything* you eat.

For columns 4 and 5, however, I want you to single out foods you consider either inappropriate or higher in calories than food you would normally allow yourself. For those foods only, write down your mood or feeling before eating and the reason you're eating this food.

After keeping the diary for a week, re-evaluate what you've written. Focus on the foods you considered inappropriate and turn to column 6. Ask yourself this question: If I had it to do all over again, would I eat the higher-calorie food today? In the same circumstances, in the same mood, is there another choice I could have—would have—made? What might it be? Write it all down in column 6. Finally, remember that the higher-calorie choice is not necessarily an inappropriate choice. What counts is the reason for your choice, the thinking behind the decision.

The point of using the Direct Action Food Diary is to heighten your awareness so that you can determine whether to make changes and what changes you could be making. Of course, awareness—being mindful of what you eat when you eat it and being able to see options—is at the heart of the weight-loss program in this book. It's the jumping-off point for the choices you make.

It's your choices, as I've often said, that ultimately determine your weight. The Direct Action Food Diary, with its expanded requirements, is aimed specifically at jolting you back into the kind of mindfulness that prompted you to take the first step toward initial weight loss. That's why it's important that you fill out the diary carefully, thoughtfully, thoroughly, and in "real-time" throughout the day—not by recapitulating from memory at day's end.

Some Scenarios

Let's say you're having dinner at a friend's home, where the entrée is fettuccine Alfredo. Ordinarily, you would not choose such a high-calorie pasta dish, but tonight you do—mostly because you're at someone's home, and you don't want to offend your host by rejecting what is served.

The fettuccine main course is followed by a rich tiramisu for dessert. It looks delicious. As you see it, there's a chance that you have already "blown" the day with the high-calorie pasta dish, so you decide to eat the tiramisu as well.

When you write up your Direct Action Food Diary that evening, you'll need to fill out all five columns for both the fettuccine

Direct Action Food Diary: When You Meet Resistance

Date/Time	Food	Hunger/Appetite Rating (0–4)	Mood/Feeling	Why am I eating this now?	Could I have made another choice?

and the tiramisu. Both are higher-calorie dishes than you would normally choose. But it's when you come to review your choices and fill out column 6 ("Could I have made another choice?") that the Direct Action Food Diary really shows its worth.

As you assess and evaluate the choices you made, it quickly becomes clear that you made one good choice and one not-so-good choice. Given the circumstances, the pasta dish, although high in calories, was a necessary and logical choice. It was the centerpiece of the meal; not eating it would have been truly insulting to your hosts, who had clearly gone to great trouble to prepare something delicious for you.

Your "reason" for eating the tiramisu, by contrast, was like letting the car slide all the way down the hill instead of catching it as it slipped and holding it fast. Now you could say that you were a victim of circumstances, and you had no choice but to surrender. But in fact, you could easily have begged off the dessert. All you had to do was say, "No, thank you."

Wouldn't that have been feasible? You could have said that because the dinner was so good and you ate so much of it, you had no appetite left for the tiramisu, delicious as it looked. In any event, rejecting dessert is hardly the same as rejecting the main course.

The point is that eating the tiramisu represented fall-from-grace thinking. You could have made another choice.

Let Them Eat Cake

Now let's suppose you're at your favorite restaurant one night, and New York cheese-cake is featured on the dessert menu. It's a dessert you love, in a restaurant that is justifiably renowned for its cheesecake, and, as it happens, you've eaten low-calorie meals all that day. So you make the choice to order the cheesecake, and you savor every morsel.

Later, as you review the Direct Action Food Diary and reflect on the choice of cheesecake, you affirm your reasons for making the choice—you wanted it and you had eaten low-calorie foods all day. Given the same circumstances today, you realize, coolly and rationally, that you would make the same choice. It was a logical choice, the right choice, not inappropriate.

Chip Choice

Imagine yourself at work, where the cheerful new receptionist keeps a bowl of potato chips on her desk—right along your route to the watercooler. Sure enough, on your way there today, you automatically dipped into the bowl and pulled out a handful of chips, almost without slowing down.

Even as you write this entry in your Direct Action Food Diary, you're aware of what was wrong about the choice. The chips themselves were not to blame. The problem was the mindlessness of grabbing a handful. Maybe if you were really hungry and were really in the mood for potato chips, this might have been an appropriate choice. But the truth is that you never asked yourself if you were hungry. You never considered whether potato chips were what you were hungry for, or whether something else might be available.

The choice of chips was inappropriate not because of the potato chips but because of the automatic nature of the "choice." It's not the number of calories that counts; it's the thinking behind the choice. The diary makes that clear.

New Awareness

Just these few examples are enough to demonstrate why it's so important to keep the Direct Action Food Diary. As you record the simple facts—meal by meal and snack by snack throughout the day—you'll raise your level of awareness and understanding.

What happens when you review the diary at the end of a week? Perhaps you'll see six foods that contain more calories than you would normally eat on your weight-loss program. And perhaps a review of the six finds two choices that were appropriate and four that were inappropriate.

The point is, now you know. You've achieved the desired result. You have a heightened awareness of what you're doing differently and why. And next time, given similar circumstances, you can make a different choice.

Along the way, you really have to stop and think every time you fill out the food diary. That in itself can be helpful. Many people find that the reason they've changed their food choices is quite simple—they haven't been paying attention.

As you do stop and think, you might find yourself applying a refreshed mindfulness to your food choices. And that's when you might find that you resume losing weight.

What looked like an insurmountable barrier may be out of the way. And your weight loss picks up its pace.

Has Anything Else Changed?

There are other possible factors, though.

Maybe the change in your eating choices is being propelled by a change in your personal or professional life. That change isn't necessarily cataclysmic or tragic, such as a death in the family. It could be something that seems innocuous and benevolent. Perhaps you just got a new assignment at work and are eagerly looking forward to getting it done.

All kinds of stress, as we saw in chapter 9, can have a profound impact on your eating behavior. As we also saw in chapter 9, that's all right, so long as you are in touch with the reasons for the changes in your eating.

Of course, when there's a change for the worse, we find many ways of trying to deal with our misery, depression, or sense of loss. Suppose you've ended a relationship or lost a partner, and you're dealing with the unhappiness of being alone. Or you're demoted on the job and your livelihood is suddenly in jeopardy. Or you may have moved, and on top of all the anxiety and confusion associated with moving, you find that a precious family heirloom has been shattered.

One way to deal with these kinds of stresses is to eat. It's all too simple: There's no need to interact with others; there's no need to think about your actions. All you have to do is open your mouth.

What's more, in our society, the fact of

your misfortune is generally regarded as a reason to eat. It is understood that you are "allowed" to eat when your life is troubled. You know how it works: a job loss, a death in the family, a spouse's sickness—if you're battered by such calamities, you owe it to yourself to find comfort in food.

This isn't necessarily a mindless or automatic use of food. It can be deliberate—and should be. The giving and receiving of food combines many emotional messages, including sharing, caring, and comforting. Your acceptance of food—or seeking it out—is also an emotional respose. The point, as always, is to be in touch with the feeling prompting the eating decision.

Good-Time Consumption

Any change, good or bad, can produce the kind of stress that makes you think of food. You may be surprised that good changes can create added pressure or stress—but it's so.

What if you marry and start a family? Suddenly, you're facing huge new responsibilities. Or you get a splendid promotion at work—and you wonder if you can handle it.

Coaching the Little League team can become a stress. If you win this season, you're under pressure to repeat the victory next season.

All these are positive events, and each one carries its payload of stress. One way to deal with that stress is eating. And that's sometimes what we do mindlessly, without even noticing.

What's Been Happening?

The bottom line of life changes? It could be the number that shows up on your bathroom scale. When that number stops going down, it's important to review your life, including your relationships, job, and living situation, to see what might be causing you the kind of stress that affects your eating habits.

Again, it isn't the food itself that's the issue. You may decide, for example, that your need for comfort is an entirely appropriate and valid reason for turning to food. So long as you make a logical decision to use food, you're still ahead of the game.

At the same time, it's a good idea to evaluate the ways in which some stress-filled events have affected different aspects of your life.

Two things in particular may have changed a lot—the amount of exercise you're getting and your degree of motivation. Let's look at those two areas.

Exercise

Re-evaluate your commitment to exercise. Has it slipped? Are you exercising less often? Less vigorously? When you go out to exercise, are you spending less time at it?

Even if you are making all the right choices in your eating, a change in the exercise that used to accompany your eating program can account for the slowdown in your weight loss.

It's always possible to find a reason not to exercise. Maybe you love to jog, but not when it's raining. Or the local exercise club has just upped its fees, and you dropped your membership because you "don't use it enough." Or perhaps your enjoyment of long walks takes a nosedive as soon as you have to put on winter clothes.

Exercise, after all, is usually something of a production. It requires special clothing, or at least a change of clothes. You often need special equipment, such as a racket, knee pads, or goggles. Sometimes, you need a team of people.

And exercise takes time. If you're putting in long hours at the office or your home obligations have increased significantly, the days already seem long enough. Fitting exercise into a busy schedule may seem like "just another thing."

Remember, though, that exercise is necessary. You might have to change to some other kinds of exercise. You might have to vary your routines to keep yourself interested. Or you might need to incorporate exercise into your lifestyle, as I've suggested elsewhere in this book, by mowing your own lawn, tending your own garden, and so forth.

You don't need a lot of exercise. But you do need some.

Motivation

Every year, the entire nation goes into a post-holiday depression on January 2. After the long period of getting psyched up for the holidays, after all the parties and late nights and family and friends and gifts and excitement, after all the champagne of New Year's Eve, the obvious next step is a long step down to exhausted disenchantment.

Your motivation for your weight-loss program may be suffering a similar letdown. You were pumped when you started the program, but it's difficult to maintain that level of intensity.

When you have been on your program for a while and have enjoyed its results, you may find that it begins to become a bit routine. The novelty wears off. The excitement abates. Instead of attacking each day with charged-up electricity, you feel you're just plodding along.

Some Cell Defiance

As I said earlier in this chapter, the very fact that you've lost weight has actually lowered your need for calories. Technically speaking, to maintain the rate of weight loss you've already experienced, you would have to eat less and less and less. Even then, the weight loss would eventually stop.

Of course, we tend to do just the opposite of eating less. All those shrinking cells are yelling "Feed me!" even louder. Your body wants to eat more—and it wants to eat higher-calorie foods.

A motivational dip is natural. No one can maintain motivation at a high intensity indefinitely. Presumably, once you've identified the change in your eating habits and the cause of the change, once you're again making the kinds of choices that contribute to weight loss, once you again see results, your motivation will also rise. But the fact is that it may not come back to its original energy level. And in a very real sense, isn't that the point? Aren't you trying to make weight control the norm? Don't you want low-calorie choices to be absolutely routine?

Don't despair! The slowed rate of weight loss is no cause for gloom. Don't evaluate your performance by the number on the scale. Think of the weight loss you have achieved, think of all the things you're doing right, think of how much better you look and feel, and applaud yourself.

Chapter 11

CHANGES

I don't even feel like I'm dieting."

This statement, in an astonished tone of voice, usually comes about the 3rd or 4th week after a person has begun the picture perfect weight-loss program.

It's the tip-off to me that the program is working. Whatever the final outcome in terms of the number of pounds lost, the program has been a success for this person.

It's a success because of what has changed and what hasn't changed. What has not changed is the person's lifestyle. What has changed is the person's relationship with food. Living the same life, going to the same job, feeling the same pressures and influences, the individual is nevertheless making new and different food choices, new and different decisions about eating. He or she is in the driver's seat—alert, aware, in control of direction and pace.

That's exactly what happened with the four individuals in our classic eating profiles in chapter 4. They still have the same jobs and the same relationships. They're in the same life situations. But they bring to their lives a new awareness about food and a new power to choose among eating options.

For these people, food is no longer the enemy. When they started the picture perfect weight-loss program, they thought of food as something to be avoided if possible—even regarded with dread. They enjoy food now, without fearing that they'll have to pay for the enjoyment with a later sacrifice, with deprivation, with dull, bland meals no one could enjoy.

Signs of Change

How did they do it? A comparison of their "before" and "after" food diaries—with portion sizes and calories approximated by our staff nutritionist—tells the story.

The "after" diaries are not "diets" prescribed by me or by our nutritionist. Instead, they represent the choices the four people made after working with all of our staff to become mindful about their food choices.

In each case, the individuals are eating the same amount of food—if not more. Yet in each case, their food diaries reflect reduced calories and much healthier eating. They're making better protein choices. Their intake of fruits and vegetables has increased dramatically. In the meantime, their consumption of saturated fats and refined carbohydrates has decreased dramatically.

And in each case, the individuals in our classic eating profiles are losing weight.

Susan: Before and After

If you are tied to a steady office job and you're required to spend a lot of time at your desk, you probably identified with Susan—the woman profiled on page 65.

Before she started the picture perfect weight-loss program, Susan considered herself to be obsessed with food. She lived in a state of constant fear of going off her diet, and at the same time, she had numerous misconceptions about what she should be eating. As a result, she forced herself to eat bland, uninteresting food that she was certain was "diet food." It was never satisfying or enjoyable; worse, it was not particularly healthy and, since it was high in calories, it was not helping Susan lose weight at all.

That has all changed. Susan doesn't fear eating anymore, and while she thinks about food, she does so deliberately, mindfully, not with horror. To her astonishment, Susan says she is "eating more than I ever did. I'm never hungry, I never feel deprived, and I'm thinner—and healthier—than I've ever been in my life."

On the next two pages you'll find two sample days from Susan's diaries. On page 270 is her diary before she started the picture perfect weight-loss program.

Things have changed, as you can see from her "after" diary on page 271.

Susan's day used to start with unsweetened grapefruit juice, which she never really liked very much but which she drank because she thought it was "burning off" fat.

What's the difference? The grapefruit juice was "only" 140 calories. But why waste calories on liquids? Besides, even unsweetened calories accumulate during the course of a day. It's much better to eat the fruit. Apart from offering much more flavor, the fruit is something to chew on, and it's fiber, which Susan needs. The fruit is also more filling, and it has fewer calories.

The "before" diary also included a dry bagel for breakfast. Susan simply assumed that, like the unsweetened grapefruit juice, it was "nutritionally correct" because it was fat-free. But she can save 340 calories over the bagel with an English muffin and jam—something she absolutely loves.

Lunch used to be dull. Susan would force herself to eat a white-meat turkey sandwich on rye for lunch on the theory that it was "dietetic." Today, she starts with a minestrone soup. It's full of beans, and beans are full of protein and fiber. The soup is also filling.

Another new lunchtime favorite is a baked potato with broccoli and salsa. These foods provide fiber as well as some essential vitamins and minerals that were utterly lacking in Susan's "before" lunch. Over all, the "after" lunch offers a nice variety of flavors and textures, is far healthier than the white-meat turkey sandwich, and is far lower in calories.

When it's time for that afternoon pick-me-up snack, Susan doesn't have to rationalize her way into utterly unsatisfying reduced-fat cookies. She munches on pretzel rods to satisfy her craving for salt, and then sucks a Tootsie Pop to satisfy her sweet tooth. It's not just tastes she's varying; the combination gives her something to chew on and something to suck on—for quite a while—thus satisfying the psychological needs to consume.

Susan's "Before" Diary—The Whole Day

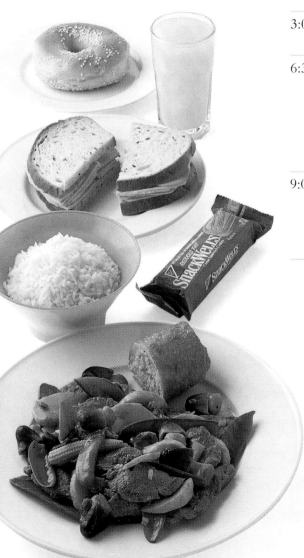

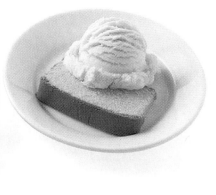

Time	Food	Calories
9:00 A.M.	Dry bagel	400
	Unsweetened grapefruit juice	140
Noon	White-meat turkey on rye with mustard	540
3:00 P.M.	Reduced-fat cookies (1 package)	210
6:30 P.M.	Chinese takeout: Steamed veggies with beef	420
	Plain rice (1 pint)	400
	½ egg roll	200
9:00 P.M.	Low-fat ice cream (¼ container)	140
	One slice low-fat cake, frozen	200

TOTAL 2,650

Susan's "After" Diary—The Whole Day

Time	Food	Calories
9:00 A.M.	Fruit cup	50
	English muffin with jam	150
Noon	Minestrone soup (1 cup)	80
	Baked potato with broccoli and salsa	180
3:00 P.M.	2 pretzel rods	70
	Tootsie Pop	60
6:30 P.M.	2 vegetable dumplings with dipping sauce	120
	Hot-and-sour soup (1 cup)	40
	Shrimp and Chinese vegetables steamed with black bean sauce	250
	Fortune cookie	30
9:00 P.M.	8 dried apricot halves	70
	2 low-calorie frozen fudge bars	60

TOTAL 1,160

Susan has always been mad for Chinese food, and nothing's easier at the end of a long day at the office than ordering takeout from her favorite Chinese restaurant. In the old days when she lived with constant "food dread," she would force herself to order a meal that was completely tasteless and not even characteristically Chinese. She was careful to stay away from salty foods and sweet sauces on the assumption that such things were fattening, but the prospect of bland beef and vegetables was so unappealing that she invariably "needed" the not-very-healthful egg roll as well. The result was a high-calorie, low-satisfaction meal that almost inevitably led to Susan's wanting more of something else.

Today, Susan buys a lot of Chinese takeout, but now she eats highly sauced, highly satisfying, very "Chinese-tasting" meals for far fewer calories than before. She has learned that the appetizers in Chinese restaurants tend to be fried and high in calories, so she makes a conscious effort to order soup or perhaps steamed vegetable dumplings instead. Her "after" food diary shows an evening when she has chosen both—but she dips the dumplings in soy and ginger, and the soup is hot-and-sour, so the taste sensations are very savory indeed.

For her main course, she chooses a seafood dish, thus saving considerable calories. It also comes with a tasty sauce, and it's accompanied by filling and nutritious vegetables. It's a much more interesting, certainly more tasty meal—and it has 580 calories less than her "before" Chinese takeout dinner.

In the past, Susan's sweet tooth was hard to control. She would treat herself to a late-night snack of low-fat cake and/or ice cream and find it awfully hard to stick to just one

slice or just half a cup. Now the treat is dried fruit, which Susan had always assumed was fattening, and low-calorie frozen fudge bars. Both are satisfying, but it's the portions that make the difference to Susan. Where before she had to struggle to limit herself to one slice of cake and a small helping of ice cream, the eight apricot halves and the two fudge bars seem more than generous.

"I'm now eating foods I used to think were forbidden," Susan says, "for fewer calories and more health benefits. I'm enjoying eating more than I ever did before, and I'm not constantly struggling to stay on a diet."

Susan goes to bed feeling well-fed and satisfied. But instead of the 2,650 calories that she used to eat in a typical day, she has consumed only 1,160 calories. That's nearly a 1,500-calorie difference—and not for one moment did she have to deprive herself or think in terms of dieting.

Stan: Before and After

Remember Stan? He was the business traveler who didn't understand the concept of moderation.

If you identified with some aspects of his high-pressure lifestyle, you probably recall his eating patterns as well. Stan was on the road as much as half the time, confronted by menus over which he had no control, and eating whenever possible to fuel himself for the next meeting, the next presentation, the next important decision. He was convinced that his way of life simply precluded control over his eating.

His lifestyle, Stan learned, was costing him. Because he was eating inappropriately—grabbing whatever was available, whenever he could grab a bite—he was pretty far along the route to overweight and ill health. Those two looming inevitabilities propelled Stan into my office to get help.

The first step was to get Stan to understand that he did have choices—wherever, whenever, and whatever he was eating. Once he understood that, the next step—making the appropriate choice—was downright easy.

Before he started the program, Stan's typical day looked like the diary on page 274.

As Stan started to make some different choices, his daily tally of calories plummeted, as you can see from the "after" diary on page 275. But he was actually *less* hungry than he had been before.

For example, consider that early-morning "bite" in the car on the way to the office. Where Stan used to munch on a 560-calorie bran muffin, he began eating a 100-calorie banana instead. He found it was just as convenient, just as easy to eat while he was driving, and just as healthy, if not more so. By 8:00 in the morning, Stan has already "saved" 460 calories.

Power breakfasts are still a big part of Stan's life. But his menu choices have changed significantly. In his "before" mode, Stan would have eggs, bacon, potatoes, and a buttered bagel, even though he'd already eaten and wasn't that hungry. These days, he orders melon, smoked salmon, and a pumpernickel roll. Adding up the banana and the power breakfast, Stan has consumed 400 calories before noon—instead of the 1,740 calories that were on his "before" menu.

Though Stan has a low-calorie morning, it's hardly a diet regimen. After the on-the-road banana, he has had a sophisticated, interesting, highly tasty meal. It's also extremely healthy—low in saturated fats and high in fiber. And with the workday just getting underway, Stan has saved an additional 880 calories. He's ahead of the game by a total of 1,340 calories—and it's just 10:00.

For lunch, Stan used to make an effort to diet—or at least to eat what he thought was a "diet" meal. Lots of people think of chicken Caesar salad as a light, healthy, low-fat lunch. Calorically, however, it's costly. A large tossed salad with shrimp and a light dressing is just as filling, much healthier, and has 450 fewer calories.

For a filling starch "hit," Stan has now replaced bland, dry bread sticks—which he thought of as diet food—with one of his favorites, a sourdough roll. That roll may be slightly more caloric than the bread sticks, but he likes the taste. And he can now well afford it. In fact, with a tasty lunch under his belt, he is now ahead by 1,780 calories.

When we explored his dinner menu, Stan and I discussed one substantive change in behavior, which he has adopted as a regular course of action. He and I refer to it as "deferring" the first drink at dinner.

Instead of a Scotch on the rocks, Stan starts with a club soda with lime. It's his assertion to himself that he is in the driver's seat of this meal. Back in his "before" mode, when Stan would quickly down his first Scotch and move on to the second, he found that he'd pretty much given up all sense of control over the menu.

The club soda, he finds, goes down just as quickly; any first drink goes down quickly, Stan finds, so it might as well be club soda. It also answers his beverage yearning and diminishes the total number of alcoholic drinks he'll

Stan's "Before" Diary—The Whole Day

Time	Food	Calories
8:00 A.M.	Bran muffin (6 oz)	560
9:00 A.M.	2 scrambled eggs	200
	3 bacon strips	300
	Hashbrown potatoes	180
	Bagel (5 oz) with 1 Tbsp butter	500
1:00 P.M.	Chicken Caesar salad, including 4 oz chicken	700
	Few bread sticks	150
8:00 P.M.	Scotch on the rocks	160
	Mozzarella and sun-dried tomatoes	300
	Penne à la vodka	650
	Roll and butter	220
	2 glasses of wine	200
11:00 P.M.	Large chocolate bar	280

TOTAL 4,400

want. For the same reason, Stan makes it a habit now to order a bottle of Italian mineral water—plain club soda would do just as well—as soon as he sits down. When he does order wine with dinner, he alternates between vino and aqua minerale—a sip of one, two sips of the other, back and forth. The result? He drinks less wine—and actually enjoys it more.

Stan also tries to start a meal with soup rather than with another kind of appetizer. His diary lists Manhattan clam chowder. It's tasty, chunky, and satisfying. Had he ordered the mozzarella and tomatoes, he knows he would also have eaten a roll or a couple of pieces of bread with it. The soup is just as filling.

Stan loves pasta, but instead of ordering a pasta with a cream sauce, he now goes for primavera style—pasta with vegetables. It's delicious, filling, full of fiber, and a saving of calories. In fact, the overall reduction in calories means that Stan can continue to enjoy his two glasses of wine and have a dessert—something he used to fight against.

Stan has just had a highly enjoyable meal. Since he had just the two glasses of wine with dinner—not Scotch *and* wine—his resolve to stay away from the minibar is still intact when he gets back to his hotel room.

Stan's "After" Diary—The Whole Day

Time	Food	Calories
8:00 A.M.	Banana	100
9:00 A.M.	½ melon	50
	Smoked salmon	100
	Pumpernickel roll	150
1:00 P.M.	Large tossed salad with shrimp and light dressing	250
	Sourdough roll	160
8:00 P.M.	Club soda with lime	0
	Large Manhattan clam chowder	200
	Pasta primavera	560
	Two glasses of wine	200
	Mixed berries and raspberry sorbet	120

TOTAL 1,890

Over time, Stan will save a lot of calories just by deferring that first Scotch and eliminating trips to the minibar. As it is, by the end of the day, he is 2,510 calories to the good over his earlier eating habits.

Here's Stan in his own words:

"I now feel as in charge of my eating as I feel about the other things in my life, like business. Actually, deciding among food choices is a lot like making business decisions. Different foods have different values to me now. There are more options than I ever knew about, and I can make informed choices.

"I feel much healthier. I'm more ener-getic. I used to feel crippled getting off an airplane. Now I feel light, eager to move. That's essential in business, because it really takes a great deal of physical energy to sustain effort and compete in today's business environment."

Diana: Before and After

Are you a parent who spends a lot of time at home with the kids?

If so, you probably identified with the profile of Diana. Before she started the program, Diana used to pick mindlessly at food throughout the day.

Diana's "Before" Diary—The Whole Day

Time	Food	Calories
8:00 A.M.	Few handfuls low-fat granola	300
8:45 A.M.	Small slice coffee cake	260
10:00 A.M.	Handful of cheese crackers	300
1:00 P.M.	Green salad with oil and vinegar	150
	4 crackers	60
	Toasted corn muffin, dry	480
3:00 P.M.	Ice cream bar	250
6:00 P.M.	Leftover macaroni and cheese (½ cup)	200
8:00 P.M.	¼ chicken (6 oz) Rice (1 cup) Vegetables (½ cup)	520
10:00 P.M.	3 chocolate-chip cookies	240

TOTAL 2,760

The "before" diary shows what used to be a typical day for her.

You can see from her "after" diary that she still picks at food all day long. But instead of doing it mindlessly, she shows some awareness of her actions. As a result, she is making better choices.

Diana can still nibble—and she does! She has a bit here, a bit there, then a real meal, then another snack. She's nibbling much the same quantities as before, but now she does it with thought. Her choices are lower-calorie choices than she was making when she kept her "before" food diary. Those choices are also far more healthful.

Obviously, her routine has changed in some ways—and so have her eating habits. She feeds her kids Cheerios for breakfast now, so when she scoops up a handful of their leftovers, she is saving a lot of calories. She isn't sacrificing much in the way of health benefits, either. While granola has a great reputation for being a healthful food, Cheerios are also a whole-grain cereal with plenty of nutrition and fewer calories.

When she wants to nibble again at 8:45 in the morning, and again at 10:00, Diana goes right to the refrigerator or the pantry. Both are stocked with foods from the Anytime List described in chapter 7, so she is confident that

Diana's "After" Diary—The Whole Day

Time	Food	Calories
8:00 A.M.	Few handfuls Cheerios	80
8:45 A.M.	Banana	100
10:00 A.M.	Few slices pineapple	40
1:00 P.M.	Salad with light ranch dressing	30
	Chocolate cake	400
3:00 P.M.	Frozen fruit bar	70
6:00 P.M.	Leftover macaroni and cheese (½ cup)	200
8:00 P.M.	¼ chicken (6 oz)	
	Vegetables (1 cup)	
	Rice (½ cup)	440
10:00 P.M.	Tootsie Pop	60

TOTAL 1,420

whatever strikes her fancy will be low-calorie. This morning, it's a banana—full of vitamins and minerals and only 100 calories. Later, at 10:00, it's fresh pineapple. She cuts off a few slices of this sweet, filling caloric bargain.

By 1:00 in the afternoon, Diana is lunching with friends. But she's not making the same food choices she used to make. Notice that there's no "diet competition" going on during this lunch. Diana used to grit her teeth and make what she thought were "diet" choices. She'd have oil and vinegar instead of dressing on her salad, bland crackers, and a butter-free corn muffin.

Now she finds she actually enjoys the light dressing that has so many fewer calories than oil. She has given up that virtuous-but-starved feeling she got from munching dry crackers and bread. Instead, she made the decision that she would enjoy chocolate cake for dessert. And that's exactly what she had—enjoying every leisurely bite while she chatted with her friends.

So far, she's had 650 calories. By this time, her "before" diary shows, her total used to be around 1,550 calories. That was well over twice the calories, yet she used to feel deprived and hungry by midafternoon.

At 3:00 P.M., Diana picks up her kids from school and takes them for a treat. Instead of the ice cream bar, she has a frozen fruit bar.

The point of the outing—enjoying a treat with her children—is maintained without wasting calories. Instead of consuming 250 calories, she's having 70.

But what does the evening hold?

Diana still got a satisfying bite to eat when the children got their meal. As her diary shows, when she fed the children their supper at 6:00 P.M., she nibbled at their leftover macaroni and cheese. And a satisfying taste it was! This is a dish she has loved since her own childhood, and she decided to have some.

Half a cup of macaroni and cheese represents only a minor calorie penalty. She no longer always "steals" a bite. But this time, she thought it through and decided it was worth it.

Later on, she has dinner with her husband. Right here, her "after" diary looks a lot like the "before" one. She eats the same chicken, rice, and vegetables she used to eat, and the same total quantity of food. But there's a difference. This time, Diana reverses the portions of rice and vegetables: She halves the amount of rice and doubles the amount of vegetables.

The "filling" effect is the same, but the calorie saving is significant. It's a small change with a big impact.

It also represents an important lesson Diana has learned. Loading up on fruits and vegetables—whether they're cooked, raw, or in the form of soup—is a great way to cut down her intake of starchy foods while helping herself to important health benefits.

Later that night, as she's fixing the children's lunches for the next day at school, Diana feels in the mood for a little something sweet. Here's another case of a small change

making a big difference—in this case, having a Tootsie Pop instead of chocolate-chip cookies. That Tootsie Pop has one-fourth the calories of the chocolate-chip cookies, and it certainly lasts a lot longer.

At the end of the day, without sacrificing either taste or satisfaction, Diana has nibbled her way to an impressive savings of 1,340 calories—nearly half her previous calorie count.

As she herself says: "I used to just grab food mindlessly—while thinking I was trying to stay away from it. But in fact, you have to develop a relationship with food rather than flee from it. I have a better 'head' for food now, and even though I still munch throughout the day, I do so mindfully and my choices are better."

Diana used to think in terms of being "good"—by depriving herself throughout the day—or "blowing it" by overindulging. That good-or-bad thinking no longer controls her choices.

"I know I can't 'blow it' because there's no such thing," Diana says. "The decision is mine. I'm not depriving myself, so if I decide to eat something that has a high number of calories, it's because I decide it. I'm not saying I'm going to change everything I do, but I'm now aware of everything I do, and I have power over it."

Doug: Before and After

Doug, the New York City detective, was the prime example of someone who eats on the run. When you look back at his food diary before Food Awareness Training, one day is enough to tell the whole story.

Even if you're not a member of the

NYPD, this may be a day that's very much like yours. It's quite typical of someone who keeps irregular hours, joins friends when they're eating, and quits work late at night.

During a typical day, Doug used to consume about 4,400 calories. You can compare his "before" and "after" days in the diary selections on pages 280 and 281.

With food awareness, Doug's social habits didn't change at all. He still goes along with the crowd when everyone else wants fast food. He still joins in when his fellow officers order takeout. He's there when the gang heads for the restaurant that serves the biggest portions in town. He still stops for a late-night snack and still starts his day at Mickey D's. The *where* and *when* of his eating haven't changed.

But the *what* is totally different today from his "before" diary.

The result? Doug is eating—and living—more healthfully. He is enjoying food even more. He doesn't feel deprived. And he feels good—lighter and more energetic.

Today, his 10:00 A.M. breakfast is hot cakes with syrup. That's nearly a 200-calorie savings over the sausage and egg biscuit he used to have, but Doug finds the new breakfast just as satisfying as the old one used to be. Plus, the source is the same: McDonald's. He doesn't have to go out of his way to get the lower-calorie breakfast.

Lunch?

It's still 2:00 before he gets around to lunch—and he's hungry. But now Doug makes different choices. He has substituted vegetable pizza for pepperoni pizza. It's just as convenient and filling, and he finds he enjoys the veggie pizza just as much. He's also aware that it's much healthier, that he gains nutrition while he loses calories.

The grapes that are dessert for lunch are a revelation. Doug has forgotten how much he likes fruit. Now that he has been reminded to eat it, he's aware also of how handy a snack it is.

Doug has always looked forward to dinner, and his "after" diary shows that Doug's dinner portions remain substantial. Obviously, he isn't depriving himself. But he has made some important choices—as reflected in his "after" diary. This time he has a healthful and very tasty shrimp cocktail as an appetizer. He follows it with a sizable platter of linguine in clam sauce, accompanied by a slice of garlic bread, his favorite, and a sesame bread stick.

Together, the appetizer, main dish, and bread are more than ample substitute for the veal parmigiana, spaghetti, and bread he used to have. But right there, he's saving 380 calories.

He still has a salad as well. But this time, instead of a high-calorie Caesar salad, he chooses a simple tossed salad with light Italian dressing at one-fifth the calorie count.

Dessert? Sure. He orders a lemon sorbet with biscotti that he finds refreshing and flavorful.

Whatever else may change, Doug can't give up stopping at the local diner when his shift is over. In days past, he would have the cheeseburger, fries, and Coke—and emerge "feeling stuffed," as he used to record in his diary. Measured in terms of calories, feeling stuffed added up to a hearty 825.

These days, he still stops by the diner. But he comes out feeling satisfied, not stuffed. His

Doug's "Before" Diary—The Whole Day

Time	Food	Calories
10:00 A.M.	McDonald's sausage and egg biscuit	530
2:00 P.M.	2 slices pepperoni pizza	1,100
	Coke	145
6:30 P.M.	2 pieces garlic bread	300
	Veal parmigiana	540
	Spaghetti	320
	Caesar salad	260
	Cannoli	280
	Cappuccino (sweetened)	100
11:00 P.M.	Cheeseburger	460
	Fries	220
	Coke	145

TOTAL 4,400

food diary tells the story. The container of pea soup, crackers, and diet drink add up to about one-fourth the calories he used to have in his "cheeseburger" days.

If you look at Doug's diary for the entire day, you can see that he hasn't changed his reasons for eating. He also hasn't changed the places where he eats or the people he eats with. But he *has* changed the foods he chooses to eat. His health is up, and his weight is down, and he feels and looks better than he ever has.

What made the difference?

Between the "before" and the "after" food diaries, there's a whopping difference of 2,350 calories. What's most amazing, however, is that Doug didn't have to change his eating patterns at all. He still joins his friends at breakfast and dinner. He still hits the fast-food places. He still has a hearty Italian dinner. But he's making different choices.

Every one of those choices is whittling away at the total calorie count. But Doug never feels like he's starving himself. And he certainly never feels like he's on a diet.

Has Doug's attitude toward food changed?

Doug's "After" Diary—The Whole Day

Time	Food	Calories
10:00 A.M.	McDonald's hot cakes with syrup (no butter)	350
2:00 P.M.	2 slices vegetable pizza	400
	Bunch of grapes	80
	Diet 7-Up	0
6:30 P.M.	Shrimp cocktail	110
	1 slice garlic bread	150
	1 sesame bread stick	40
	Linguine with red clam sauce	480
	Tossed salad with light Italian dressing	50
	Lemon sorbet and biscotti	170
11:00 P.M.	1 pint pea soup	160
	Pack of crackers (4)	60
	Diet ginger ale	0
	TOTAL	**2,050**

One thing certainly has.

"I'm constantly reading labels now," he says. "I've stopped using food as a crutch just to fill myself up. Of course, I still eat good-size portions, but my weight is gradually going down, and I've changed the way I deal with food."

Doug's new consciousness is even catching on around the squad room. "People realize there are health issues here. If you're a New York City detective, blood pressure can be a real problem, and we're all beginning to see that what we eat can make a difference."

Doug thinks his new consciousness— awareness—is the key. "Nobody waved a magic wand to make this happen," Doug says. "I was pretty skeptical. Believe me, I'm a detective, so I don't believe anything anybody tells me. But I've seen the visual demonstrations, and I've seen the proof in my own case. It's just simply a question of choice."

A Question of Choice

Not a diet, not a prescribed regimen, nothing forbidden, nothing required. Just . . . choice.

All four of the individuals that I've profiled came to a new awareness about food, about nutrition, about their own reasons for eating what they ate. That new awareness empowered them to choose from an expanded range of options.

In most cases, these individuals made different food choices. Sometimes, they did not. The choice was theirs, and they always knew why they were making it and what it would mean.

But notice this: Their lifestyles remained the same. If you're a New York cop, you can't tell your sergeant that you'd like to change your hours so you can eat more healthfully. If you're a mom with kids at home, you can't ask them to finish their leftovers so you won't be tempted to clean their plates. An office worker who is tied to her desk can't tell her supervisor that she needs a 3-hour exercise break. And a hard-driving, multi–time-zone executive traveler can't beg off an essential negotiation in Los Angeles just because it interferes with his meal plan.

All of them could make different food choices, however—and they did. The circumstances in which they made their food choices remained the same. The people they dealt with and the realities they faced remained the same. But in all four cases, their relationships with food changed. And what a difference that has made to their weight, their health, their appearance, and their lives.

Chapter 12

GUILT-FREE DINING OUT

*I*f you're on a diet, few things are more terrifying than dining out at a restaurant. Either you're afraid you won't be able to resist the temptation of delicious foods and will go "off" the diet, or you're worried that if you avoid forbidden foods in favor of the dieter's typical meal of dry-broiled fish and salad—no dressing, please—everyone you're with will know you're dieting. There will follow the inevitable expressions of surprise, support, dismissal, encouragement, or interest—all of which you'd just as soon live without.

The alternative, of course, is to stay home.

But that is not an alternative. Life goes on, and part of life is going out to restaurants. Whether it's taking the kids to the local fast-food place for a snack after the game, or grabbing lunch for yourself when you're out shopping, eating out is a fact of your existence.

And so it should be. One of life's pleasures is enjoying the world's vast variety of tastes and styles and traditions and innovations in eating. Another of life's pleasures is not having to prepare food, cook it, serve it, or clean up after it. Of course you're going to dine out. The issue for the weight-conscious is dining out without being done in.

Into Not-Forbidden Territory

Fortunately, as a reader of this book, you already know how to make food choices no matter where you are. You're not on a diet. No foods are forbidden to you, and no foods are required. You don't have to reduce portion size or weigh and measure the food you're eating, or eat at certain times of the day or night. Rather, you just need to make mindful decisions about what to eat.

Menus everywhere offer an array of options. All you have to do is find and choose the low-calorie, healthful option. Eating out adds only one parameter to the equation: finding and choosing the low-calorie, healthful option that maintains the essence of the restaurant, whether it is a particular ethnic cuisine or the inventiveness of a certain chef.

With that as your guideline, you can go to any restaurant in the world without fear. Whether you're dining on a Big Mac or a Mandarin banquet, at your daily lunch spot or a once-in-a-lifetime destination, you can make the choices that allow you to both enjoy the restaurant experience and still lose weight.

283

Managing Menu Madness

In the pages that follow, I've reproduced partial listings of menus from a number of well-known New York restaurants, including some of my favorites. I've highlighted the menu choices that are lower-calorie, more healthful, and still characteristic of the reason people go to the restaurant in the first place. I've chosen New York both because it's the place I know best and because it has some of the world's most justly famous restaurants. If you can see how to make the low-calorie choices in these places, you should be able to do it anywhere.

Following the New York restaurants, I've included some comments about choices in renowned restaurants in other parts of the country. I'll also show you how to select low-calorie choices at some of the nationwide chains of restaurants—such as the Olive Garden and Red Lobster—and even at the fast-food restaurants that dot the world's landscape.

All the menu choices—from a sandwich at Subway to the lobster roasted with young artichokes and wild mushrooms "en cocotte" at Le Cirque 2000—are based on the same principles that have been articulated throughout this book.

1. You're looking for the lowest- or lower-calorie choice at all times. Of course, in restaurants, your choices are always circumscribed by the scope and variety on the menu. As you look through the menus in this chapter and see the choices I've made, you may notice the same food checked off as a good choice in one restaurant but not in another. That probably means that the restaurant where it is checked off has only a few low-calorie choices—among which this one stands out—while the restaurant where it is not checked off has lots of other low-calorie choices, so you can do better with something else.

For example, a platter of soft-shell crabs might be a top pick if it were the only seafood on a menu, but in a restaurant in which there are many other fish choices, soft-shell crabs, which are typically sautéed in butter, would move down the scale of desirability. If there are lower-calorie fish dishes on a menu, you can choose those instead.

2. I consider not just the amount of fat in a dish but the kind of fat as well. A pesto sauce may be as high in fat as a cream sauce, but the fat it contains derives from vegetable sources—pine nuts and olive oil, which qualify as "good fats"—versus the "bad" saturated fat from animal sources in a cream sauce.

3. Proteins from fish and shellfish, from soy products, and from any food of the bean group are preferable to proteins from meat, poultry, and dairy.

4. I encourage you to eat fruits and vegetables anywhere, as they offer the greatest caloric bargain. They also give you the most rewards in terms of needed vitamins, minerals, and fiber.

5. Most desserts are high in calories. But if part of the reason you're eating out is to splurge, go ahead. On the other hand, if eating out is something you do all the time, think twice about dessert.

Finally, remember that nothing is forbidden. Ever. You needn't make special requests of the restaurant kitchen—unless you choose to. There's no need to confine yourself to certain kinds of foods or methods of preparation. In any restaurant anywhere, you can make a reasonable choice for weight loss and for enjoying what you came for. A menu simply offers choices. The choosing is up to you.

The Calorie-Added Factor

Women who routinely eat in restaurants or buy take-out food have higher-calorie diets than those who often eat at home, according to a study at the University of Memphis. The study points to the conclusion that eating in restaurants tends to be a high-calorie occupation.

How can you keep the calorie count low if you eat out a lot? In addition to making mindful choices from restaurant menus, here are some other strategies.

- When you know you'll be dining out or getting takeout, try to adjust the day's other meals accordingly. Don't starve yourself in anticipation of that meal. But try to make lower-than-usual calorie choices throughout the day.

- When you're ordering, consider getting two appetizers instead of an appetizer and an entrée. Often the entrée is more than you want to eat—but because it's on your plate, you end up finishing it anyway.

- If you frequently eat out, consider these "routine" meals rather than "special" meals. If you have customer lunches 5 days a week, or a take-out dinner most evenings, these are routine events. What's the difference? If we look upon dining out as a special event, we tend to indulge. But if dining out is routine, it meansyour low-calorie choices need to be routine. Other times, there will be abundant opportunities to sample special foods.

A Careful Reading

To a great extent, choosing well comes from reading a menu well. Of course, you already know how to read a menu. What I mean is reading it from the vantage point of a person who is conscious of nutrition and mindful about options.

It helps to know the meaning of common menu terms. Pan-seared means the food has been cooked fast in a small amount of fat over very high heat. A primavera dish (primavera simply means "spring") has vegetables in it. Poached means that the food is cooked in liquid just below the boiling point.

Just as important, you should evaluate whether the high-calorie ingredient shown on the menu is central to the dish or just a peripheral accompaniment. That can be the deciding factor when making your choices.

As you look through the menus that follow and read my comments, be aware of these subtle nuances. Reading "between the lines" of a menu can give you important information for your decision-making.

And remember, you've gone out to a restaurant for a complete meal, possibly one consisting of several courses. That means that you probably want to consider what you want to eat for all of the courses at one time. If you think about the whole meal at the beginning, you can strike a balance among appetizers, main courses, and side dishes.

Fancy French Food:
Le Cirque 2000

New York City's Le Cirque offers haute cuisine at its most "haute." From its location in a landmark building to its fabulous circus setting to the nightly roster of VIPs in attendance to the superb food, Le Cirque is what a lavish restaurant experience is supposed to be.

Although French cuisine is hardly known for being low in fat, Le Cirque's menu offers many low-calorie selections, which I've highlighted in the menu to the right. The lowest-calorie items are the seafood dishes listed under the rotisserie and grill section. These are prepared with the same attention to taste and presentation as the most elaborate and unusual dishes. That means that if you do choose one of those lowest-calorie dishes, it will likely be mouth-wateringly delicious, simple though it is.

You'll also find a profusion of Le Cirque "inventions" that are lower-calorie. Among the appetizers, there are 10 choices that are seafood or vegetables—nearly half the total.

Among the entrées, however, you're in somewhat treacherous waters. Nearly all have sauces, and of course all sauces have some fat. This is a French restaurant, after all! But in general, the main course choices that I've highlighted are interesting and characteristically French, and all are certainly lower-calorie options.

Note that vegetables are an integral part of just about every checked main course (although they must be ordered separately if you choose something from the grill).

If you want to splurge on a dessert, this might just be the place to do it. The pastry chef is world famous.

Appetizers

"Fruita de Mer," Shellfish and Oysters

Terrine of Foie Gras and Baby Lettuce

Cassolette of Baby Vegetables with Black Truffles

Spirale of Assorted Smoked Fish served with Baby Lettuce

Jumbo Lump Crab Meat with Guacamole, Peas, and Tomatoes

Foie Gras Sauté

Seared Sea Scallops and Shrimp with Curry Sauce and Vegetable "Beggar's" Purse

Carpaccio of Tuna with Riviera Salad

Lobster Salad "Le Cirque"

Artichoke or Asparagus

Mesclun Salad

Lasagne with Wild Mushrooms, Spinach, and Summer Truffles

Risotto with Lobster, Coral, and Rosemary

Ravioli with Wild Greens served with Tomato Sauce

Gazpacho with Buffalo Mozzarella and Basil

Fish Soup

Consommé with Foie Gras Ravioli

Prosciutto

Smoked Fish Plate

Smoked Salmon

Beluga

Osetra

Sevruga

Main Course

"Paupiette" of Black Sea Bass in Crispy Potatoes with Braised Leeks and Barolo Sauce

Cod Filet, seared with Cassolette of Fresh Beans, Octopus, Cockles, Mussels, and Champagne Broth with Parsley

Halibut Filet, grilled with Braised Shiitake Mushrooms, Baby Bok Choy, and Leeks with Almond and Ginger Sauce

Le Cirque 2000

Lobster, roasted with Young Artichokes and Wild Mushrooms "en Cocotte"

Striped Bass Rosace, steamed in Lemongrass served with Caviar and Lemon Sauce

Red Snapper, roasted with Niçoise Vegetables and Piperade Sauce

Salmon, broiled with Crispy Fennel, Artichokes, Tomato Salad, and Lemon Vinaigrette

Black Angus Tenderloin with Marrow, Red Wine Sauce, and Gratin of Vegetables

Chicken Fricassee with Ginger, Scallions, Sweet Peppers, Onions, and Mushrooms

Duck Magret, roasted with Seasonal Fruit, Savoy Cabbage stuffed with Leg Confit, Foie Gras, and Herbs

Rack of Lamb, roasted and glazed with Bar-becue Sauce, a Vegetable Tartlet, and Roasted Creamer Potatoes

Sweetbreads and Veal Kidney with Shallot Confit and Caramelized Endive

Veal Chop, sautéed "au Jus" with Wild Mush-rooms

From Our Rotisserie and Grill

Black Angus Steak

Chicken Diable

Cote de Porc

Paillard du Jour

Spit-Roasted Pigeon

Tuna Steak

Dover Sole

Flounder "Le Cirque"

Filet of Red Snapper

Salmon Filet

Braised Veal Shank

Chateaubriand

Cote de Boeuf

Roast Chicken

Roast Duck

New Signatures of Le Cirque

Chocolate Extravaganza
Five Exquisite Chocolate Fantasies Seductive Enough to Rival Your Wildest Dreams

Adam's Apple
Warm Caramelized Apples on a Crispy Puff Pastry Cloud

Kalamansi Lace with Jivara Milk Chocolate

Rainbow
Terrine of Spring Fruit with Almond Cream

Tropical Island
Crispy Layer of Coconut Tuile, Coconut Cream, and Pineapple Sorbet Enrobed Thinly in White Chocolate

Hot Apricot Strudel
Served with Chocolate Cream

Berry Berry
Layers of Crispy Almond Phyllo, Strawberry Mousse, and Fresh Strawberries

Cherry on Top
Cherry Mousse, Griottines, and Crème Brûlée Custard—Everything You Love in Life!

Classic Le Cirque Desserts

Crème Brûlée
The Legendary Crème Brûlée of "Le Cirque"

Le Cirque Stove
Mini Chocolate Stove over a Chocolate Coffee Opera Cake

Chocolate Fontaine
Chocolate Sponge, Chocolate Ganache, and Fresh Raspberries Wrapped in Phyllo Dough

Chocolate Fondat
Warm, Creamy Chocolate Cake served with Candied Orange

Jacques' Napoleon
Very Light, Crispy Puff Pastry, layered with Vanilla Cream

Banana Clown Hat
Light, Crispy Puff Pastry filled with Vanilla Cream, Caramelized Bananas, and Soft Ice Cream

Soufflé
Traditional Chocolate or Fruit-Flavored Soufflé

Bomboloni
Warm Brioche filled with Vanilla Cream

Assortment of Homemade Sorbets

Refined, Simple, Elegant: Japanese Cuisine at Nobu

One of New York's trendiest and re-spected restaurants, located in the fashionable Tribeca district, Nobu is the signature creation of chef Matsuhisa Nobuyuki, in partnership with Robert DeNiro and restaurateur Drew Nieporent. The atmosphere—in a setting of oiled wood and cherry blossom stencils—is "casual chic," while the culinary innovations dazzle.

For the weight-conscious, at Nobu as at any Japanese restaurant, some basics apply.

The Japanese cuisine is one of the health-iest and lowest-calorie cuisines on Earth. For proof, look at all the "recommended" selec-tions I've highlighted in this menu. All tem-pura dishes, however, are deep-fried and are therefore high-calorie. But virtually all soups and salads are excellent choices, and so are just about all sushi, sashimi, and other fish choices.

As for noodles, which are not the best choices for weight loss, they are nevertheless characteristically Japanese and offer interesting tastes. Note that udon is a wheat-based noodle, while soba is buckwheat or buck-wheat with yam.

Given these guidelines, a great deal of Nobu's menu—indeed, of any Japanese menu—offers excellent low-calorie choices, as you can see from all the highlights on the menu. There is a range of fish dishes—cooked and raw—as well as all the salads and soups.

For dessert, Nobu's highlighted choices are the sorbets, fresh fruit, and a unique of-fering—red watermelon soup.

Nobu Special Hot Dishes

Rock Shrimp or Scallop with Yuzu Sauce served on Lime Stone Lettuce

"Anti-Cucho" Peruvian Style Spicy Chicken Skewer

Sea Urchin Tempura

Eggplant Miso

Asparagus with Egg Sauce and Salmon Eggs

Mushroom Salad

New Zealand Mussels with choice of Special Matsuhisa Sauce

Broiled Yellowtail Collar

Matsuhisa Shrimp and Caviar

"Toro-Rosa" Broiled Toro with Spicy Miso

Chilean Sea Bass with Black Bean Sauce

Toro "Hagashi" Special

Rock Shrimp Tempura with Ponzu and Chili Pepper Creamy Spicy Sauce

Baby Abalone with Light Garlic

Arctic Char grilled medium rare with Crispy Baby Spinach

Tuna Tempura

Creamy Spicy Crab

Spicy Sour Shrimp

Halibut Cheeks with Wasabi Pepper Sauce

Squid "Pasta" with Garlic Sauce

Creamy Spicy Shrimp

Seafood "To-Ban" Yaki

Toro "To-Ban" Yaki

Shrimp and Lobster with Spicy Lemon Sauce

Fresh Lobster with Wasabi Pepper Sauce

Nobu Special Cold Dishes

"Kumamoto" Oysters with Maui Onion Salsa

Salmon Kelp Roll

Tiradito "Nobu Style"

Ceviche

Nobu

Shiromi Usuzukuri (Whitefish with Ponzu)

Sashimi Salad with Matsuhisa Dressing

Lobster Salad with Shiitake Mushroom and Nobu Spicy Lemon Dressing

Toro Tartar with Caviar

Salmon Tartar with Caviar

Tuna Tataki with Ponzu

Hot-Miso "Chips" Tuna or Scallops

Salmon Skin Salad

Sea Urchin in Spinach

"Ceviche" South American Style with Fresh Lobster

Fresh Yellowtail Sashimi with Jalapeño

Baby Spinach Salad with Fresh Fluke Sashimi

Morohelya Pasta Salad with Fresh Lobster

Yellowtail Tartar with Caviar

Monkfish Pâté with Caviar

New Style Sashimi

Matsuhisa Specialty

Black Cod with Miso

Kushiyaki

Beef

Chicken

Scallops

Shrimp

Squid

Vegetable

Dinner Entrées

(Served with Miso Soup and Rice)

Fillet of Salmon with Teriyaki Sauce

Scallops with Pepper Sauce

Scallops with Spicy Garlic

Tempura Dinner

Sashimi Dinner

Sushi Dinner

Chicken Teriyaki

Chicken with Pepper Sauce

Tenderloin of Beef with Teriyaki Sauce

Salmon Anti-Cucho

Salads

Field Greens with Matsuhisa Dressing

Shiitake Salad

Kelp Salad

Oshitashi (Spinach)

Combination Sunomono

Soup

Miso Soup

Mushroom

Akadashi

Clear Soup

Desserts

Red Watermelon Soup
Served with yellow watermelon shiso sorbet

Bento Box
A warm chocolate soufflé cake with shiso syrup and green tea ice cream

Coconut Rice Pudding
With yuzu brandy tuile and dried currant sauce

Yuzu Cheese Crème Caramel
Served with pistachio tuile

Yuzu Roll
White chocolate yuzu mousse covered with milk chocolate and hazelnuts served with yuzu sauce and green tea ice cream

Ice Cream or Sorbet
Served with yuzu biscotti

Fresh Seasonal Fruit
Served with sorbet

Infused Seasonal Fruit Sake

Veggies Galore:
Zen Palate

Vegetarian restaurants, once thought of as the province of health-food advocates, have come into their own. In fact, many restaurants these days offer a special vegetarian menu or a vegetarian section on their main menu. But it's often in "pure" vegetarian restaurants that the most interesting and innovative vegetarian cooking takes place.

New York's Zen Palate, which has three locations in Manhattan, is one of those real veggie restaurants. Zen Palate offers a beautiful—and serene—architectural setting and a lengthy and inventive menu. Some of its dishes are macrobiotic, some create meatlike foods out of soy and vegetables—the mini vegi-loaf or basiled vegetable ham—and many are Asian in origin and style. From tasty morsels like steamed vegetable dumplings to such main dishes as eggplant in garlic sauce, shepherd's pie croquettes, and the house salad, there is something for every taste. Most of the dishes are low-calorie, and all are very good for you. (There's no need to show the menu because all the choices are great!)

Here, as in other vegetarian restaurants, you can enjoy many of the most important characteristics of dining out—a pleasant atmosphere, elegant service, and the enjoyment of not having to cook. And all the while, you're eating very, very healthful low-calorie foods. It can be done!

Catch the Heartbeat:
Heart-Healthy
Haute Cuisine

Talk about positive trends: Drew Nieporent's Myriad Restaurant Group operates Heartbeat, offering sophisticated "health food" in a glossy midtown setting. The mission is to place organic, heart-healthy ingredients center stage, to have highly trained chefs prepare the food, and to flavor the food boldly without added fats. As for the sommelier, he is a tea steward rather than a wine steward.

Not surprisingly, just about everything on this menu is highlighted—except for the few chicken and meat options and a couple of risottos and rice side dishes. And the only reason I've left *those* off the list is because there are so many other low-calorie, high-health choices available.

In fact, at a place like Heartbeat, with so many good choices, you can afford to be particularly meticulous about what you order. That's why I have not checked the Asian pear salad, for example. Even though its pecans are heart-healthy, the blue cheese forms a major part of the dish. You might just as well avoid that appetizer in favor of any other.

On the other hand, I have checked the rice and beans side dish—precisely because it is a side dish. In such a moderate portion, the starchy rice calories are pretty much counterbalanced by the protein benefits of the beans.

Heartbeat

Dinner

Organic vegetables consommé with sage dumplings

Simple green salad with lemon herb vinaigrette

Sliced raw tuna with radish salad and wasabi-yuzu

Roasted roots and baby green salad

Asian pear salad with tamari pecans and maytag blue cheese

Shrimp, shellfish, and calamari with vine-ripe tomato broth

Mackerel ceviche with lemon and chervil sauce

Chilled oysters on the half shell with osestra caviar

Grilled tofu with scallion salad and barley miso

Tamari seared shrimp and scallops

Pistachio roasted baby chicken with vegetable mushroom hash

Coriander seared duck breast with roasted parsnip and sweet potato sauce

Pan seared skate with parsley root and garlic broth

Pan roasted monkfish in spicy shellfish broth

Miso salmon with sweet pea sauce

Steamed black bass with saffron artichoke broth and boluga lentils

Sweet onion risotto with pan roasted vegetables and mushroom syrup

Fillet of natural beef tenderloin with wild mushrooms and baked yukon potato

Pan seared trout with sweet pea and summer corn pancakes

Grilled rack of lamb with kumquat chutney and roasted yukon potatoes

Grilled and roasted vegetables with texmati rice and beans

Sides

Wilted Greens

Grilled and roasted vegetables

Roasted onion risotto

Brown rice

Broccoli rabe

Baked yukon potatoes

Vegetable mushroom hash

Rice and beans

Dessert

Bowls of fresh organic berries with goat's milk yogurt and organic honey

Plates of sliced tropical fruits with assorted housemade sorbets

Matcha green tea ice with spiked yellow water-melon

Assorted housemade sorbets

Indulgences

Baked granny smith apple with anise flan and walnut crisp

Spiced sautéed pineapple and passion fruit with lime-fennel sorbet and vanilla beet sauce

Three-chocolate parfait with sorbet and cocoa bean florentine

Warm maracaibo chocolate gratin with bing cherry gelato

Plate of assorted sweets

The Mediterranean Concept

Researchers have long recommended the Mediterranean diet as a good path to health and longevity. Milos Restaurant, of Montreal and New York, has built its menu on the concept of the Mediterranean style of eating—and the menu makes a point of explaining it all to you in careful detail. The fish menu, for example, will tell you the origin of the fish, its taste, and its preparation. As you can see from the highlighted selections, I recommend *all* the grilled fish that are available.

Milos prides itself on dealing with small suppliers—family-owned fishing companies in the Mediterranean and independent North American fishermen who work off Florida and Nova Scotia. Freshness, of course, is the key. And Milos balances its seafood offerings with equally meticulous choices in vegetables, legumes, and fresh fruit.

Milos's emphasis on fresh fish and fresh vegetables and its highly informative menu make it a model restaurant for mindful eaters.

First Course

Milos Special
Paper-thin zucchini, eggplant, and saganaki cheese, lightly fried.

Greek Spreads
Taramosalata, ktipiti, tzatziki, skordalia.

Fava
Cultivated on the volcanic earth of Santorini, pureed, served with French shallots and olive oil.

Mushrooms—Poland
Oyster mushrooms charcoal-grilled.

Peppers—Holland
Grilled red and yellow peppers.

Octopus—Tunisia
Sushi-quality octopus, grilled.

Calamari
Rings of fresh and tender calamari, lightly fried in fresh oil.

Calamari
Grilled whole stuffed with feta served over spinach.

Shrimp
Our famous charcoal-broiled jumbo shrimp.

Crab Cake
95% crabmeat and 5% Maryland spices served with kastorian beans.

Sepia
An Aegean delicacy from the squid family, on the charcoal.

Marides—Greece
Fresh sea smelts, fried in fish oil.

Anchovies—Agadir
Fresh anchovies, deliciously deep-fried in fresh oil.

Sardines—Portugal
Fresh grilled sardines, with extra virgin olive oil, lemon, and oregano.

Scallops—Canada
Sea scallops charcoal-grilled on the skewer with Vidalia onions.

Estiatorio Milos

Soft Shell Crab—Maryland
Live, specially selected, lightly fried.

Oysters
A variety of North American oysters. According to seasonal availability.

Salads

Tomato Salad
The authentic Greek salad, prepared with vine-ripe tomatoes.

Mixed Field Salad
Organic greens with extra virgin olive oil and balsamic vinaigrette.

Arugula Salad
Arugula, Feta cheese.

Green Salad
Hearts of romaine with a picante dressing and fresh dill.

Whole Fresh Fish, Live Lobster, and Shrimp

From our own North American waters to the seas of our forefathers, Milos presents the world's finest fish (line-caught), live lobster, and shrimp, grilled on the charcoal.

Red Snapper—Pensacola
White fish, moist and sweet.

Black Sea Bass—North Carolina
Wild bass, tender and flaky.

Pompano—Florida
Unique, meaty, and very flavorful dish.

Loup de Mer—Mediterranean Bar loup
Most sought-after fish in Europe.

Royal Dorado—Mediterranean
Very delicate white fish of the Dorado family.

Paegeot—Greece
Firm and tasty snapper.

Dover Sole—Holland
Fresh sole, the Dover variety, served on the bone.

Solette—Mediterranean
Baby sole, pan-sautéed, on the bone.

Sargos—Greece
"Sar Vrais," the European name of this very tasty white fish.

St. Pierre—Mediterranean
Extremely elegant taste and texture.

Barbouni (Rouget)
Firm and full-flavored fish. Fried, on the bone.

Lobster—Nova Scotia
Deep sea lobster, on the charcoal.

Lobster Salad
Nova Scotia lobster, grilled and prepared with Metaxa brandy, endive, and fennel.

Langouste—Peloponnese
Grilled Mediterranean lobster.

Langoustine
Live Mediterranean langoustine, on the charcoal.

Yellow Fin Tuna
Sushi-quality, seared in red wine vinegar over a bed of baby beet leaves.

Swordfish
Marinated on the skewer with onions, peppers, and tomatoes.

Arctic Char—Iceland
Flavorful pink sea trout from the Arctic.

Side Dishes

Horta

Seasonal Vegetables

Mixed Vegetables

Yukon Gold Potatoes

Mixed Grilled Vegetables

The Menu with Everything: Union Square Cafe

An instant classic since it first opened in the heart of what would become New York's newest "hot" neighborhood—home to Silicon Alley—the Union Square Cafe offers a range of deliciously prepared food in a grown-up but casual atmosphere.

Although the menu choices are highly inventive, the range is what might be called basic New American. Not surprisingly, most of Union Square's salads and soups, fish dishes, and vegetable accompaniments are good choices for the weight-conscious. Since these choices represent just over half the total choices on the menu, that leaves you plenty of room to maneuver.

Of course, a little bit of grated Gruyère or some extra-virgin olive oil adds a few calories to some dishes, but not enough to put the foods out of the lower-calorie range. Even a dollop of high-calorie balsamic butter shouldn't disqualify the sautéed salmon with corn, spinach, and shiitake mushrooms. By contrast, where the seared skate would normally be a good choice, in this case it is accompanied by fried artichokes and mashed potatoes—a bit too much to qualify as lower calorie.

Appetizers

Fettuccine with Lobster, Basil, Sweet Peas, and Mushrooms

Maine Crabmeat and Artichoke Tortelli with Roasted Tomato-Oregano Butter

Spaghetti all'Amatriciana with Tomato, Basil, Guanciale, and Pecorino Toscano

Squash Blossom Fazzoletto-Homemade "Handkerchief" Pasta with Marjoram and Salsa di Zucchini

Braised Artichoke, Radicchio, and Fennel Ragout with Summer Herbs and Toasted Foccacia

Terrine of Spiced Duck Foie Gras with Peach-Cherry Chutney and Toasted Brioche

Union Square Cafe's Fried Calamari with Anchovy Mayonnaise

Sheep's Milk Ricotta Gnocchi with Lemon-Spinach Cream

Salad and Soup

Bibb and Red Oak Leaf Salad with Grated Gruyère and Dijon Vinaigrette

Union Square Cafe Greens Salad with Garlic Croutons and Oregano Vinaigrette

Spinach and Portobello Salad with Fennel, Shaved Parmigiano, and Balsamic Vinaigrette

Union Square Cafe

Yellowfish Tuna Carpaccio with Baby Zucchini Salad, Extra Virgin Olive Oil, Lemon, and Fleur de Sel

Arugula and Oven-Roasted Tomato Salad with Ricotta Salata and Lemon Vinaigrette

Union Square Cafe Black Bean Soup with Lemon and Australian Sherry

Main Courses

Pan-Roasted Poussin with Frisée-Frittata Salad, Italian "Fries," and Balsamic Jus

Chili and Sage-Rubbed Hanger Steak with Sautéed Swiss Chard and Macaroni and Cheese

Yellowfin Tuna Burger with Ginger-Mustard Glaze, Grilled Red Onions, and Creamy Cabbage Slaw

Greenmarket Vegetables in Lemon-Herb Nage with Quinoa, Basmati, and Red Rice Pilaf

Seared Skate with Tartar Sauce, Fried Artichokes, and Horseradish-Mashed Potatoes

Sautéed Salmon with Sweet Corn, Spinach, Shiitake Mushrooms, and Balsamic Butter

Sizzled Soft-Shell Crabs in Tomato-Basil Nage with Pea Shoots, Oyster Mushrooms, and Vidalia Onions

U.S.C.'s Grilled Marinated Fillet Mignon of Tuna with Gingered Vegetables and Wasabi-Mashed Potatoes

Crisp Lemon-Pepper Duck with Peach-Cherry Chutney, Glazed Carrots, and Three Grain Pilaf

Grilled Lamb Chops Scotta Dita with Potato-Gruyère Gratin and Sauteed Insalata Tricolore

Grilled Smoked Black Angus Shell Steak with Mashed Potatoes and Frizzled Leeks

Herb-Roasted Organic Chicken with Tomato and Tapenade Gratin and Italian "Fries"

Vegetables and Condiments

Hot Garlic Potato Chips

Sautéed Broccoli Rabe "Mama Romano Style"

Union Square Cafe's Mashed Potatoes with Frizzled Leeks

Fagioli alla Toscana—Simmered White Beans with Savory Herbs, Extra Virgin Olive Oil, and Pecorino

Crostini di Fegatini—Grilled Sourdough Toasts with Chopped Chicken Livers, Juniper, and Sage

Creamy Polenta with Mascarpone, Toasted Walnuts, and Crumbled Gorgonzola

Sautéed Spinach with Lemon and Extra Virgin Olive Oil

Grilled Slices of Sweet Red Onion

Steak:
Smith and Wollensky

It's hard to think about dining out in New York City and not think of steak houses, and it's hard to go into a steak house and not order steak. But let's suppose you've been invited, or you're there on business at a customer's request, or it's your spouse's choice. Is there anything on a steak-house menu that would qualify as low-calorie and healthful?

The answer is yes. Plenty. Most steak houses typically offer a few key seafood dishes as well, so you can order fish and still be in keeping with the character of the restaurant—one of my criteria for the choices on these menus.

Smith and Wollensky is a New York classic of world renown with satellites in Miami, New Orleans, Las Vegas, Chicago, and Washington. Just about any of its appetizers, almost all its seafood and side dishes, and even its fresh berries dessert are lower-calorie, healthy choices that are entirely in keeping with the style of the place.

Smith and Wollensky

Appetizers

Wollensky's Special Salad
Shrimp Cocktail
Fresh Lump Crabmeat Cocktail
Lobster Cocktail
Prosciutto di Parma with Melon
Smoked "Pastrami" Salmon
Asparagus Vinaigrette
Smith and Wollensky's Famous Split Pea Soup
Soup du Jour

Dinner Classics

Sliced Steak Wollensky
Sirloin
Filet Mignon
Filet au Poivre
Prime Rib of Beef
Triple Lamb Chops
Veal Chop
Veal New York/Milan
Chopped Steak
Lemon Pepper Chicken
Grilled Chicken Breast
Calf's Liver

Butcher's Specials
Double Sirloin (for two)
Château Briand (for two)

Seafood

Lobster
Grilled Salmon
Lemon Pepper Tuna
Grilled Swordfish
Maryland Crab Cakes
Stone Crabs
Fish du Jour
Soft Shell Crabs

Sides

Vegetable
Asparagus
Baked Potato
Hashed Browns
Onions Rings/Fried Zucchini

Dessert

Fresh Berries

Eating Extravaganza: Tavern on the Green

Another quintessentially New York eatery is the world-famous Tavern on the Green, right smack-dab along the western edge of Central Park, which serves as a front lawn.

The setting is a glitzy, theatrical extravaganza, complete with crystal chandeliers, hand-carved mirrors, and stained glass. The menu has everything. Note the offer to "simply grill" any available fish and serve it "with an organic field green salad." For dessert, Tavern's sorbets are a good bet.

Tavern on the Green

Cold First Courses

Tomato Gazpacho
Avocado, Spanish Olives, and Chopped Egg

Bruschetta

Prosciutto di Parma
Fresh Figs

Gulf Shrimp Cocktail
Duet of Sauces

Daily Selection of Oysters on the Half Shell
Mignonette and Cocktail Sauce

Fruits de Mer Platter
Lobster, Oysters, Clams, Shrimp, Crab, and Mussels with a Quartet of Sauces

Organic Field Greens Salad
Sherry Shallot Vinaigrette

Caesar Salad

Caviar
Beluga or Osetra Caviar served with Blini, Crème Fraiche, and Melted Butter

Hot First Courses

Corn Chowder

Crisp Fried Calamari
Cajun Remoulade Sauce

Sautéed Crabcake
Horseradish Coleslaw, Creamy Sweet Corn Sauce

Barbecued Baby Back Ribs

Sautéed Foie Gras

Pasta

Orecchiette
Mussels, Basil, Cherry Tomatoes, Fresh Cranberry Beans

Spaghetti alla Chittara
Plum Tomato and Basil Sauce

Ravioli
Ricotta, Sundried Tomatoes, Peas, Prosciutto

Risotto Frutti di Mare
Bay Scallops, Calamari, Rock Shrimp, Clams, Spinach, Tomatoes

Seafood

Seafood Salad
Marinated Shrimp and Calamari, Sundried Tomato, Pinenuts, and Basil

Seared Salmon
Chanterelles, Champagne Cream with Tossed Pea Shoots and Asparagus Tips

Pan-Roasted Striped Bass
Calamata Olive Mashed Potatoes, Warm Gazpacho Sauce, Haricots Verts

Fish May Be Simply Grilled and served with an Organic Field Green Salad

Side Dishes

French Fries

Mashed Potatoes

Creamed Spinach

Haricots Verts

Mangia Italian: Elio's, Mezzogiorno

Everybody loves Italian food, and here are two of New York's best. Elio's is one of the great old standbys of the City. Located on the super-fashionable Upper East Side, it is packed nightly with celebrities from the worlds of entertainment, politics, publishing, culture—you name it.

Mezzogiorno is located in the chic heart of Soho and attracts a mostly neighborhood crowd—youthful, dynamic, very much in vogue.

From the masters of Italian cuisine, of course, the world got pasta, olive oil, and the idea of cooking with cheeses—all high-calorie choices. But Italians have also long celebrated fish and vegetables, opening a world of possibilities for the weight-conscious.

At Elio's, for example, nearly all of the soups and many of the appetizers are excellent choices. Note especially the shrimp and white bean salad, roast peppers and anchovies, and mussels salsa verde. These are quintessentially Italian in taste and definitely healthy and low-calorie. Among pastas, all but those with meat are okay choices, although the pasta with pesto and the risottos will be somewhat higher in calories. The pasta primavera, however, is an excellent choice here. And Elio's main-course menu offers a range of seafood and vegetable dishes as well.

Mezzogiorno specializes in pizza—a difficult choice for the calorie-conscious. As you can see from the menu, I've selected 4 pizzas out of 13. That's a pretty good batting average if you love pizza. As with Italian menus in general, there are sufficient vegetable and excellent fish choices among the "primi piatti" and "secondi piatti" selections that you can enjoy both the taste of Italy and a low-calorie meal at the same time.

One menu item in particular that is unique to Mezzogiorno is orata, a flaky white fish that is flown in fresh daily from Italy. It is cooked in a wood oven and served boneless. It's delicious, low-calorie, healthful, utterly Italian, and a special treat. Top off such a meal with one of several lower-calorie desserts available on the Mezzogiorno menu, and you've taken yourself back to Italy.

Elio's

antipasto

roast peppers and anchovies

mozzarella di bufala

asparagus or artichokes

raw mushroom salad with fennel and
parmesan

prosciutto di parma and melon

bresaola valtellina

beef carpaccio with salsa verde or truffle oil

vitello tonnato

shrimp and white bean salad

seafood salad

mussels salsa verde or with white wine

clams oreganate

stuffed mushrooms

minestrone

tortellini in brodo

stracciatella fiorentina

spaghetti sugo di carne

spaghetti filetto di pomodoro

spaghetti primavera

spaghetti puttanesca

spaghetti alle vongole

spaghetti frutti di mare

fettuccine amatriciana

paglia e fleno

pasta al pesto

tortellini

penne lucifero

risotto porcini secchi

risotto frutti di mare

fried calamari

grilled gamberoni

zuppa di pesce with saffron and lobster

swordfish or tuna

fish of the day

filetti di pollo francese

chicken scarpariello

chicken ortolana

liver veneziana or grilled

scaloppine piccata

scaloppine marsala

saltimbocca

milanese capricciosa

cotoletta ripiena

nodino alla salvia

broiled veal chop

veal or beef paillard

steak

fried zucchini

broccoli or spinach aglio e olio

rugola, radicchio, and endive

special salad, chopped

organic lettuce salad with gorgonzola

Mezzogiorno

Antipasti

Mozzarella di bufala con pomodoro e basilico

Prosciutto di Parma con melone

Grigliata mista di verdue di stagione
Mixed grilled vegetables with flavored oil

Carpaccio di tonno agli aromi mediterranei
Tuna carpaccio with Mediterranean flavors

Insalate

Insalata tricolore (endive, radicchio, arugula)

Insalata Mezzogiorno (celery, mushrooms, parmesan, artichokes)

Insalata Contadina (truffled fresh pecorino cheese, pear, walnuts, mesclun salad)

Costa Smeralda (shrimp, crab meat, avocado, radicchio)

Insalata Siciliana (arugula, orange, grapefruit, red onion, peppered pecorino)

Pantesca (tuna fish, tomato, capers, potatoes, red onion, olives)

Primi Piatti

Penne alla Bisanzio
With fresh tomato, basil, and mozzarella

Pappardelle con gamberetti e verdure
With shrimp, asparagus, string beans, leeks, cherry tomatoes

Linguine nere sciué sciué
Black linguine in spicy sauce

Rigatoni con melanzane e ricotta salata
With eggplants, tomato sauce, ricotta, shaved aged ricotta

Trenette prezzemolate con vongole e olive alla maniera sarda
With clams and olives Sardinian style

Fusilli ai capperi, olive, peperoncino delle Lipari
With sundried tomatoes, capers, olives, fresh hot pepper

Risotto del giorno
Risotto of the day

Raviolo dello chef del giorno
Ravioli of the day

Lasagna del giorno
Lasagna of the day

La minestra regionale del giorno
Regional soup of the day

Secondi Piatti

Vitello tonnato "classico"
Sliced cold roasted veal in tuna sauce

La tagliata alla Robespierre
Sliced sirloin steak with arugula and pepper-corns

Milanese con insalatina di campo
Veal milanese with field salad

La Paillard di vitello alla piastra
Veal paillard grilled on a steel plate

La nostra insalata Pollanca (versione estiva)
Chopped chicken salad, mache, corn, celery, apples, raisins in zesty lemon sauce

Carne cruda alla tartara tradizionale
Steak tartare of beef hand cut with complete seasoning (egg optional)

Grigliata mista mare al salmoriglio
Grilled seafood combination with salmoriglio sauce

Pollastrino al forno con patate e verdure
Roasted fresh poussin with potatoes and vegetables

Pesce del giorno
Fish of the day (cooked in our wood-burning oven)

Le Pizze

(*From our wood-burning oven*)

Selvatica
With pesto, pine nuts, tomato, mozzarella

Marinara
With tomato, garlic, anchovies

Pugliese
With tomato, onions, pecorino

Bianca al prosciutto crudo, rucola
White pizza with prosciutto, fontina, arugula

Margherita
With tomato, mozzarella, and basil

Ai carciofi
With artichokes, mozzarella, tomato

Zucchine e pomodori secchi
With zucchini and sundried tomatoes

Ai 4 formaggi
With four cheeses

Bicolore
Half margherita, half gorgonzola

4 stagioni
With 4 sections

Ortolano
With fresh grilled seasonal vegetables

Ai funghi
With wild mushrooms

Piccante
With spicy sausage

Stromboli
With olives, capers, hot pepper, anchovy, tomato, mozzarella

Cestino di focaccia
Focaccia bread basket

Today's Specials

Antipasto

Grilled portobello mushrooms and endive

Pasta

Maccheroni crudaiola sauce

Ravioli

Black ravioli filled with shrimp in a spicy tomato sauce

Lasagna

Lasagna Bolognese

Risotto

Risotto with zucchini and scallops

Main

Orata roasted in our wood-burning oven

Minestra

Pasta e fagioli

Dolce

Bavarese al melone

Desserts

Tiramisu

Misto bosco al vino rosso
Mixed berries marinated in red wine

Torta di ricotta con salsa alla pesca
Ricotta cheesecake with peach sauce

Pesche marinate con gelato di vaniglia
Marinated peaches with vanilla ice cream

Torta di gianduia con puree di pere
Hazelnut chocolate cake with pear sauce

Crema gratinata ai lamponi e zucchero di canna
Crème brûlée with raspberry and raw sugare cane

Sorbetto di arance sanguigne
Sicilian blood orange sorbet

Affogato al caffè
Vanilla ice cream with hot espresso

Cantuccini col Vin Santo
Almond biscuits with glass of sweet dessert wine

Greeks Bearing Gifts: Molyvos

People are taking a fresh look at Greek cuisine, and restaurants like Molyvos are one reason why. Their beautiful room makes you feel as if you're in a Greek fishing village, and the food is simultaneously traditional home-style and elegantly refined.

As is true of all Mediterranean cuisine, Greek cuisine offers lots of fish and vegetables. Beans are a major protein source for the people of the region, and they take in "good fat" with all those wonderful olives. So it's no wonder I've ticked off a number of choices at Molyvos—from their "little bites," through soups and appetizers hot and cold, to entrées and side dishes, to salads and even pastas.

Note the offer to prepare all fish specials "simply grilled with olive oil and lemon." That's the way you'll want to ask for it.

Salads

Greek Garden Salad

Shredded Romaine

Cretan Bread Salad

Octopus Salad

Lighter Entrées and Sandwiches

Molyvos Wrapped Lamb Sandwich

Greek Seafood Pilaf

Charred Lamb with Mixed Greens

Penne Pasta with Eggplant and Tomato

Grilled Chicken Paillard

Seafood Farfalle Pasta

Grilled Steak Sandwich

Entrées

All fish specials are available simply grilled with olive oil and lemon and a side of horta.

Wood-Grilled Whole Fish
Lemon, Oregano, and Extra Virgin Olive Oil

Crispy Cod Fillet
Skordalia and Marinated Beets

Aglaia's Moussaka
Casserole Layers of Eggplant, Potato, and Tomato; Spiced Ground Lamb and Yogurt Bechamel

Lamb Yuvetsi
Braised Savory Marinated Lamb Shanks baked in clay pot; Orzo, Tomatoes, and Kefalotyri Cheese

Grilled Atlantic Salmon
Fricassee of Fennel, Potatoes, and Sweet Onion with Lemon and Dill

Wild Striped Bass Plaki
Roasted with Tomato, Garlic, Onions, and Red Wine

Lemon and Garlic Roasted Chicken

Molyvos

Souvlaki
Fruitwood-Grilled Rosemary Skewered Tenderloin of Beef and Vegetables; Chickpea Rice

Side Dishes

Chickpea Rice

French Fries

Beets with Garlic Sauce

Rustic Roasted Potatoes

Steamed Wild Greens

Baked Giant Beans with Tomato, Onion, Fennel, and Dill

Soups

Roasted Tomato Soup
Trahana Pasta, Oregano, and Feta

Chicken Magiritsa
Velvety Chicken Soup finished with Egg, Lemon, and Dill

Cold Appetizers

Grilled Marinated Sardines
Roasted Peppers, Baby String Beans; Smashed Greek Fava and Olive Oil

Greek Fava
Mashed Yellow Split Peas topped with Chopped Arugula, Spring Onion, and Capers

Sampling of Traditional Greek Spreads
Eggplant Salad, "Caviar" Mousse, and Cucumber Yogurt with Garlic

Beets and Gigantes
Red Beets and Marinated Giant Beans with Garlic Sauce

Hot Appetizers

Saganaki
Haloumi Cheese, Ouzo, and Lemon

Vegetable Dolmades
Tender Grape Leaves filled with Rice, Tomato, and Herbs

Grilled Baby Octopus
Fruitwood-Grilled with Olive, Fennel, Lemon, and Oregano

Baked Gigantes
Giant Beans, Tomato, Onion, Fennel, and Dill

Keftedes with Trahana
Small Meatballs made with Bulgur Wheat Pasta and Zucchini, served with Tzatziki

Little Bites

Taramosalata
"Caviar" Mousse

Grilled Marinated Sardines
Roasted Peppers, Baby String Beans; Smashed Greek Fava and Olive Oil

Marinated Olives
House Marinated Olives with Garlic, Olive Oil, and Herbs

Tyro-keftedes
Cheese Fritters Scented with Mint

Tzatziki
Rich Sheep's Milk Yogurt with Cucumber, Garlic, and Mint

Grilled Country Greek Sausage
Homemade Sausage Scented with Fennel, Orange, and Coriander

Greek Fava
Mashed Yellow Split Peas topped with Chopped Arugula, Spring Onion, and Capers

Feta Cheese from Dodoni
Feta Cheese with Oregano drizzled with Olive Oil

Melitzanosalata
Roasted Eggplant Salad with Garlic and Lemon

Beets with Skordalia
Red Beets, Marinated Giant Beans with Garlic Sauce

Spinach Pie
Spinach, Leeks, and Feta wrapped in House-made Phyllo

Keftedes with Red Sauce
Small Meatballs with Tomato and Spices

One of America's Favorite Cuisines— Chinese: Shun Lee

In a city rich with Chinese restaurants—and boasting one of the nation's largest and liveliest Chinatowns—Shun Lee stands out. Located just opposite the Lincoln Center for the Performing Arts, the restaurant's elegant setting plays host to some of the world's most important performing artists. As is true of all Chinese cuisine, Shun Lee's menu has an abundance of healthy vegetables and tofu. Chinese chefs are masters at cooking both. Whether or not you've tried Chinese-style tofu before, this is the place to make new discoveries about how it can be prepared and served.

Shun Lee also offers a "Spa Cuisine" menu, but you don't need to order from that to find Chinese taste in low-calorie choices. Instead, focus on the usual seafood and vegetables, try the tofu, and, if possible, avoid anything described as "crispy."

In many Chinese restaurants, it's a good idea to pass over the appetizers, since so many of them are deeply fried. On the Shun Lee menu, however, there are numerous interesting appetizer choices.

Hot Appetizers

Vegetable Spring Rolls
Spring Rolls
Honey Baby Ribs
Shanghai Steamed or Pan-Fried Dumplings
Vegetable Steamed Dumplings
Scallion Pancakes
Szechuan Wonton
Chicken Soong or Spicy Chicken Soong
Baby Little Neck with Black Bean Sauce
Scallops steamed with Noodles in Garlic
Crispy Shrimp Balls
Grilled Scallops
Giant Prawns in Black Bean Sauce
Barbecue Spare Ribs
Soft Shell Crabs

Cold Appetizers

Hacked Chicken
Hot and Sour Cabbage
Tangy Spicy Kidney
Shrimp with Mint Leaf and Coriander
Jelly Fish
Hunan-Style Calamari

From the Gardens

Triple Fragrance
Sugar snap peas, lotus root, fresh water chestnuts; these refreshing vegetables lightly sautéed with ginger.

Buddha's Delight
A mixture of fresh water chestnuts, Chinese mushrooms, bamboo shoots, snow peas, tree mushrooms, ginkgo nuts, dried bean curd, Chinese cabbage, and carrots.

Dry Sautéed String Beans
Fresh string beans sautéed with minced garlic pickle.

Shun Lee

Baby Eggplant Szechuan Style
Baby eggplant, fresh ginger, garlic, and scallions delicately simmered in spicy Hunan sauce.

Broccoli Sautéed in Spicy Hunan Sauce
Fresh broccoli cooked in a spicy barbecue sauce.

Vegetable Duck Pie
Crispy vegetables served Beijing style. Layers of vegetable pie crispy fried; served with Chinese pancake, scallions, and Hoisin sauce.

Mo-Po Beancurd
Tender soybean curd cooked in a tangy spicy sauce.

Lily in the Wood
Tender Chinese cabbage heart and black mushrooms simmered in a light chicken broth and cooked until tender.

Shun Lee Specialties

Beijing Duck

Rack of Lamb, Szechuan Style

Whole Sea Bass Braised in Hot Bean Sauce

Dry Shredded Crispy Beef

Szechuan Duck Liver

Prawns on Banana Leaves with Curry Sauce

Szechuan Scallops with Bean Curd

Chef Man's Salmon Fillet

Shredded Beef with Leeks and Hot Pepper

Baked Lobster Cantonese Style

Seafood

Beijing Prawns

Curry Prawns

Prawns with Garlic and Scallions

Heavenly Sea Bass Fillet

Crispy Sea Bass, Hunan Style

Lobster in Szechuan or Black Bean Sauce

Sizzling Scallops

Neptune's Net

Casserole Specials

Steak and Eggplant
Sliced tender filet mignon sautéed with shredded eggplant in Szechuan sauce.

Red Cooked Pig's Knuckles and Ox Tails
This authentic Shanghai delight is for the true connoisseur. Chunks of pig knuckles and ox tails stewed in soy sauce and red wine, then slowly simmered for three hours till done to perfection.

Beancurd Family Style
Soft beancurd simmered with Szechuan hot pepper, leeks, garlic, and soy sauce in a casserole.

Tingling Curry Chicken
Large chunks of tender chicken cooked with curry and five spices in a tingling spicy sauce.

Lobster with Cellophane Noodles
Chunks of Maine lobster with shell simmered in lobster broth with cellophane noodles, slowly cooked with ginger, scallions, and rice wine.

Spa Cuisine

Steamed Eggplant with Garlic

Whole Wheat Noodles with Vegetables

Grilled Chicken Breast with Sautéed Chinese Vegetables

Cantonese Style Steamed Chicken with Broccoli and Mushrooms

Steamed Prawns in Garlic Sauce

Charcoal-Grilled Salmon with Sautéed Szechuan Vegetables

Steamed Lobster with Noodles in Garlic Sauce

Hunan Chicken

Sautéed Prawns with Garlic and Hot Pepper

Norwegian Salmon Lightly Sautéed with Chinese Vegetables

Whole Seabass poached with Ginger and Scallion

From the Sub-Continent: Nirvana

You think you've attained Nirvana when you catch the view of Central Park and upper Manhattan from this restaurant's 15th floor aerie. This is the oldest Indian restaurant in the country, and it serves classic Indian food. It offers a great chance to have your fill of protein from legumes in the form of the lentils and chickpeas that are a mainstay of Indian cuisine.

All the lentil dishes, the condiments, vegetable dishes, and fish specialties make fine choices, and Nirvana offers two breads that are both whole grain and low in fat.

Soups

Mulligatawney Soup
Made with rich meat stock, vegetables, curry, and herbs.

Vegetable Soup
A delicate blend of seasonal vegetables, lentils, fresh herbs, and other seasonings.

Breads Made to Order

Tandoori Roti
Unleavened whole wheat bread baked in the tandoor.

Tandoori Paratha
Multi-layered unleavened whole wheat bread baked in the tandoor.

Onion Naan
Bread stuffed with chopped onions and baked in the tandoor.

Garlic Naan
Bread stuffed with chopped garlic and baked in the tandoor.

Potato Paratha
Whole wheat bread stuffed with spiced potatoes and fresh herbs.

Cheese Naan
Tandoor-baked bread with homemade cheese and spices.

Nirvana Minced Meat Paratha
Whole wheat bread stuffed with minced meat, fresh herbs, and spices.

Nirvana Poori
Giant puffed bread.

Condiments

Tamarind Chutney
Sweet-and-sour chutney of tropical tamarind fruit.

Mango Chutney
Sweet chutney of sliced mango.

Lemon Achar
Fiery-hot lemon pickle with exotic spices.

Nirvana

Chili Achar
Fiery-hot chili pickle with exotic spices.

Coriander Chutney
Freshly made chutney of coriander leaves.

Assorted Condiments
An assorted platter consisting of Mango Chutney, Lemon Achar, and Chili Achar.

Side Dishes

Vegetable Raita
A cool blend of creamy yogurt and fresh vegetables, seasoned with mild spices and herbs.

Nirvana Dal of the Day
Lentils cooked with spices and fresh herbs—a different type each day.

Spinach Bhaji
Fresh spinach gently cooked with spices and fresh herbs.

Vegetarian Cuisine

Chana Allo Masala
Chickpeas and potatoes sautéed with a blend of spices and fresh herbs.

Dal Kodu
Lentils cooked with Bengali squash, spices, and fresh herbs.

Dal Shabji
Lentils cooked with mixed vegetables, fresh herbs, and spices.

Aloo Chop
Breaded Bengali-style potato fritters prepared with spices and fresh herbs.

Dal Shag
Lentils cooked with fresh spinach, spices, and herbs.

Vegetable Bhaji
A delicate blend of fresh vegetables sautéed with spices and herbs.

Vegetable Masala
Mixed fresh vegetables cooked with a blend of spice and fresh herbs.

Okra Masala
Fresh okra sautéed with onions, tomatoes, spices, and herbs.

Peas Paneer
Moist pieces of homemade cheese braised with green peas and fresh herbs in a spicy sauce.

Spinach Paneer
Cubes of homemade cheese gently cooked with fresh spinach and aromatic spices.

Vegetable Biryani
Fresh vegetables cooked with fragrant basmati rice, saffron, raisins, and almonds.

Vegetable Cutlet
Mixed vegetable patties prepared with spices and fresh herbs.

Vegetarian Dish of the Day
Fresh vegetables cooked with spices and herbs—a different dish each day.

Fish Specialties

Fish Cutlet
Fish patties prepared with a blend of spices and fresh herbs.

Fish Masala
Delicate fish fillets sautéed with onions, tomatoes, chilis, spices, and fresh herbs.

Shrimp Biryani
Shrimp cooked with fragrant basmati rice, saffron, and almonds.

Shrimp Dopiazi
Juicy shrimp sautéed with sliced onions, spices, and fresh herbs.

Around the United States

Some of the most interesting menu innovations of the day come from regional chefs using local ingredients and inspired by local traditions. And some of the finest restaurants in the world are spread out across the United States. To prove to you that you don't have to order "plain salad, please" when you're traveling cross-country, to demonstrate conclusively that it's possible to eat low-calorie, healthful choices that are the best a great chef anywhere has to offer, here are some top picks from some of the country's most renowned restaurants and most important chefs.

Miami: Joe's Stone Crab

Stone crab is what you came for, but the fact is that at a place like this, all the fish is so fresh and of such high quality that it's worth it to try something unusual—pompano, perhaps, or yellowtail or grouper.

For an appetizer, Joe's is a great place to go for baked oysters or conch salad—things hard to find elsewhere. Note also their excellent selection of vegetables including grilled veggies, black beans and rice, and baked sweet potato.

Berkeley: Chez Panisse

This restaurant offers the mother of all fresh-ingredient, good-for-you, fabulous-tasting menus. At Chez Panisse, everything is interesting, and lots of dishes qualify as low-calorie.

Start with watercress and fennel salad with king salmon rillette, then move to grilled California sea bass with squash and cherry tomato and marjoram vinaigrette, and end with white nectarine sherbet with raspberry sauce.

Seattle: Wild Ginger

There are plenty of choices in this pan-Asian emporium. For something a bit different, try Buddah's won ton soup with vegetarian dumplings, Jeem's chili prawns in the chef's own special sauce, and the Pike Place Market satay. All the vegetables are delicious; be sure to have a side order of wild mushrooms with pea pods.

Chicago: Charlie Trotter's

How about white corn grits with porcini mushrooms, stinging nettles, fennel, and mushroom juices? Or steamed Maine halibut with lobster stew brandade, preserved cucumber, and sorrel sauce? Or braised artichoke with roasted eggplant, hen of the woods mushrooms, turnips, artichoke, and white bean puree? After one of these, you'll probably want to cleanse your palate with celery and lemon mint sorbet.

Chicago: Morton's

A landmark of the heartland, now with satellites across the country, Morton's offers wonderful fresh seafood along with its signature steaks and an exceptional selection of vegetables. I would order the sautéed wild mushrooms or maybe black bean soup for an appetizer and the farm-raised salmon for a main course.

Las Vegas: André's

At André's, bet on seared ahi tuna Napoleon with eggplant caviar or maybe the Dover sole veronique—that is, with white grape sauce. Note, too, that the restaurant offers a special vegetarian choice.

Boston: Legal Shellfish

With so much delicious, high-quality fresh fish available, there is an enormous range of choices. I love anything from the raw bar and would be happy taking the fish of the day—whatever it might be. Legal even offers a light clam chowder and boasts a superb assortment of fresh vegetables.

Dallas: Mansion on Turtle Creek

The new cuisine of the Southwest offers interesting tastes you can certainly enjoy in lower-calorie dishes—like the warm lobster taco with yellow tomato salsa and jicama salad, or the tiny spinach and crabmeat salad with yellow tomatoes, hearts of palm, and burnt honey mustard dressing. Another fine selection is the bronzed sea scallops on potato puree and green bean salad with sherry-walnut vinaigrette. Or go for the mouth-burner with the adobo seafood enchilada on avocado chilaquiles. Hot!

Atlanta: Float Away Café

Lovely fish and vegetables abound at the Float Away. Try Georgia organic baby greens with black truffle vinaigrette, then a seared Irish salmon with wilted leek and cucumber salad. Low-calorie desserts abound, too: espresso granita, nectarine soup, and blackberry sorbet.

New Orleans: Emeril's

"Pork fat rules," says television's favorite chef, but even in Emeril Lagasse's own restaurant, it doesn't rule exclusively. What about the olive-oil roasted portobello mushroom, or Portuguese-style steamed clams and mussels? Or get the unforgettable pan stew of organic vegetables.

Philadelphia: Le Bec Fin

There are lots of interesting fish selections at this Philadelphia landmark. How about tuna ceviche, a roasted monkfish flavored with orange in a saffron bouillon, or an intriguing layered smoked salmon terrine served with a cucumber salad and caviar? A vegetarian menu is also offered, or try the capuccino di champignons—not coffee, but a wild mushroom soup.

Los Angeles: Spago

Trend-setting, celebrity-studded Spago—an L.A. superstar that has branched out across the country—offers such interesting low-calorie choices as marinated hamachi sashimi with yuzu, wasabi, and pumpkin seed oil, and roasted turbot with Provencal ratatouille, basil potato puree, and yellow pepper nage.

Houston: Brennan's

Vichyssoise without the cream? Gumbo without the roux? Brennan's offers distinctive dishes with a low-calorie slant. Also try their blackened redfish served with crawfish étouffée broth. In addition to these choices, Brennan's boasts a "light" menu as well.

Nationwide Chains: The Sit-Down Restaurants

Between haute cuisine and fast food are the moderately priced sit-down restaurants that you can find in just about every corner of

Are You Programmed to Inhale Calories?

Some experts believe that the proliferation of fast food and the pervasive advertising about food are, in effect, helping "program" children to eat high-calorie food. And with fast food now being served in school cafeterias, the programming may get even worse.

In our ancestors' environment, where food was more scarce and people burned a lot of calories in daily exercise, it made sense that our bodies were "programmed" to store up food energy. "In an environment where food was scarce and calorie expenditures were high . . . being programmed to eat high-calorie food was adaptive," notes Kelly Brownell, a Yale professor of psychology, epidemiology, and public health and an obesity expert. But these days, adds Dr. Brownell, "there's no scarcity, and we expend far fewer calories."

Now that we've entered an era when many people get enough food but not enough physical activity, we need fewer daily calories. But evolution hasn't yet caught up with the environmental change, notes Dr. Brownell. In fact, he says that catch-up "takes thousands or millions of years."

We should be cutting back on calories through our own mindful decision-making. Instead, we are often pressured to do just the opposite.

With convenience foods and fast-food restaurants all over the place, and with the food industry spending billions to promote eating all the time, Dr. Brownell says that "it's difficult to be optimistic about the future." Among children he has noted record levels of obesity. At the same time, he has seen "phenomenal sales of snack foods, fast foods, and soft drinks."

---

the land. With their extensive menu selections, generous portions, and emphasis on families, they offer an easygoing dining experience. Best of all, somebody else is doing the cooking.

The Olive Garden

Although many of the Olive Garden's appetizers are high in calories, the mussels di Napoli and the minestrone are fine. We can't recommend the pasta e fagioli, normally a good choice for nutrition and weight control, because it contains beef.

The best lower-calorie choices are the linguine marinara, the angel hair pasta pomodoro, and the shrimp primavera. Not surprisingly, these dishes are also featured on the Olive Garden's low-fat "Garden Fare Selections."

Red Lobster

The Red Lobster chain has an absolutely huge menu—which means there are a number of good choices for the weight-conscious. Most main dishes come with a salad or a potato and vegetables, but they also are accompanied by Cheddar Bay Biscuits, which are high in calories. A nice feature is that you can combine two or more fish items from the menu, or order one of the restaurant's combo dishes—like the Chesapeake Bake or the Outer Banks Sampler. Where your choice is blackened or fried fish, the blackened version is the lower-calorie choice.

T.G.I. Friday's

The multi-page menu at Friday's is devoted mostly to fried foods, chops, and tidbits for dipping. But the soup-and-salad combination looks good for the weight-conscious person, if the soup of the day is a bean, vegetable, or seafood base—anything other than a cream soup.

As for salads, there are three fat-free options among the dressings. Any of these go fine on the house salad.

The Veggie Wrapper is the lower-calorie choice among sandwiches, and among main dishes, stick to salmon dishes, the Broken Noodles pasta with vegetables, or the Seafood Medley. Or try these choices from the More Good Stuff menu: fresh vegetable medley, salad and baked potato combination, and the garden burger.

Fast Food

They're everywhere. From Moscow to Melbourne, from Cairo to Copenhagen, fast-food restaurants cover the globe. Here at home, fast food anchors malls, highway service centers, airports, train stations, and bus depots—not to mention downtowns and suburban centers everywhere.

Fortunately, many of the major fast-food franchises are becoming as nutrition-conscious as their patrons. Of course, a focus on low-fat items does not always mean low-calorie, but as the review that follows makes clear, there's an increasing number of good choices for the weight-conscious at many fast-food restaurants.

Wendy's

The Wendy's chain—known nationwide and around the world—has made a substantive and successful effort to expand its menu from

Hold the Fries

In most fast-food restaurants, a large order of french fries will cost you some 470 calories and 20 grams of fat. The king-size or supersize fries have as many as 590 calories and, in the case of Burger King, a grand total of 30 grams of fat—12 of them saturated fat! (At McDonald's, the supersize serving has "only" 26 grams of fat, 4.5 of them saturated.)

Those are the sizable drawbacks for anyone trying to lose weight. But what about the health effects?

Typically, french fries are fried in trans fat–laden shortening. A by-product of the hydrogenation process, trans fat does not show up on the nutritional listings. And that's unfortunate, since trans fat is a major contributor to heart disease.

burgers and chili to the "nutritionally correct." In fact, it is not difficult to get yourself a healthy, low-calorie meal from the Wendy's menu.

Start with the range of choices at the salad bar. If it won't take you from A to Z, you can at least go from B(roccoli) to W(atermelon). Then figure in the very impressive list of condiments, not to mention the several choices in low-fat and low-calorie dressings. Combine it all with perhaps a hot baked potato, and you have yourself a highly nutritious, low-calorie lunch or dinner.

If it's a sandwich you crave, your best bet is the Garden Veggie Pita.

Taco Bell

While Mexican cuisine in general can offer a dazzling array of bean dishes, the fast-food menu of Taco Bell focuses more on meat and cheese dishes adapted to American tastes. A few items, however—the Bean Burrito, the Veggie Fajitas, even the Mexican rice—are good low-calorie choices. And the very good selection of condiments means you can season whatever you get to taste—from mild to hot.

Koo Koo Roo

Koo Koo Roo, currently found only in California, Florida, and Nevada, is a chain based on a concept of healthier eating. Its main dish is a skinless, flame-broiled chicken. As a policy, the chain eschews deep frying and microwaving, and it offers fresh salad ingredients and fresh fruits. Above all, it offers an unusual variety of very good side dishes that include vegetables, grains, and beans. Some 20 of them are low-calorie.

Our office nutritionist, who oversaw this review, said she was actually "impressed" by Koo Koo Roo's offerings. Particularly interesting, she thought, were the baked yam, Italian vegetable plate, three-bean salad, vegetable soup, and 12-vegetable salad with low-fat dressing—not to mention the fresh fruits! All of these are excellent choices for their low-calorie, high-health attributes.

Subway

Found in 71 countries and all over the United States, Subway is making an effort to

How about a Smoothie?

Doesn't a smoothie sound like the perfect health drink? Now, there are a number of fast-food outlets that tantalize you with various offerings in blended fruit. What could be more delicious than a variety of fresh fruits in a cool, tall drink?

Sounds perfect indeed—until you count the calories.

For example, a standard 24-ounce blend of papaya, peach, banana, orange sherbet, coconut, and ice weighs in at 552 calories. Compare that to a 15-ounce chocolate shake at 360 calories or a tall glass of ice-cold Diet Pepsi at zero calories.

Bottom line? Why waste calories on liquids? For both weight control and your health, you're better off eating the fruit—with all its fiber intact—and drinking a low-calorie beverage.

Question the Crazes

As you look around for places to eat, it helps to be a little wary of food fads. Certain foods have a tendency to soar in popularity—sometimes with good reason, sometimes not.

Take bagels, for instance. In the 3 years from 1994 to 1997, bagel sales increased fivefold across the United States. Many people got the impression that they are the ultimate low-fat breakfast food.

As you've seen from the food demonstrations in this book, popular perception is worth questioning. Bagels are, in fact, high in calories. A fresh-baked bagel, typically weighing some 6 ounces, will cost you an estimated 480 calories.

Another fast-food craze is the "wrap"—a sandwich alternative that stuffs rolled-up flatbread with meats, cheeses, salad, and dressing. Airlines serve wraps in coach class, and a number of fast-food chains—including Wendy's, Au Bon Pain, Taco Bell, and Long John Silver's—have concocted their own lines of wraps.

But is this "new" fast food a healthful, low-calorie alternative?

Maybe not. While a wrap's "stuffing" may be a healthy potpourri of vegetables, the dressing that makes the wrap palatable tends to be high-fat and high-calorie. For example, Au Bon Pain's Southwestern Tuna wrap has 950 calories, nearly two-thirds of them from fat!

---

expand its nutrition-conscious offerings. Unique among fast-food restaurants, so far as I can determine, it offers a number of tuna and seafood sandwiches made with light mayonnaise.

Seafood, tuna, and "veggie delite" are all available on subs with the light mayo. Veggie delite also comes as a salad, and Subway provides fat-free salad dressings—French, Italian, or Ranch—to go with it.

Dining Up

Many intrepid travelers face the challenges of dining *up* as well as dining *out*.

Of course, I'm referring to airplane food. And I'm sure you've heard it insulted in just about every imaginable way. The problem is, airplane food is a kind of hybrid of fast food and wannabe gourmet dishes. And that marriage of opposites sometimes makes for some high-calorie creations that seem to be drowning in cheese or cream sauces.

But thanks to increasing demands from passengers, more airlines have become aware that they must extend their range of catering ideas if they are going to meet the needs of many of their customers. One of the most impressive in the area of innovation is TWA. Today, TWA offers upon request a range of vegetarian and seafood meals, "light" snacks, and even low-calorie dressings for its servings of salad. Not only are these choices lower in calories and more healthful than the standard airline fare, that are also *interesting* meals—well-prepared and with a surprising range of ingredients.

If you request a vegetarian meal at the time you make your reservation, you may be served any one of a number of interesting selections. The rotating lineup of vegetarian hot lunches and dinners includes vegetarian chili with rice, spinach, and carrots; a vegetarian stew with couscous and sunflower seeds; and a stuffed pepper with rice, vegetable, and raisin filling served with curried rice and ratatouille. All these choices come with salad, fruit, and a roll.

The airline also provides seafood dishes on request. The fisherman's seafood platter consists of crab claws, shrimp, and smoked salmon. The accompaniments include zucchini slices and a pasta salad with olives and red peppers.

If it's a short flight, you might only get a snack—but that can be a vegetarian selection, too. One vegetarian snack includes fresh fruit and crackers. Another, the harvest fruit plate, includes pineapple, kiwifruit, strawberries, seedless black grapes, and cottage cheese topped with a lemon leaf and mint.

While TWA is just one airline, many others are also offering lower-calorie, healthier food. Sometimes, it's true, it may be necessary to make a bit more effort to get the food you want. It's always wise to ask about meal choices at the time you make your reservation, or before your arrival at the gate.

But the effort will be worth it. For the weight-conscious, it means that you no longer have to resign yourself to eating the standard fast food of frequent flyers. If you need to travel often, and you also like to make low-calorie food choices, now you can do both.

Food Fest

So what did we learn here?

Simply this: You can eat healthful, low-calorie, *enjoyable* meals in any restaurant anywhere in the country. The choice is yours. This is what I've taught executives, actors, politicians—any number of my patients who must travel for their careers—not to mention those of us who eat out only on occasion. If they can do it, so can you and I.

Chapter 13

WANT TO LOSE POUNDS?
THROW OUT SOME DIET BOOKS

If you thought this was a "diet book" when you picked it up, I hope you're now convinced otherwise.

As you can tell, I simply don't believe that diets can help you lose weight permanently. They rely too heavily on prescribing exactly why, when, what, or how much you should eat. As I've realized from working with people who really do lose weight—and do keep it off—we simply need to change our relationship with food, so we make mindful decisions about what we eat.

But diets abound, and so do diet books. Celebrity-authored diet books are all the rage. Protein diets are popular. And in recent years, many people have wondered about the long-term success of the Zone.

So, what's wrong with these diets?

That's the question that people ask me over and over again. After all, they're supposed to "work," and if people go on a diet, and it doesn't work for *them*, they feel as if they're at fault.

No fair!

I don't care if you've been on one diet or a hundred. If a diet hasn't worked for you, that's not your fault. In the long run, diets don't work. And there are sound nutritional, lifestyle, and even psychological reasons why they may not help you keep weight off permanently.

What's Wrong with Diets?

With the help of my staff nutritionist, Phyllis Roxland, I've examined some of the most popular diets, many of which have been promoted in popular books. Some flaws immediately become apparent when you look at what the proponents of these diets are saying.

We've looked at the most prominent of the current crop of diet books. For each, we answer two questions: Is the diet healthy? and Will you lose weight by following it? We also include a typical meal from each.

By "a healthy diet," we mean two things. The diet should first supply adequate amounts of essential nutrients—protein, vitamins, and minerals. Second, it should decrease the risk of such diet-related diseases as cancer, heart disease, diabetes, and osteoporosis.

During the last 2 decades, research has made it clear that the healthiest diet is one that includes a variety of vegetables, fruits, whole

315

grains, and protein from vegetable rather than from animal sources. Despite these findings, most of the books focus on carbohydrate restriction while allowing liberal quantities of animal protein and fats.

It's important not to lump together all protein foods or all fats. There is a distinction between animal and vegetable protein, between beans or veggie-burgers, for example, and cheese or steak. Similarly, not all fats are equal. Butter and bacon should not be equated with olive oil and nuts.

Fish is probably the only animal food worth including in your diet because it's a good source of essential fatty acids.

But even if fish is a good source of these "good fats," nuts, seeds, and vegetable oils are probably the best sources.

The Atkins Approach

According to Robert C. Atkins, M.D., your fastest route to weight loss is paved with lots of protein and fat—and no carbohydrates.

Dr. Atkins' New Diet Revolution describes this "bacon-cheeseburger-hold-the-bun" diet. It restricts carbohydrates more stringently than any of the other low-carb diets we looked at—every food, every meal, every day. In fact, because of the strict limits on fruits, grains, and many vegetables, it's nearly impossible to meet your needs for vitamins, minerals, and fiber on the Atkins diet without resorting to supplements.

What the Atkins diet does is simple: It puts the dieter into a state of ketosis. Ketones are substances that form when fat is broken down for energy but not completely burned, or metabolized. The Atkins diet is based on the theory that if you restrict carbohydrate, the body will turn to its fat stores for energy. If you subscribe to this reasoning, then the presence of ketones in the urine "proves" that body fat is being broken down.

There are two things wrong with this. First, biochemists are not certain that the ketones in the blood or urine are products of broken-down body fat or of dietary fat—that is, of the high fat content of the Atkins diet.

Second, ketones are not normally present in the blood or urine. They are typically seen in uncontrolled diabetes, starvation, or after following a very low carbohydrate diet for at least 2 days. (At least some carbohydrate is necessary for the complete metabolism of fat.) It's probably safe to say that a mild degree of ketosis, from time to time, won't hurt you, but we aren't sure about the long-term effects of being in a constant state of ketosis. If you have type 1 diabetes, are pregnant or thinking about becoming pregnant, or have gout or a family history of gout, you should *absolutely not* be on a ketogenic diet.

Another possible effect of the Atkins diet is its lowering of the brain chemical serotonin, one of the body's main controllers of mood and appetite. Serotonin needs some carbohydrate to keep on working. It's no wonder, therefore, that people on very low carb diets often feel down, depressed, cranky, irritable, or all of the above.

What's more, people invariably find that once they "go off" the low-carb diet, they virtually binge on carbohydrate foods. Whether low serotonin levels are to blame for this effect is not yet proven, but they tend to show up in Atkins dieters.

The Atkins Attack on Weight

Will you lose weight on the Atkins diet? Probably. But the calorie intake on the diet can be very high, so many doctors and nutritionists suspect that much of the weight loss is water. Certainly, diets high in protein and fat are dehydrating.

Even taking dehydration into account, though, it's safe to assume that at least some of the weight loss is from fat. After all, nobody carries around 20 to 30 pounds of extra water! So yes, you can lose weight on the Atkins diet—at least temporarily.

But, apart from ketosis—which can be dangerous—and possibly low serotonin levels—is the Atkins diet healthy?

Not in our view—and not in the view of most health care professionals. Our concern, of course, is with the high intake of animal protein and fat, which can increase the risk of many diseases.

Certainly, some of the effects of the high-fat, high-protein diet can be mitigated if you get most of your protein from such foods as fish and soy products, and most of your fat from the likes of olive or canola oil or nuts, for example.

But let's face it: The vast majority of Atkins dieters are there for the meat, cheese, and butter. Who can blame them? On a diet this restrictive, there needs to be some compensation. And what could be more tempting than these rich foods that are almost always forbidden on any other diet?

Are You a Carb Addict?

Most health professionals, myself included, will tell you that you can't be addicted to a nutrient like carbohydrate. Sure, there may be some superficial similarities between the thoughts and behaviors of drug addicts and dieters/bingers. But the differences between them are substantial—and fundamental. Yet Doctors Richard F. Heller and Rachael F. Heller—in their book titled *The Carbohydrate Addict's Lifespan Program*—clearly imply that people who are "hooked" on carbs can get "unhooked" somehow.

A Day of Atkins Dining

What follows is a day in the life of an Atkins dieter. In our view, this is a diet that will catch up with you sooner rather than later, as you add back the pounds and put a heavy burden on your body's functioning. For all meals, there are no limits on portion size.

Breakfast
Fried eggs, sugarless sausages

Lunch
Chef's salad with ham, cheese, chicken, egg, and sugar-free dressing

Dinner
Shrimp cocktail with mustard and mayonnaise dressing, clear consommé, steak, green salad with sugar-free dressing, diet Jell-O with whipped heavy cream sweetened with artificial sweetener

They propose a diet that's based on the intricacies of insulin secretion. Two meals a day consist of protein and low-carb vegetables—very much like the diet proposed by Dr. Atkins. Unlike Dr. Atkins, however, the Hellers give you one meal a day when you can eat anything you want, as long as the meal is consumed within a 60-minute time frame. The "reward" meal can be either breakfast, lunch, or dinner. Your choice.

The Hellers' diet also allows you to eat whatever amount of food you want, both at the two low-carbohydrate meals and at the "reward" meal.

Obviously, this low-carbohydrate diet is easier to follow than the Atkins diet, and it can be nutritionally adequate—depending, to a great extent, on what you eat at your "reward" meal. But the liberal use of meat, poultry, and dairy products can put you at risk for such diseases as cancer, heart disease, and osteoporosis. And while you may indeed lose weight—depending on your calorie needs and your prior eating habits—your choice of foods at the "reward" meal will play an important role in how much you lose and how long you keep it off.

The Power of Protein

Michael Eades, M.D., and Mary Dan Eades, M.D., in their book *Protein Power*, recommend another kind of low-carb, high-protein diet. They allow you a daily ration of 25 to 30 grams of carbohydrate, to be distributed evenly throughout the day. Obviously, that requires very stringent portion control on fruits, grains, and vegetables.

The authors assure dieters not to worry about fat. They even put butter on their list of "good fats." They also urge you to be as liberal as you want with steak, eggs, bacon, and the like without fear of heart disease. The reason, say the authors, is that the liver will not manufacture cholesterol from these foods unless they're eaten together with starch or sugar.

That's a dubious proposition in itself, but it also fails to take into account the risk of other diseases, like cancer or osteoporosis, associated with a high intake of animal foods.

Protein Power contends that vegetarian diets are monotonous—an ironic claim given that every meal in the book can be prepared with the tasty vegetarian products available today. Moreover, the authors claim that "the

What the Hellers Propose

Here are samples of two of the prescribed daily meals in Dr. Richard F. Heller and Dr. Rachael F. Heller's "carbohydrate addict" program. If you're on this program, there's no limit on the amounts you can eat at each meal.

Ham and cheese omelette or scrambled eggs and bacon

Herb-baked chicken, green salad with dressing, Pink Heaven (whipped heavy cream and a low-carb preserve)

Three Eades Meals

Want a sampling of the *Protein Power* diet? Here are three high-protein meals. Note that, on this diet, you can eat all you want of the high-protein or high-fat foods like chicken, turkey, cheese, and bacon. But you're supposed to restrict your intake of fruits to the amounts specified.

Sliced chicken on salad with vinaigrette dressing
½ apple

Smoked turkey and cheese sandwich on 1 slice of light bread
Lettuce, tomato, sprouts
½ cup strawberries

Double-patty burger—no bun—with bacon, cheese, lettuce
Greens in vinaigrette dressing
1 peach

---

most serious deficiency that vegetarians face is protein malnourishment." That's not ironic—it's untrue. Studies long ago proved that soy protein, which makes up most of the meat substitutes available today, is of equal quality with animal protein.

Will you lose weight with *Protein Power*? Probably—again, depending on your calorie needs and what you were eating before.

Is it healthful? It can be, but the choice is really up to you. You can eat as much as you want of the high-protein, high-fat foods in the meals, while you're allowed to have only certain prescribed amounts of the fruits that provide fiber, vitamins, and minerals. Again, a high intake of animal foods can increase your risk of cancer, heart disease, and osteoporosis.

Zone Mastery

Mastering the Zone is a book and a rigid diet plan by Barry Sears, Ph.D. When you truly master the Zone, you also master quite a number of very strict rules on eating.

Virtually everything about this diet is carefully calculated and regulated. Dr. Sears tells people when to eat, what to eat, and how much they can eat. Your protein, carbohydrate, and fat allowances are carefully apportioned in "blocks." You pick foods from those blocks and make sure they're distributed among three meals and two snacks every day.

The proportional relationships among protein, carbohydrate, and fat are predetermined. Those proportions must remain the same whether you're having a full meal or just a snack. So even if you're having very small portions of certain foods, the proportional relationships are still supposed to apply.

No food exceptions are allowed, and there are no concessions to mood, circumstance, or degree of hunger. It's practically a medical prescription.

The Zone is carefully reasoned, and it builds upon what scientists know about the biochemistry of weight loss. The diet is designed to create a hormonal balance that will maximize fat loss while supposedly keeping your energy level up and your hunger level down. It may indeed work for some people, but it does so at the sacrifice of your relationship with food. Look at the sample meals and you'll see why.

Because the Zone is low in calories and fairly low in carbohydrates, you will most likely lose weight on it. And it can be healthful, although a lot depends on which options you select from your daily "blocks" and plug into meals and snacks.

The downsides are that it doesn't help you change your overall relationship with food and that it is so rigidly controlled. You can never have just a frozen yogurt on the Zone, or a piece of fruit, or a bowl of pasta. You would have to have a specific portion of each, and you would be required to eat it together with a well-regulated portion of protein and portion of fat.

Bust That Sugar Habit

The team that helped create the "Sugar Busters" diet and wrote the book of the same name includes H. Leighton Steward; Sam S. Andreas, M.D.; Morrison Bether, M.D.; and Luis A. Balart, M.D. Some have nicknamed this the "hamburger and hot dog diet," and again, it allows for high consumption of protein and fat.

The diet is based exclusively on the glycemic index. As I noted earlier, the glycemic index reflects the rate at which sugar enters into the bloodstream. For purposes of weight loss, the slower the rate of entry—and the lower the glycemic index—the better.

To ensure that the diet favors low-glycemic-index foods, the authors exclude all refined carbohydrates. You can, however, consume liberal amounts of animal proteins and fats. That alone detracts from the healthfulness of the Sugar Buster diet.

In addition, some of the food recommendations don't always make sense. For example, you are not allowed to have beets, carrots, a ripe banana, or a piece of watermelon. But chocolate bars are fine as long as they contain 70 percent cocoa, and ice cream is welcome as long as it has a very high fat content. Com-

A Meal and Snack in the Zone

The meal and snack below are representative of the portion sizes you must restrict yourself to on the Zone diet. At every meal and snack, the ratio among the three food groups—protein, carbohydrate, and fat—must be 40-30-30. The "blocks" apportion food for each of the groups.

Zone meal		Zone snack	
3 blocks protein	3 oz chicken	1 block protein	1 oz lean meat
3 blocks carbohydrate	¾ pita bread	1 block carbohydrate	⅓ pear
3 blocks fat	½ Tbsp peanut butter	1 block fat	1 macadamia nut

Sayonara to Sugar

The Sugar Busters diet can be nutritionally adequate, depending on your choices. But this diet can also increase your risk for disease, again depending on your choices. If you eat foods like those in the sample meals below, you may get most of your required nutrients, even if you don't lose weight. But other meals include not only meat and butter but also ice cream and chocolate bars. If someone does lose weight on this diet, I'd hate to think what the individual was eating before!

Breakfast
Eggs, Canadian bacon, whole grain toast

Lunch
Ham and Swiss on whole wheat, mustard, lettuce, tomato

Dinner
Pork chops, red kidney beans cooked with ham chunks, brown rice cooked with chicken broth, ½ steamed artichoke dipped in melted butter

mercial peanut butter, on the other hand, is not permitted because of its very small quantity of added sugar. (The authors make no mention, however, of the artery-clogging hydrogenated fat in the peanut butter.)

My quarrel with Sugar Busters is that the authors let you eat an entire cow, pig, or deer if you want to, but they don't let you flavor it with teriyaki sauce or accompany it with a sweet pickle or cole slaw. The moral is, you can have as much protein and fat as you can stomach, but don't even think about the second half of that artichoke!

Suzanne Says Do This

Suzanne Somers recommends a form of food combining that she has dubbed "Somersizing." She has promoted Somersizing in at least two books, *Suzanne Somers' Eat Great, Lose Weight* and *Suzanne Somers' Get Skinny on Fabulous Food,* both written by Somers and coauthors.

Somers has figured out that since protein, fats, and carbohydrates are digested at different rates, combining them "improperly," as she puts it, will halt digestion. Poorly digested food, she goes on to claim, is more likely to be stored as body fat.

There's just one problem with this neatly logical explanation. It has no basis in fact. Undigested food cannot be absorbed from the intestine into the bloodstream, let alone stored as fat.

Yet on the basis of this false assertion, Somers prescribes a stringent eating plan. She specifies that fat can be eaten together with protein, but not with carbohydrates. Fruit must be eaten by itself as a separate meal, while foods containing sugar and white flour must be eliminated. Somers calls them "funky foods."

Some odd discrepancies crop up in the Somersizing program. Somers puts banana, pumpkin, and winter squash on the same list as white flour. So these foods are to be eliminated from your diet. She lists beets and carrots with white sugar, so they have to go as well!

Somers also wants you to eliminate what she calls bad combo foods from your diet. These are foods that contain small amounts of carbohydrate in addition to protein and fat and that therefore cannot be neatly placed into any other category. Bad combo foods include nuts, olives, tofu, and soy milk, among others.

Ironically, the amount of carbohydrate in a serving of tofu or olives, for example, is insignificant—½ to 2 grams—and is much lower than the amount of carbohydrate found in many of the foods Somers allows. As these examples and many others suggest, her "bad combo foods" are very healthful. Many nutritionists—Phyllis among them—wish people would actually eat more of the foods that are on Somers's banned list.

The misinformation in the book is sometimes startling. The glycemic index, Somers tells us, "rises corresponding to the level of hyperglycemia caused by eating carbohydrates. The higher the glycemic index, the higher the level of hyperglycemia."

This is just one example of many misstatements. Hyperglycemia, or too much sugar in the blood, is usually seen in diabetics. Normal individuals maintain their blood sugar ranges regardless of what they've eaten. The glycemic index of a food—not of a person—does not change and is not influenced by high blood sugar, low blood sugar, or anything else in the body.

To put this another way, if Somers were correct in her assumptions, everyone's blood sugar would be off the charts. We'd have sugar crystals in our veins after eating a rice cake or a carrot, both of which have a high glycemic index.

I think my favorite, however, is the author's claim that fruit is not a healthy choice for dessert because "if you mix fruit with other foods, it can lose its nutritional benefit." What's more, says Somers, fruit "spoils in the stomach (and) . . . can trap the energy of other foods and cause unnecessary storage of fat."

Some Somers Strategies

Any weight loss on the Suzanne Somers program is the result of reducing your intake of total calories or carbohydrates. Yet Somers proposes many recipes and meal menus that she believes can help control glycemic index. Following are two samples of Somersizing meals (though we've omitted the full recipes that are in her book).

Greek Salad, Frank's Amazing Chicken, Cheesecake Bar

Steamed Artichoke with Lemon-Dill Dip, Parsnip Garlic Ravioli with Mushroom Ragout, Mountain of Lemon Meringue Pie

Somers suggests, instead, various rich cakes and pies that make wonderful desserts, in her view. Recipes for these desserts are included in the book. There's nothing wrong with cakes and pies, but to say that fruit can "lose its nutritional benefit" or "trap the energy of other foods" or "cause fat" is not just dead wrong, it's downright absurd.

The Home Run Hitters

Despite my obvious skepticism—and criticism—of a number of programs and books that promote diets, I have found two books that are authoritative and helpful. They are *Food for Life,* by Neal Barnard, M.D., and *Eat More, Weigh Less*, by Dean Ornish, M.D.

Here are two books that, in my view, are worth their weight in gold. Both doctors recommend a low-fat vegetarian diet of whole grains, beans, vegetables, and fruit. Only to nonvegetarians does this style of eating seem restrictive. In fact, I've found that the meals can be both varied and tasty.

Certainly, the ways of eating discussed by both Dr. Barnard and Dr. Ornish are healthful. It's also highly likely that you will lose weight if you follow the advice in these books and eat the recommended foods. Their favorite foods are low in fat and high in fiber, enabling you to feel satisfied on a relatively small number of calories.

On either Dr. Barnard's or Dr. Ornish's program, you could dine on generous portions of black pepper polenta with bell pepper sauce and shiitake mushrooms. On the side, you could have Italian bean salad along with tossed greens—then finish off your meal with melon sorbet.

Want more alternatives? Dr. Barnard and Dr. Ornish might suggest fixing a stuffed baked potato; a salad of broccoli, potato, and chickpeas with lemon-tarragon dressing; and peaches cooked in red wine.

And if you've done your homework in this *Picture Perfect Weight Loss* book, you know that these menus contain the kinds of healthful, low-calorie choices I recommend for everyone.

Chapter 14

WHAT YOU'LL LOSE, WHAT YOU'LL GAIN

When the gentleman I'll call Philip first came to see me, he was 76 years old and had a sad story to tell. Having spent a lifetime as a high-powered and highly successful executive at a major corporation, he had long looked forward to a retirement in which he and his wife of 45 years would together enjoy the things they loved: music, travel, the theater, gourmet dining.

But shortly after the retirement dinner and the cash-in of the stock options, Philip's wife became ill with cancer. For the past 3 years, he had acted as virtually a full-time nurse, at his wife's side during difficult and exhausting chemotherapy and radiation treatments. Philip had to watch helplessly as the cancer reduced a once vibrant woman into a frail, suffering shadow of her former self. The loss of his wife, just a few months before Philip walked into my office, had left a gaping hole in the middle of his life.

His suffering was visible—and it took a toll on his body. Philip was thick through the middle, obviously carrying more weight than was comfortable. His face was pasty-looking, with fleshy jowls, and he moved laboriously,

as if weighed down by his sadness. What's more, he had gout, diabetes, heart disease, and high cholesterol.

Philip had a simple but strange request to make. "I want to lose 20 pounds," he told me. "I expect to live only 2 more years, and I would like to be 20 pounds thinner for those 2 years."

So convinced was Philip of the length of time left to him—so resigned to it—that he initially resisted subjecting himself to the complete physical exam that is a prerequisite for any patient of mine. "It's not worth it," Philip said of the exam. "It's a waste of time. I'll only be around for 2 more years."

That was 10 years ago. Today, Philip typically starts his day with a brisk walk—outdoors if weather permits, on the treadmill in his apartment if it does not. He bought the treadmill when he decided there was more to life than playing cards with his cronies at the club every afternoon. He still plays cards, but it isn't the only thing he does in the afternoons. As a former businessman, he volunteers his accumulated business wisdom to small start-up companies in the inner city, and lately he has been perfecting his computer skills.

Most evenings are spent out—at a concert or a play, or perhaps having dinner with friends at one of New York's hot new restaurants. That is, when he isn't traveling. Last year, there was a museum trip along the Nile. This year, he's planning to join a group for a vacation in England.

Of course, Philip lost the 20 pounds he wanted to lose—in fact, he lost 40. What he gained, however, was nothing less than a fresh start on a whole new time of life.

Seeing the Light—Mary

I said at the beginning of this book that weight loss needs to be something that happens while you're still getting on with your life. But it is also true that changing your relationship with food can make your life richer in any number of ways. It isn't just pounds you lose; it's the baggage of being tied to a "diet," or feeling you must avoid certain situations, or depriving yourself of things you love.

What you can gain, very often, is the real you.

At the age of 26, Mary was not just one of the shiest people ever to walk through the door of my office, she was simply a closed book. Quiet, modest, diffident, she joined one of the office support groups and almost never said a word. Privately, she also began to see the office psychologist. Quietly, she hired a personal trainer to work with her in her own apartment. She showed up punctually for her appointments, answered all my questions succinctly, and paid close attention to the nutri-

tion demonstrations. Yet it wasn't until the 4th or 5th week of the program that she even began to lose weight.

Slowly, as Mary changed more aspects of her relationship with food, more and more pounds began to disappear. The exercise began to take effect, toning and sculpting her muscles. The therapy began to take effect, too, as Mary was seen to smile in her support group, then to laugh out loud. And as Mary began to see results, the world began to see the real Mary.

This once-shy person began to venture comments that were both funny and insightful. As her appearance changed, she began to get compliments, and soon she was buying a new wardrobe.

Mary took her exercise regime out of the privacy of her home and into the public arena of a gym, where she quickly and easily made friends—even though the sport she took up was boxing! At work, she was promoted to a job of greater responsibility, for more money, requiring travel to exotic overseas locations. It was like watching a butterfly emerge from its chrysalis, like seeing the true Mary break out of her shell.

Today, 35 pounds thinner, Mary still comes to the office—between trips to Bangkok and Taipei and Singapore. She continues to see the therapist, and she does some form of physical activity for "at least an hour" five times a week—whether it's a workout in the hotel gym, or a brisk walk through the streets of a foreign capital, or a jog around the reservoir in Central Park.

She loves her new job, loves the travel, loves the one-on-one contact with customers. She's good at it. The personality that burst forth when she changed her relationship with food and lost weight is one customers feel comfortable with, while Mary herself now finds it easy to be outgoing, to listen to the concerns of others, to take charge of problems and find solutions. In the same manner, she has taken charge of her food choices and her way of eating.

Eat Yourself Thin—Jennifer

Jennifer came to my office with an actress friend who didn't want to come alone. She didn't take weight loss as seriously as her friend, but was happy to provide some moral support. Then she stepped on the scale.

In her twenties, Jennifer had been lithe and slim. She was now approaching 50, and she had steadily put on weight—but not a whole lot, she figured. She thought she weighed about 140. Until she stepped on the scale.

When Jennifer saw the number 163, she was horrified. She signed up for the program and set about changing her relationship with food.

As CEO of her own company, Jennifer ate almost all her meals out. She was constantly entertaining customers, and one way they like to be entertained is by dining at lavish New York restaurants. When she did prepare her own food, Jennifer tended to the extravagant—"my Italian background," she explained—serving lots of olive oil, lots of pasta, and huge portions.

Jennifer changed her relationship with food, but she did not—could not—change her lifestyle. She still entertains customers four or five nights a week and just about every day at lunch. She still cooks for pleasure when she's on her own.

She still eats huge portions, too, but now she enjoys cooking low-calorie, healthful dishes. Identifying those choices in restaurants, she eats them with gusto. And today she prefers walking to the restaurant, taking the stairs whenever possible, and making exercise a comfortable and regular part of her routine.

Jennifer went from 163 pounds to 128. That was less than she'd weighed at any time during the 5 years before she came to see me. In fact, she weighs less now than at any time since her twenties.

Her business continues to be hectic and exhausting, and there's no letup in the amount of entertaining she must do. But Jennifer has more energy for it at 128 pounds than at 163—and more desire, in her own words, to "rock 'n' roll."

Picture This:
The Weight Is Over

Of course, I am not promising you that you will add years to your life, or that a funny and fabulous new personality will emerge. And I can't promise that you will become thinner than you've *ever* been when you change your relationship with food. What I am promising is that a changed relationship with food will add benefits to your life even as it subtracts pounds and takes away your fear of regaining weight.

Knowledge is power, as the saying goes, and the knowledge you gain from this book can give you the power you need to change the most constant, necessary, and ongoing relationship that you have—your relationship with food.

First of all, the knowledge you take from these pages should give you a realistic sense of just what is an appropriate goal for you. Genetic predisposition and even psychological factors can affect your weight. Therefore, for the person you are, there's an appropriate weight at which you'll look and feel your best. That's the goal you want to aim for and maintain.

Second, the nutritional knowledge you glean from the book's Food Awareness Training provides the essential tools you'll need to get to that goal and stay there. I'm sure that the visual demonstrations are burned into your brain. Now, more often than not, when you see one kind of food that you might have eaten impulsively, you also see vivid images of the other, appealing lower-calorie choices. And if you don't remember, or if the images start to fade, the pictures in this book will always be right here.

Looking Beyond

Gaining an understanding of how to read nutrition labels and learning to look behind the "low-fat" or "low-sugar" labels to the calorie numbers are equally important. So is an awareness of the wide range of foods that you may have been surprised to find are not at all "forbidden."

Further, what you've learned in these pages doesn't end when you close the book. You now have a basis on which you can build. As new studies provide new information on nutrition, you're equipped to assess what they mean. As new food products come on the market, you know enough to be able to determine if they should be added to your own personal list of options.

All this knowledge puts your weight in your own hands. Quite literally. The hand that reaches for Cheerios instead of Grape-Nuts, club soda before Scotch and soda, fish rather than meat has been empowered by mindfulness.

What's more, when you have undertaken the program in this book, you have the power forever. Once you have gone through Food Awareness Training and have become a mindful eater in the driver's seat of your food choices, you possess all the tools you'll ever need to maintain an appropriate weight for the rest of your life.

You'll look it, and you'll feel it—not just in a sleeker appearance, but also in self-esteem and self-confidence. It's all mutually enhancing—and mutually renewing. The better you look and feel, the greater your confidence. The greater your confidence, the better you'll look and feel. Simply put, the more you succeed, the greater your power to succeed.

Gaining by Losing

I promise you that a changed relationship with food—combined with regular physical activity—will make you a healthier person. What's more, the soundness and fitness that come from healthy eating and regular exercise invariably coincide with a more cheerful and positive attitude, with a higher energy level, and even with clearer thinking and a stronger sense of well-being. For the rest of your life, the quality of your life will be better.

It's a lot to gain.

And you don't have to go hungry, look or act like you're "on a diet," give up your favorite foods, abstain from alcohol, join a gym, or be afraid you'll gain back the weight you shed.

Isn't it time you started changing your relationship with food? After all, what have you got to lose?

Index

Underscored page references indicate boxed text and tables.
Boldface references indicate photographs.